KU-091-839

IMPORTANT PRESCRIBING INFORMATION

All doses recommended in this book are, unless stated otherwise, based on an average (70 kg) adult. Doses suggested are those typically suitable for critically ill patients. Individual patients may, however, require more or less than the doses stated to achieve the optimal therapeutic effect.

Every effort has been made to ensure the accuracy of the information contained in this book, particularly that relating to drugs and drug doses. It is, however, the responsibility of the prescribing practitioner to ensure that all drug prescriptions are correct, and neither the authors nor the publishers can be held liable for any errors.

If in doubt seek advice from a pharmacist or consult the British National Formulary (BNF).

Intensive Care

Commissioning Editor: Michael Parkinson
Project Development Manager: Janice Urquhart
Project Manager: Nancy Arnott
Designer: Erik Bigland
Illustrations: Cactus

CHURCHILL'S POCKETBOOKS

Intensive Care

Simon M. Whiteley MB BS FRCA
Consultant, Intensive Care, St James's University
Hospital, Leeds, UK

Andrew Bodenham MB BS FRCA
Consultant, Intensive Care, The General Infirmary
at Leeds, Leeds, UK

Mark C. Bellamy MA MB BS FRCA
Consultant, Intensive Care, St James's University
Hospital, Leeds, UK

SECOND EDITION

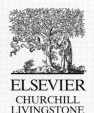

ELSEVIER
CHURCHILL
LIVINGSTONE

EDINBURGH LONDON NEW YORK OXFORD
PHILADELPHIA ST LOUIS SYDNEY TORONTO 2004

CHURCHILL LIVINGSTONE
An imprint of Elsevier Limited

First edition 1996
Second edition 2004
    Reprinted 2005

ISBN 0 443 07258 2

British Library Cataloguing in Publication Data
A catalogue record for this book is available from the British Library

Library of Congress Cataloguing in Publication Data
A catalogue record for this book is available from the Library of Congress

Note
Medical knowledge is constantly changing. Standard safety precautions must be
followed, but as new research and clinical experience broaden our knowledge,
changes in treatment and drug therapy may become necessary r appropriate.
Readers are advised to check the most current product information provided by
the manufactacturer of each drug to be administered to verify the recommended
dose, the method and duration of administration, and contraindications. It is the
responsibility of the practitioner, relying on experience and knowledge of the
patient, to determine dosages and the best treatment for each individual patient.
Neither the Publisher nor the editors assume any liability for any injury and/or
damage to persons or property arising from this publication.
The Publisher

Printed in China

PREFACE

This small book follows other successful titles in the Churchill's pocketbook format. It is not intended to compete with the many already well-established texts in the field of intensive care, but is intended to present a distillation of sensible practice and ideas.

Every new doctor who is resident in the intensive care unit will be faced with a large variety of clinical problems to be solved. This book is therefore based on the common problems the authors are asked about on a regular basis, most of which can be easily solved by following simple rules. The aim has been to use the minimum of space by avoiding excessive detail, and no apology is made for repetition, or for what may on occasion appear a didactic approach. Information related to the specialist areas such as paediatric and cardiothoracic intensive care has been specifically excluded, although the general principles described are equally applicable in those areas.

In many countries there are increasing moves to rotate trainees from different specialties, without previous intensive care experience, through intensive care. The hope is that this guide will prove timely and useful in this respect.

In the six years since the first edition of this book was published there have been a number of changes in intensive care. We have incorporated these changes in this new edition. As a result we have extensively revised the text and included a number of new or revised figures. The overall format however remains the same. We hope that this edition will continue to provide new trainees in intensive care with safe, sensible and practical advice.

S. M. W.
A. B.
M. C. B.

CONTENTS

6. Gastrointestinal system

7. Renal system

8. Metabolic and endocrine problems

ABBREVIATIONS

A&E accident and emergency

ACE angiotensin converting enzyme

ACN acute cortical necrosis

ACT activated clotting time

ACTH adrenocorticotrophin hormone

ADH antidiuretic hormone

AF atrial fibrillation

AIDS acquired immune deficiency syndrome

ALI acute lung injury

APTT activated partial thromboplastin time

ARDS adult respiratory distress syndrome

ARF acute renal failure

ASB assisted spontaneous breathing

AST aspartate aminotransferase

ATLS Avanced Trauma Life Support

ATN acute tubular necrosis

AV arteriovenous; atrioventricular

ANCA antineutrophil cytoplasmic antibodies

BAL bronchial alveolar lavage

BIPAP biphasic positive airways pressure

BNF *British National Formulary*

BSA body surface area

CCU coronary care unit

CFM cerebral function monitor

CK creatinine kinase

CMV controlled mandatory ventilation; cytomegalovirus

CO cardiac output

COPD chronic obstructive pulmonary disease

CPAP continuous positive airway pressure

CPDA citrate, phosphate, dextrose, adenosine

CPP cerebral perfusion pressure

CRP C-reactive protein

CSF cerebrospinal fluid

CT computerized tomography

CVA cerebrovascular accident

CVP central venous pressure

CVS cardiovascular system

CVVHD continuous venovenous haemodialysis

CVVHDF continuous venovenous haemodiafiltration

CVVHF continuous venovenous haemofiltration

CXR chest X-ray

DI diabetes insipidus

DIC disseminated intravascular coagulation

DKA diabetic ketoacidosis

DVT deep venous thrombosis

EBV Epstein–Barr virus

ECF extra cellular fluid

ECG electrocardiogram

ECMO extracorporeal membrane oxygenation

EDTA ethylenediamine tetra-acetic acid

EPO erythropoietin

ERCP endoscopic retrograde cholangiopancreatography

ETCO$_2$ end-tidal carbon dioxide

FBC full blood count

FDP fibrin degradation product

FFP fresh frozen plasma

FRC functional residual capacity

GCS Glasgow Coma Scale

GCSF granulocytic-colony stimulating factor

GFR glomerular filtration rate

GH growth hormone

GIT gastrointestinal tract

GTN glyceryl trinitrate

HDU high dependency unit

HELLP haemolysis, elevated liver enzymes, low platelets

HIT heparin-induced thrombocytopenia

HIV human immunodeficiency virus

HR heart rate

HUS haemolytic uraemic syndrome

ICP intracranial pressure

ICNARC Intensive Care National Audit and Research Centre

ICU intensive care unit

IHD ischaemic heart disease

INR international normalized ratio

IPPV intermittent positive pressure ventilation

ISS injury severity score

LDH lactate dehydrogenase

MAP mean arterial pressure

MH malignant hyperpyrexia

MODS multiorgan dysfunction syndrome

MRSA methicillin-resistant staphylococcus aureus

NG nasogastric

NIPPV non-invasive ventilation

NSAID non-steroidal anti-inflammatory drug

PA pulmonary artery

PACS patient-controlled analgesic system

PACU post anaesthesia care unit

PAF platelet activating factor

PAFC pulmonary artery flotation catheter

PAOP pulmonary artery occlusion pressure

PCA patient-controlled analgesia

PCP *Pneumocystis carinii* pneumonia

PCR polymerase chain reaction

PE pulmonary embolism

PEA pulseless electrical activity

PEEP positive end expiratory pressure

PEG percutaneous endoscopic gastrostomy

PT prothrombin time

RAST radioallergosorbent tests

RRT renal replacement therapy

RTS revised trauma score

RV right ventricle

SAGM sodium chloride, adenosine, glucose, mannitol

SAPS Simplified Acute Physiology Score

SARS severe adult respiratory syndrome

SCID severe combined immune deficiency

SDD selective decontamination digestive tract

SIADH syndrome of inappropriate antidiuretic hormone

SIMV synchronized intermittent mandatory ventilation

SIRS systemic inflammatory response syndrome

SV stroke volume

SVR systemic vascular resistance

SVT supraventricular tachycardia

T3 tri-iodothyronine

T4 thyroxine

TEG thromboelastogram

TIA transient ischaemic attack

TIPSS transvenous intrahepatic portosystemic shunt

TISS transvenous itrahepatic

TNF tumour necrosis factor

TO4 train of four

TPA tissue plasminogen activator

TPN total parenteral nutrition

TRALI transfusion-related acute lung injury

TSH thyroid stimulating hormone

TT thrombin time

TTP thrombotic thrombocytopenic purpura

U&Es urea and electrolytes

VCJD new variant Creutzfeldt–Jakob disease

VF ventricular fibrillation

VPB ventricular premature beat

VRE vancomycin-resistant enterococci

VSD ventricular septal defect

WCC white cell count

ORGANIZATIONAL ISSUES

INTRODUCTION

Modern intensive care originated during the poliomyelitis epidemics of the 1950s when tracheal intubation and positive pressure ventilation were applied to polio victims, leading to a substantial reduction in mortality. The patients were managed in a specific part of the hospital and received one-to-one nursing care, features which still largely define intensive care units (ICUs) to this day. From these beginnings, there was a gradual development until the ICU was a recognizable component of most general hospitals.

In the early days of intensive care, patients were often young and previously fit, with only single organ failure. If they survived, a full functional recovery could be anticipated. Today, patients are increasingly elderly, often with complex pre-existing medical problems, and frequently develop multiple organ failure with much more limited prospects of survival. This, together with the realization of the large costs involved in providing intensive care, typically £1500 per day, has led some to question how intensive care should be provided in the future.

There is little doubt, however, that intensive care medicine has an established role in modern health care. Critical illness may arise from a variety of disease processes, but the pathophysiological changes that result lead to common patterns of organ dysfunction. By recognizing these patterns and understanding the interactions between different organ systems, intensive care teams can improve the outcome of critically ill patients. The role of intensive care therefore includes:

- resuscitation and stabilization
- physiological optimization of patients to prevent organ failure
- facilitation of complex surgery
- support of failing organ systems
- recognition of futility.

DEFINITIONS

Traditional definitions of intensive care units (ICUs) and high dependency units (HDUs) attempt to separate the functions of each.

Intensive care unit (ICU)

An area for patients admitted for the treatment of actual or impending organ failure, especially those requiring assisted ventilation. There is usually at least one nurse per patient and a doctor assigned solely to the intensive care unit throughout the 24-hour period.

High dependency unit (HDU)

An area for patients who require more intensive observation and interventions than can be performed on a general ward, but who do not require assisted ventilation. Nursing levels are generally between those of an ICU and a general ward. There is not usually dedicated medical cover.

There are, however, difficulties with such definitions. In many smaller hospitals for example, the ICU, HDU and coronary care unit (CCU) are often combined in one area, with nursing and medical staff working flexibly as required. Post anaesthesia care units (PACUs) or recovery rooms, which provide high dependency care, may be used to ventilate patients when the ICU is full. Many patients with chronic respiratory disease are now ventilated on respiratory wards, either via face/nasal masks or by long-term tracheostomy.

It is increasingly recognized, therefore, that the level of medical and nursing care received by individual patients should not be a function of their physical location, in an ICU or on the ward, but a function of their clinical condition. This has led to the classification of levels of care for critically ill patients based solely on need.

LEVELS OF CARE FOR CRITICALLY ILL PATIENTS

Critically ill patients can be classified according to the level of medical and nursing care required (Table 1.1). Patients should be

TABLE 1.1 Levels of critical care

Level 0	Patients whose needs can be met by ward-based care in an acute hospital
Level 1	Patients at risk of their condition deteriorating (including those recently moved from higher levels of care) whose needs can be met on a normal ward with additional advice or support from the critical care team
Level 2	Patients requiring more advanced levels of observation or intervention than can be provided on a normal ward, including support for a single failing organ system.
Level 3	Patients requiring advanced respiratory support alone or basic respiratory support together with support for at least two organ systems

Specialist care is recorded by attaching one of the following letters as a suffix:

N, neurosurgical; C, cardiac; T, thoracic; B, burns; S, spinal injury; R, renal; L, liver; A, other specialist care.

nursed in an area capable of providing the appropriate level of care. While level 2 care may be provided in an HDU or ICU, true level 3 care can only be provided in a suitably equipped intensive care unit. It is important to appreciate that these levels of care are not discrete entities but represent a continuum and patients may move between levels as their condition changes. (See Identification of patients at risk, below.)

CRITICAL CARE OUTREACH

Outreach is a new concept in critical care. Traditionally, intensive care staff have tended to stay in the ICU and await the referral of patients from other areas by the attending medical staff. It is increasingly recognized, however, that the ICU staff have much to offer critically ill and potentially critically ill patients outside the ICU. This has led to the development of critical care outreach teams.

Outreach teams generally consist of a senior member of both medical and nursing staff from the ICU. They provide a liaison service and an immediate point of contact between the ICU and other areas of the hospital. Their role includes:

- identification of patients at risk
- prevention of further deterioration and the need for subsequent ICU admission
- support for level 1 care on the wards
- education and the promotion of critical care skills
- identification of patients unlikely to benefit from ICU admission
- facilitation of discharges from higher levels of care back to the ward.

IDENTIFICATION OF PATIENTS AT RISK

The levels of care required by critically ill patients described above are not absolute discrete entities, but represent a continuum, with patients moving up and down the levels of nursing dependency as their condition changes. It is important that patients who are at risk of deteriorating and requiring increased levels of care are identified early and the appropriate interventions instituted.

A number of scoring systems have now been developed to help staff to detect those patients who are at risk. These are based on the principle that patients develop abnormal physiological parameters as their condition starts to deteriorate. The scoring system can be administered by any member of the ward medical or nursing staff and,

TABLE 1.2 Typical early warning scoring system

Score	3	2	1	0	1	2	3
Heart rate		<40	41–50	51–100	101–110	111–130	>130
Systolic BP	<70	71–80	81–100	101–199		>200	
Resp. rate		<8		9–14	15–20	21–29	>30
Temp.		<35	35.1–36.5				
CNS				A	V	P	U
Urine output last 4 hours	<1 ml/kg	<1.5 ml/kg	<2 ml/kg		>10 ml/kg		

A, alert; V, responds to voice; P, responds to pain; U, unresponsive.

TABLE 1.3 Typical response to early warning scoring system

Ward area	Score >3	Call outreach team
High dependency area	Score >3	Call responsible medical staff
	Score >5	Call outreach team/ICU
Any area	Score >10	Call outreach team/ICU

if appropriate, the intensive care (outreach) team can be called. An example of a typical early warning scoring system is shown in Table 1.2. The response triggered by the scoring system is shown in Table 1.3.

Once contacted, the outreach team may be able to offer advice and support ward staff in the care of the patient at ward level (level 1 care) or may arrange transfer of the patient to an area capable of providing a higher level of care (HDU or ICU) if appropriate. Occasionally the outreach team may, in consultation with the patient, relatives and other medical staff, decide that a patient is unlikely to benefit from intensive care and that admission would not be appropriate.

ADMISSION POLICIES

The aim of intensive care is to support patients while they recover. It is not to prolong life when there is no hope of recovery. Sometimes difficult decisions have to be made about whether or not to admit a patient to intensive care, as there is often a shortage of intensive care beds and a requirement to use the available resources responsibly. To aid such decisions, some units have written admission policies. For example:

Typical admission policy

Requests for admission
- Patients who, in the opinion of the ICU consultant, are likely to benefit from a period of intensive care will be admitted to the ICU. Patients in whom further treatment is considered futile will not normally be admitted.
- Requests for admission should be made by contacting the ICU consultant on call. Requests should normally come from a consultant who has seen the patient immediately prior to making a referral.
- In the case of elective surgery where the admission of the patient can be foreseen a request should be made at least 24 hours prior to surgery. The bed should be confirmed prior to commencement of anaesthesia.

Bed management issues
- All problems related to availability of beds will be dealt with initially by the ICU consultant on call, who is in a position to make decisions about the potential admission and the needs of the patients already in the ICU.
- If there are no beds immediately available, the continued provision of care at an appropriate level to the patient remains the responsibility of the staff in attendance, supported where possible by the ICU outreach team.
- Where no ICU bed is available the ICU consultant may be able to give advice as to the location of other available ICU beds; however, his or her prime responsibility is to patients already in the ICU.

Joint responsibility
- All patients will be admitted under the care of a named ICU consultant and the ICU team will assume responsibility for the patient's care. (Responsibility may be shared jointly with the admitting team.)

Discharges
- Will be arranged by the ICU staff in conjunction with the responsible consultant. In cases of emergency, however, patients may be discharged by the consultant on call for the ICU.

The difficulty with all admission policies is that it is impossible to predict with accuracy which individual patients stand to benefit from admission to intensive care. On this basis, patients are often admitted for a trial of therapy to see whether they will stabilize and improve over time.

Inevitably, on occasion, truly hopeless cases will be admitted. For example, patients from the resuscitation room, or those who have suffered catastrophic complications during surgery, may be admitted even though they are likely to die. This allows the relatives time to visit and the bereavement process to be better managed. Medicolegal considerations may also be relevant in this context. Admission policies need, therefore, to be sufficiently flexible to allow the admission of what may seem, on occasion, like inappropriate cases.

PREDICTION OF OUTCOME

The difficulties outlined above have led to a wealth of work, using scoring systems, to predict the outcome of patients treated in intensive care. This generally involves the collection of a large amount of data from many patients, stratification of the data to produce a risk score, and then the application of the risk score to individuals. There are, however, major difficulties with this approach:

- There is, as yet, no satisfactory diagnostic categorization for intensive care patients. Often the problems relating to intensive care admission bear little relation to the original presenting complaint or diagnostic category.
- Although patients may survive to leave the ICU, there is a significant mortality on the wards, and later at home, after leaving intensive care. Many studies use 28-day mortality as an end point. It has been suggested that 6 month or 1 year outcomes of mortality and measures of morbidity (quality of life measures) are better end points.
- Scoring systems may accurately model population outcomes, but are unreliable for prediction in individual cases.

The APACHE II score, for example, takes into account both acute physiological disturbances and the chronic health of the patient. While the APACHE score correlates well with the risk of death for the intensive care population as a whole, it does not accurately predict individual mortality. There have been attempts using computer modelling to improve the accuracy of outcome prediction in individual patients. The Riyadh Intensive Care Program, for example, uses daily scores as a basis on which to predict those patients in which further treatment is futile. This approach has, however, failed to gain widespread support.

In practice, most units use simple clinical decision-making to determine which patients to admit to the ICU. In many cases, unless the outlook is truly hopeless, patients will be admitted for a trial of treatment. Instantaneous judgements regarding the continuation or withdrawal of treatment from patients in the operating theatre, resuscitation room or on the wards are often difficult. Senior staff should be involved from the outset. Increasingly, lawyers and clinical ethicists are being involved in the most difficult decisions.

APACHE II SEVERITY OF ILLNESS SCORE

The acute physiological and chronic health evaluation tool, APACHE II, is the most widely used severity of illness scoring system in intensive care. A score is assigned to each patient on the basis of:

- worst physiological derangement, occurring in the first 24 hours of admission (Table 1.4)
- age (Table 1.5)
- chronic health status (Table 1.6).

Notes on completing APACHE II scores

In many ICUs, APACHE data are collected by audit clerks and entered into electronic databases often as part of a much larger data set. You may, however, be expected to calculate scores on your patients and you should understand the process:

APACHE II score = acute physiology score (A) + age score (B) + chronic health score (C).

- Score the worst value for each parameter in the first 24 hours.
- Where results are not available, score as zero. But this does not mean that you do not have to try to find the result first!

Oxygen

$FiO_2 > 0.5$: calculate the alveolar–arterial oxygen difference or $(A-a)DO_2$ expressed in kPa:

alveolar oxygen = $FiO_2 \times$ (atmospheric pressure – SVP water) – $PaCO_2$
alveolar oxygen = $FiO_2 \times (101-6.2) - PaCO_2$

therefore

$$(A-a)DO_2 = (FiO_2 \times 94.8)-PaCO_2-PaO_2.$$

The result of this gives the A–a gradient, which is then scored from the APACHE table:

Score	+4	+3	+2	+1	0
Result	>66.6	46.7–66.5	26.7–46.5		<26.7

$FiO_2 < 0.5$: simply score the PaO_2 in kPa.

Score	0	+1	+2	+3	+4
PaO_2 (kPa)	>9.3	8.1–9.3		7.3–8.0	<7.15

Serum HCO_3

Only use bicarbonate when there are no blood gases available. Otherwise score the arterial pH.

Glasgow Coma Scale (GCS)

A number of approaches to this are adopted in different units. Either (a) assign the assumed GCS the patient would have if not artificially

TABLE 1.4 APACHE II
A: Acute physiological derangement score sheet

Score	+4	+3	+2	+1	0	+1	+2	+3	+4
Core Temp. (°C)	>41	39–40.9		38.5–38.9	36–38.4	34–35.9	32–33.9	30–31.9	<29
Resp. rate	>50	49–35		34–25	24–12	11–10	9–6		<5
MAP	>160	130–159	110–129	24–34	79–109		55–69	40–54	<39
Oxygen If FiO₂ >0.5 use A-a gradient	>66.6	46.7–66.5	26.7–46.5		<26.7				
Oxygen If FiO₂ <0.5 use PaO₂ (kPa)					>9.3	8.1–9.3		7.3–8.0	<7.3
Serum HCO₃ (mmol/l) or arterial pH	>52 >7.7	41–51.9 7.6–7.69		32–40.9 7.5–7.59	22–31.9 7.33–7.49		18–21.9 7.25–7.32	15–17.9 7.15–7.24	<15 <7.15
Sodium (mmol/l)	>180	160–179	155–159	150–154	130–153		120–129	111–119	<110
Potassium (mmol/l)	>7	6–6.9		5.5–5.9	3.5–5.4	3–3.4	2.5–2.9		<2.5
Creatinine (µmol/l) (score double in ARF)	>309	169–306	125–168		53–124		<53		
Hb (g/dl)	>20		16.7–19.9	16.6–15.4	153–10		9.9–6.7		<6.7
White blood count (× 1000)	>40		20–39.9	15–19.9	3–14.9		1–2.9		<1
Glasgow Coma Scale					Score 15 minus actual GCS				

**TABLE 1.5 APACHE II
B: Age points**

Score	0	+2	+3	+5	+6
Age	44	45–54	55–64	65–74	75

**TABLE 1.6 APACHE II
C: Chronic health score**

For patients with severe organ system insufficiency or immune compromise assign scores as shown.
Condition must have been evident prior to this hospital admission and conform to the definitions below.

Category	Score
For non-operative or emergency postoperative patients	+5
For elective postoperative patients	+2

Definitions

CVS New York Heart Association Class IV.

Respiratory Chronic restrictive, obstructive or vascular disease resulting in severe exercise restriction, i.e. unable to climb stairs or perform household duties, or documented chronic hypoxia, hypercapnia, secondary polycythaemia, severe pulmonary hypertension or respiratory dependency.

Renal Receiving chronic dialysis.

Liver Biopsy-proven cirrhosis and documented portal hypertension, episodes of past upper GI bleeding attributed to portal hypertension or prior episodes of hepatic failure/encephalopathy/coma.

Immunity Decreased resistance to infection, resulting from immunosuppressive therapy, chemotherapy, radiation, long-term or recent high-dose steroids, or has a disease that is sufficiently advanced to suppress resistance to infection, e.g. leukaemia, lymphoma, AIDS.

sedated, or (b) as patients who are ventilated, paralysed and sedated, will have a GCS of 3, score as $15 - 3 = 12$ (see below). Ask what the usual practice is in your unit.

Chronic health points

This can provide a significant loading to an APACHE score. Apply only according to the criteria on the scoring chart, which imply established organ system impairment.

Problems with APACHE II

There are a number of problems with the APACHE II score:

● Patients with an APACHE II score > 35 are unlikely to survive. However, the score is a statistical tool based on populations and

scores for individuals cannot be used to predict outcome. Some
patients, for example those with diabetic ketoacidosis, may have
marked physiological abnormalities, but generally get better
quickly.

- The score is based on historical data, and as new interventions are
  developed the data become obsolete.
- Lead-time bias results from the stabilization of patients in the
  referring hospital prior to transfer. This artificially lowers the score
  for the patient arriving at the referral centre.
- The GCS component is difficult to assess in patients receiving
  sedative or neuromuscular blocking agents. There is an important
  difference between a GCS 3 due to head injury and due to the
  effects of drugs.
- The physiological components are based on adults. They do not
  translate to paediatrics. For children the 'Prism' score is usually
  used instead.

ALTERNATIVE SEVERITY OF ILLNESS SCORING SYSTEMS

APACHE III score

The APACHE II score has now been superseded by an updated
APACHE III score. Five new variables have been added (urine output,
serum albumin, urea, bilirubin and glucose), while two variables
(potassium and bicarbonate) have been removed. In addition, the GCS
and acid–base balance components have been altered. A complex
matrix grid scoring system is used, with a maximum score of 299.

SAPS

The Simplified Acute Physiology Score (SAPS) is similar to APACHE
and is used more commonly in mainland Europe. It utilizes 12
physiological variables assigned a score according to the degree of
derangement.

TISS

The Therapeutic Intervention Score System (TISS) assigns a value to
each procedure performed in the ICU. The implication is that the more
procedures that are performed on a patient, the sicker they are. It
depends on the doctor, however, as different physicians will have
different thresholds for carrying out many procedures. The score is,
therefore, not good for comparing outcome between patients or between
different units but is useful as a general guide to the type of care and
resources likely to be needed by patients on an individual unit.

NATIONAL AUDIT DATABASES

Although severity of illness scoring systems cannot currently predict the outcome of individual patients, they are useful for comparing the outcome of large groups of patients, for example from different units. By comparing the severity of illness scores together with diagnostic codes from different units, so-called case mix adjusted outcome data can be produced. There are increasing moves to collect and maintain national databases of intensive care patients both for this purpose and as a research tool. The Intensive Care National Audit and Research Centre for England and Wales (ICNARC) and the Scottish Intensive Care Society Audit group have national ICU databases that can provide case mix adjusted outcome data.

DISCHARGE POLICIES

Discharge policies are just as hard to define as admission policies (above). Patients may be discharged in the following circumstances:

- The patient's condition has improved to the extent that intensive care is no longer required and is therefore inappropriate.
- The patient's condition is not improving and the underlying problems are such that continued intensive care is futile. In such cases it is imperative that the general ward staff, the patient's family and, where possible, the patient agree that such decisions are appropriate and that the decision is clearly documented.

Wherever possible, patients should only be discharged during normal daytime hours. There is some evidence that patients who are discharged from intensive care outside these hours are at greater risk of subsequent deterioration and readmission. For patients whose condition is improving and for whom discharge is considered, two questions should be asked, as follows.

1. When are patients fit to be discharged?
In simple terms, patients are fit for discharge from intensive care when they no longer require the specialist skills and monitoring available on the ICU. This generally means that they have no life-threatening organ failure and that their underlying disease process is stable or improving. Table 1.7 gives some guidance.

2. Where is the patient to be sent?
This will depend at least in part on the patient's underlying diagnosis, current condition, and where the patient came from in the first place.

TABLE 1.7 Criteria for discharge from ITU

Airway	Adequate airway and cough to clear secretions (if inadequate, tracheostomy and suction, see below)
Breathing	Adequate respiratory effort and blood gases May be on oxygen (e.g. from face mask) Not requiring CPAP or non-invasive ventilation (unless discharged to HDU or respiratory unit, see below)
Circulation	Stable, no inotropes
Neurological function	Adequate conscious level Adequate cough and gag reflexes (if inadequate, e.g. bulbar palsy or brain injury may need tracheostomy to make airway safe and allow suction)
Renal function	Renal function stable or improving Not requiring renal support unless discharged to renal unit
Analgesia	Adequate pain control

Some patients, especially elective postoperative surgical patients, may be fit enough to go straight back to a general ward. Others may, because of continuing organ dysfunction or other problems, require closer monitoring, supervision and nursing care and may go back to an HDU. Increasingly patients with chronic respiratory disease or those who are slow to wean from a ventilator may be transferred to a respiratory HDU capable of providing CPAP and non-invasive forms of ventilation.

Patients who have been transferred from another ICU for specialist treatment or because of lack of beds may be discharged back to the referring hospital. In general, patients should be returned to their referring hospital as soon as possible, if only for the sake of relatives who may find travelling difficult. (See Transporting patients, p. 360.)

ICU FOLLOW-UP CLINICS

Traditionally, outcome studies in intensive care have focused on mortality. Recently there has been increased interest in the morbidity that may occur in survivors of intensive care and many units now run ICU follow-up clinics. Typically, patients who have survived are seen 2 or 3 months after discharge. As well as providing an opportunity to assess a patient's physical and emotional well-being after ICU admission, it gives patients an opportunity to reflect and give feedback on their experiences.

INTRODUCTION TO INTENSIVE CARE

INTRODUCTION

Setting foot in an intensive care unit for the first time can be quite a daunting experience. The patients are obviously very sick and some will die. There may be large arrays of unfamiliar monitoring and therapeutic equipment at the bedside. The following pages are intended to help you survive and keep out of trouble during your first few days on the ICU. Remember, if in doubt ask someone.

THE MULTIDISCIPLINARY TEAM

The care of patients in intensive care is increasingly complex, and the specialization of medical staff precludes all care being provided by a single individual or team. The critically ill patient is cared for in a central area, where he or she receives optimum care and input from a number of different specialties. A major role for junior and senior medical staff in intensive care is the co-ordination of all aspects of patient care, and in particular the maintenance of good lines of communication between the different teams involved.

Many nursing, paramedical and technical staff are involved in the care of patients on intensive care. It is important to remember that all these people have skills and experience that you do not. Do not be afraid to ask for advice. If you treat them as colleagues you will get more from them.

Nursing staff

Many nursing staff in the ICU are very experienced and very knowledgeable. You should see them as allies. Listen to and carefully consider their advice. Remember also that nurses have their own job to do, which is demanding and time consuming. They are not there to run about after you. Therefore if you can get something you need – get it, and clear up your own mess after you!

Physiotherapists

Physiotherapists provide therapy for clearance of chest secretions. They have an important role in helping to maintain joint and limb function in bed-bound patients, and in mobilizing patients during their recovery. They can often provide help with the respiratory care and management of patients on general wards who are struggling to maintain adequate respiratory function and who might otherwise require admission to intensive care. Again, listen to their advice.

Pharmacists

The nature of intensive care is such that patients will often be on many medications. There is, therefore, a great potential for drug interactions and incompatibility of infusions. In addition, many drug doses need modification in the presence of hepatic and renal failure. The pharmacist will generally review prescriptions and is a ready source of advice on all therapeutic matters.

Dieticians

All patients in intensive care require some form of nutrition. While basic nutritional support can be provided by standard regimens, many hospitals now have nutrition teams including dieticians who will tailor regimens to each patient's particular requirements.

Technicians

A large number of technical staff are involved in supporting the ICU. These include laboratory technicians, renal technicians who manage haemodialysis machines, and equipment service engineers. Cultivate a good relationship with all these people. They can be an invaluable source of help.

DAILY ROUTINE

The daily routine on the ICU will vary a little from unit to unit. There are typically one or two main business ward rounds during the day, which members of the multidisciplinary team may attend. You may well be expected to see and assess the patients prior to the ward round and then to present your findings and action plan to the ward round. There may also be additional ward rounds during the day as other clinicians and/or results become available (e.g. microbiology).

INFECTION CONTROL

Patients receiving intensive care are, to a greater or lesser extent, immune-compromised and are at greatly increased risk of hospital-acquired (nosocomial) infection. This immune compromise may result directly from the underlying disease process, as a non-specific response to critical illness, or as a side effect of a treatment. In addition, multiple vascular catheters and invasive tubes that penetrate mucosal surfaces effectively bypass host defence barriers and increase the risk of invasive infection. While patients are most at risk from their own microbiological flora, particularly that associated with the gastrointestinal tract, they are also at risk from organisms transferred

from other patients (cross-infection). You must therefore be
scrupulous about following infection control procedures.

Before entering the ICU

Before entering the ICU leave your jacket or white coat outside.
White coats in particular tend to be dirty and can carry
microbiological flora from one patient to the next. Neck ties also have
a habit of dangling in all sorts of places; tuck them out of the way. If
you are going to stay on the ICU all day it is a good idea to wear
surgical blues to prevent problems with contamination of clothes. This
not only reduces the risk of cross-infection but saves on your laundry
bills as well!

Before approaching a patient

Simple measures are the best way to reduce infection risks. Therefore,
before you go near a patient in the ICU, you should:

- Wash your hands thoroughly. If your hands are already socially
  clean, you can use an alcohol disinfectant rub, which is equally
  effective.
- Put on a disposable plastic apron.

Moving between patients

When you have finished with the patient, remove your plastic apron
and wash your hands or use alcohol disinfectant rub before leaving the
bed space.

  Do not share equipment between patients in the ICU. For example,
stethoscopes are generally provided at each bed space. You should not
use your own, which might be a vehicle for cross-infection.

Barrier nursing

Some patients may be isolated because they have a serious infection
or are colonized with an antibiotic-resistant organism that might be
transmitted to other patients or even on occasions to members of staff.
These patients will be barrier nursed, the basic principles of which
are:

- Do not enter unnecessarily.
- Wear an apron.
- Wash your hands and put on gloves.

Other precautions such as the wearing of masks and gowns will
depend on the particular nature of the problem. Instructions for
entering the room are generally displayed on the door, and the nurses
will help.

- Remove protective aprons, etc. before you leave the room.
- Wash your hands before you leave the room and use alcohol rub once outside the room.

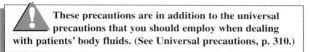

These precautions are in addition to the universal precautions that you should employ when dealing with patients' body fluids. (See Universal precautions, p. 310.)

Reverse barrier nursing

Some patients are at particular risk from infection because they are immune-compromised as a result of drug therapy, radiotherapy or immune disease, including HIV infection. These patients will often be in a side room and barrier nursed to help protect them. The precautions are generally similar to the above. Ask nursing staff for advice if unsure.

ASSESSING A PATIENT

Each patient in the ICU needs to be seen and assessed at least twice a day. Many conventional aspects of history taking and examination are either inappropriate or impracticable. This can seem daunting to the new trainee, particularly given the large amount of information available from charts, monitors and equipment at the patient's bedside. It is best to develop a system for condensing information easily so that you can assess the patient and work out a plan.

History

Make sure you know the detailed history of the patient. It is particularly important when admitting a new patient to avoid overlooking important facts. Although the history may often not be available from the patient, there is generally a lot of information available from the notes, from other doctors, nurses or the referring hospital. If in doubt, telephone the referring team. Take time to speak to family and friends to ascertain pre-existing health, physiological reserve and attitudes to life support.

Patient's chart

Looking at the patient's chart next is an extension of the history. It can be scanned for general trends in the patient's condition since arrival in intensive care, or examined more closely to give a guide to progress over the preceding 24 hours. Important things to note from the chart are:

- Haemodynamic stability:
  - trends in haemodynamic variables such as pulse, blood pressure, CVP, pulmonary artery pressures, cardiac output, inotrope requirements and evidence of adequate organ perfusion (e.g. conscious level, renal output, lactate).
- Respiratory function:
  - type and mode of ventilation, levels of respiratory support
  - progress made in weaning
  - blood gases.
- Gastrointestinal and renal function:
  - adequate volume and quality of urine
  - plasma and urinary electrolytes
  - fluid intake
  - nutrition – parenteral or enteral?
  - overall fluid balance.
- CNS function:
  - conscious level, sedation and analgesic requirements.
- Evidence of infection:
  - temperature and white cell count.

Examining the patient

Once you have put together the information available from the history and the patient's chart you should examine the patient carefully.

> ⚠ **Before examining a patient, introduce yourself and explain what you are going to do, even if the patient appears unconscious. Remember that hearing may be the last sense to be lost under anaesthesia or sedation.**

You should examine the patient in the normal way. However, you will need to assimilate information available from the monitoring at the same time. For example:

- Cardiovascular:
  - pulse, blood pressure, CVP, wedge pressure and cardiac output
  - heart sounds
  - evidence of adequate perfusion
  - cold and sweaty versus warm peripheries
  - core–peripheral temperature gradient
  - peripheral oedema
  - line sites clean or evidence of infection.
- Respiratory:
  - trachea central, air entry bilateral and equal, breath sounds, added sounds

— check position and adequacy of chest drains, endotracheal tubes, etc.
— check type and adequacy of ventilation and ventilator settings
— the CXR should be considered an extension of the physical examination in intensive care patients.

- Abdomen:
  — soft or tender, distended
  — bowel sounds present
  — bowels open
  — diarrhoea
  — enteral or parenteral feeding.
- Renal:
  — urine output
  — fluid balance.
- CNS:
  — level of consciousness
  — consider stopping all sedative/analgesic drugs to assess neurological status
  — does the patient make purposeful movements of all four limbs to command or stimulus?
  — for painful stimulus press on nail bed or supraorbital ridge (other sites cause bruising)
  — intracranial pressure and cerebral perfusion pressure.
- Limbs:
  — adequate perfusion (especially after injury)
  — evidence of swelling, tenderness, DVT or compartment syndrome.
- Wounds:
  — surgical wounds, and trauma sites, inspection for adequate healing
  — evidence of infection or discharge
  — surgical drains, volume and nature of drainage.

Special investigations

When you have examined the patient, you should go back to the patient's chart and records and check on anything that you have missed. Also review the patient's important haematology, biochemical and microbiology investigations and other investigations including CXRs and other radiological investigations.

Prescription charts

Review the patient's drug, fluid and nutrition prescription chart. Particularly check that routine stress ulcer prophylaxis and DVT prophylaxis is appropriately prescribed. Are current prescriptions appropriate to the patient's needs? In particular, are antibiotics still needed? Do any prescribed drugs require plasma level monitoring? Are any of the prescribed drugs likely to interact?

Finally, make sure that you have spoken to nursing staff and other people involved in the care of the patient. Ask for their assessment of problems and priorities, which may be different from your own.

FORMULATING AN ACTION PLAN

Daily problem list

When you have finished assessing the patient, record your examination findings and any important results in the medical notes. Summarize your findings by making a brief list of the current problems; for example:

- Increased WCC and CRP. Catheter-related sepsis?
- Haemodynamically unstable. Increasing inotrope requirements. Adequately filled?
- Urine output deteriorating, rising creatinine. Needs renal referral.

Formulate an action plan

Using this approach you can prioritize problems and formulate a plan of action. In practice this should be done in consultation with the consultant looking after the ICU. The action plan should include the following:

- Action targeted against problems identified.
- Integrated plan for each organ system requiring support.
- Ventilation and/or weaning plan.
- 24-hour fluid intake and fluid balance including nutrition.
- Changes to drug therapy.
- Further investigations required.

Communication

When you have finished with the patient and detailed your findings and plans in the medical notes you should tell the nursing staff and others involved in the patient's care what is planned. In particular:

- Leave detailed instructions and parameters for the manipulation of drugs such as inotropes, which are generally titrated to response (e.g. what is the target mean blood pressure?).
- Discuss any major changes in therapy or new problems with the referring consultant team.
- Finally, you should keep the relatives informed of progress. (See Talking to relatives, p. 24.)

MEDICAL RECORDS

The nature of intensive care is such that many different individuals are
involved in the care of the patient. At the same time, the patient's
condition may change rapidly, requiring frequent changes in therapy.
If everyone is to keep up with the patient's progress, accurate,
contemporaneous note-keeping is essential. It is also worth bearing in
mind that medicolegal cases frequently arise where patients have
suffered trauma or complications from medical and surgical treatment.
You should record:

- Daily examination and progress notes.
- Interventions and procedures.
- Complications of procedures, which must be recorded accurately
  and honestly. Complications do occur and, providing you have
  followed correct procedures, they do not imply negligence. (Failure
  to record them or act appropriately upon them does!)
- Results of important investigations.
- The patient's chart is often used to record blood gases,
  biochemistry, haematology and microbiology results. This is a legal
  document and therefore the results do not need to be routinely
  copied into the medical notes. Important positive and negative
  findings, however, particularly those which carry either diagnostic
  or prognostic significance or which directly affect management,
  should be transcribed.
- It is useful to record the content and outcome of discussion with
  the patient's relatives, so that other staff do not give conflicting
  advice or opinions.

Occasionally because of the pressure of work in the ICU it may not be
possible to make full notes at the time, for example when admitting
and resuscitating a very unstable patient. It is crucial, however, that
notes are written at the earliest opportunity, and the fact that they have
been written retrospectively recorded.

CONFIDENTIALITY

The patient's medical condition and treatment are matters of
confidentiality. While it is generally accepted in intensive care that
relatives should be kept informed of what is going on, you must
respect the patient's wishes and confidentiality at all times. Therefore:

- Make sure you know to whom you are talking before giving out
  any information.

- Avoid discussing a patient's condition on the telephone. You do not know who is on the other end of the line. The press have been known to telephone and not admit who they are. If a relative lives too far away to make it to the hospital, offer to telephone them back on a previously agreed number.
- Never make any comment to journalists. Refer them to your hospital press liaison officer or your consultant.
- Occasionally the police may request information about a patient or request a blood test. Remember that your first duty is to the patient, no matter what he or she may have done. If in doubt, refer them to your consultant.

TALKING TO RELATIVES

The relatives of critically ill patients may well ask to speak to a doctor about the patient's condition, or you may ask to speak to them. Discussions with relatives should generally take place in a quiet room away from the patient's bedside.

- Do not talk over the patient, who may be aware of the surroundings and able to hear. (Hearing is the last sensory modality to be lost with sedative drugs.)
- Do not talk standing in the corridor; use a side room away from other families.
- Avoid talking to large groups of relatives. Speak to key members of the family and encourage them to explain things to other relatives.
- It is always advisable to take a nurse with you so that he or she knows what has been said. The relatives will probably only retain a fraction of what has been said to them, and the nurse can reinforce what you have said later. The nurse may also offer comfort and moral support to the patient's family.
- Adjust the explanation of events to the level of intelligence/ experience of the relatives and avoid medical jargon and abbreviations.
- It is always sensible to be as honest as possible with relatives and not to be overoptimistic about the ability of intensive care to turn around desperate situations. There are inherent uncertainties about the outcome of any particular disease and it is best to be cautious rather than giving 'exact' probabilities of survival.
- Do not criticize medical or nursing colleagues' management of the patient. It is all too easy, with the benefit of hindsight, to see where things went wrong, but you may have done no better yourself on the wards without all the facilities and expertise available to the

ICU. Difficult questions or decisions should be referred upwards to the consultant in charge.

- Do not let family members push you into making statements that are not true. This is particularly important concerning prognosis. Don't agree with statements like 'He is going to be all right isn't he Doctor' if it is not true.
- Record in the medical notes what has been said to the family. This ensures continuity and prevents misunderstandings.
- Accept that relatives will not always absorb bad news the first time they hear it. Time and repeated explanations may be required. (See Breaking bad news, p. 367.)

CONSENT TO TREATMENT

Consent is a difficult area in intensive care. Patients will often have had no opportunity to discuss intensive care treatment prior to admission. They are admitted to ICU on the presumption that they would wish to undergo life-sustaining treatments, if given the choice. The validity of obtaining consent from third parties (e.g. spouses, partners, other relatives, etc.) is questionable in this context. Nevertheless, it is often still considered normal practice to do so, and many relatives expect it.

When is consent required?

Patients in the ICU will have repeated interventions performed, for example, tracheal suction, arterial and venous line insertion, and passage of tubes into various orifices. Most units would not seek specific consent for these procedures, but you should always explain to the patient, and the relatives if present, what you are going to do.

For more significant invasive procedures like returning to theatre for relaparotomy, tracheostomy, or insertion of intracranial pressure monitoring, it is usual to seek formal consent whenever possible.

Patients requiring intensive care are usually unfit to give consent. Despite the legal invalidity of 'informed consent' from relatives, it is good practice to inform them that such procedures are to take place and inform them of the likely risks. Most hospital consent forms have a section for third party assent and it is usual practice to obtain it. If the relatives are not present then it is courteous and avoids conflict to obtain assent over the telephone. If nothing else, it ensures relatives are kept informed and provides an opportunity for an update on the patient's condition. Relatives do not respond well to news of the death of a patient in the operating theatre when they did not know that an operation was planned and time would have allowed for a telephone call!

It is unusual for relatives to refuse consent, but it may occur on occasions, in which case the medical staff are left with the difficult decision of whether or not to carry on against the relatives' wishes. With an adult it can be argued that relatives have no right to intervene. In a child under the legal age of consent (16 years) application may be made for the child to be made a ward of court, and the court's consent to treatment obtained. If there is any difficulty with consent, seek senior help. If there is dispute, application may have to be made to the courts for a ruling.

COMMON PROBLEMS RELATING TO CONSENT

Jehovah's Witnesses

Jehovah's Witnesses have religious objections to receiving transfusions of blood or blood products. Where these views are declared it is usual practice to discuss with the patient what therapy he or she will and will not accept, and then to obtain a written disclaimer. The patient should then be managed in the appropriate way but *without* the use of blood products. The situation in intensive care is difficult if the patient is unable to express his or her view at the time; if there is sufficient evidence of the patient's religious beliefs, these should be respected.

The situation with children is different. The child should be brought under the protection of the courts and a life-saving blood transfusion should be given.

(See Blood transfusion, p. 204, and Management of Jehovah's Witnesses, p. 209.)

Advance directives

An increasing number of people are writing so-called advance directives to outline what treatment they would or would not wish to have performed in the future in the case of them being unfit to make this decision at the time. The best known scenarios for such directives come from patients who are human immunodeficiency virus (HIV)-positive with acquired immune deficiency syndrome (AIDS) and patients with progressive dementia. In the case of HIV patients the directive may take the form of a request that they are not admitted to intensive care for assisted ventilation in the case of severe opportunistic pneumonia. At the time of writing, the exact legal status of such documents in the UK is still under discussion. It seems reasonable, however, that if such decisions are properly documented, then they should be respected. This may make the doctor's role in clinical decision-making very much easier.

Organ donor cards

These are a form of advance directive. People outline their wishes regarding potential organ donation by carrying signed organ donor cards and registering with the national donor registry. (See Brainstem death and Organ donation, p. 371.)

HIV testing

The ethical guidelines on HIV testing are clear. Patients should not be tested for HIV infection without informed consent, which is taken to include adequate counselling both before the test and after a positive test result. The situation in intensive care is therefore difficult, as it is unlikely that informed consent can be obtained.

An HIV test does not generally alter the management of, for example, a severe opportunistic infection, therefore an HIV test should not usually be performed until the patient is over the acute illness and adequate informed consent can be obtained. Any decision to test a patient for HIV without consent should therefore be made by a consultant and can normally only be justified if there is likely to be direct and immediate clinical benefit to the patient.

> ⚠ **You should not perform an HIV test for the benefit of staff who consider that they may be at risk from blood contamination. Universal precautions should be adopted for all patients to avoid occupational risk. If you receive a needle-stick injury or are contaminated with infected blood you should follow your local occupational health guidelines. An assessment of the risk of HIV exposure will be made and, if appropriate, postexposure prophylaxis prescribed. This is very effective when started within 4 hours of possible exposure.**

Consent for postmortem examination

Issues relating to consent for postmortem examination and the retention of tissue from deceased patients have generated significant attention lately. These are addressed in Chapter 16, page 369.

BASIC PRINCIPLES

SEDATION

The ICU can be a very frightening place for patients. They may have little control over their surroundings and may be repeatedly subjected to invasive, often painful procedures. In order to reduce pain and distress, patients are generally sedated. The intention is both to ensure patient comfort, and to enable nursing and medical procedures to be performed safely. Comfort encompasses a number of areas of different importance to each patient:

- tolerance of endotracheal intubation, assisted ventilation, invasive catheters, etc.
- analgesia (painful wounds, limbs, viscera)
- reduced awareness of frightening or noisy environment
- amnesia for unpleasant procedures
- promoting 'natural' sleep patterns.

In addition, sedation may play a therapeutic role by, for example, reducing cerebral oxygen consumption or myocardial work.

Ideal sedative agent
The ideal sedative agent for use in ICU probably does not exist. All sedative agents cause some degree of cardiovascular instability in critically ill patients. Longer-acting agents can be given by bolus, but may accumulate and do not allow rapid change in response to alterations in a patient's condition. Shorter-acting agents can be given by infusion, are less likely to accumulate and allow rapid change in depth but can be difficult to titrate.

In general, single agents are not effective, and combinations of drugs are used. The principle employed is similar to that of 'balanced anaesthesia'. By combining the benefits of more than one class of agent, satisfactory levels of sedation can be achieved at much lower doses than could be achieved using either agent alone, thus allowing some of the adverse effects of individual agents to be reduced. A typical combination is that of an opioid (e.g. fentanyl) together with a benzodiazepine (e.g. midazolam). This combination provides analgesia, sedation and anxiolysis. The advantages and disadvantages of these agents are shown in Table 3.1. Many units now use the intravenous anaesthetic agent propofol as a primary sedative agent in combination with an opioid analgesic.

Choice of agents
The choice of agents will depend on local protocols and the clinical condition of the patient. If the balance of a patient's problem is pain, then analgesia is the main requirement. Epidural anaesthesia, other

TABLE 3.1 Advantages and disadvantages of opioids and benzodiazepines for ICU sedation

	Advantages	Disadvantages
Opioids	Respiratory depression Cough suppression Some sedative effects Analgesic	Nausea and vomiting Delayed gastric emptying and ileus Potential accumulation Respiratory depression Potential cardiovascular instability Withdrawal phenomenon
Benzodiazepines	Hypnotic Anxiolytic Amnesic Anticonvulsant	No analgesic activity Unpredictable duration of action Potential cardiovascular instability Withdrawal phenomenon

regional anaesthetic techniques and patient-controlled analgesia (PCA) may be useful. (See Postoperative analgesia, p. 299.) If the balance of the patient's problem is agitation, then the main requirement is for sedative or anxiolytic agents. Tables 3.2 and 3.3 provide a guide to commonly used drugs.

Other agents worthy of note include clonidine and ketamine.

Clonidine

(50–150 µg i.v. bolus 4–6 hourly)
(0.2–2 µg/kg/h i.v. infusion)

Clonidine, an α_2 agonist at presynaptic terminals, has general sedative effect. The main side effect is hypotension and a small test dose is usually given to assess the effect on blood pressure. If tolerated, doses can be increased. Produces little respiratory depression and can therefore be used safely in patients where agitation is hindering weaning from mechanical ventilation. Can be given orally. No particular problems associated with withdrawal. The use of an α_2 agonist as a primary sedative agent is increasing. It is particularly useful for managing withdrawal phenomena following withdrawal of alcohol or other sedative drugs. Dexmedetomidine is a similar class of drug licensed for ICU sedation in the USA.

Ketamine

(0.5–1 mg/kg i.v. bolus)
(0.2–2 mg/kg/h i.v. infusion)

TABLE 3.2 Common analgesic agents

Drug	Dose	Notes
Morphine	2–5 mg i.v. bolus 10–50 µg/kg/h	Cheap, long acting Good analgesic, reasonable sedative Standard agent for PCAS and postoperative pain Metabolized by liver, active metabolites accumulate in renal failure
Fentanyl	2–6 µg/kg/h	Shorter acting than morphine Good analgesic, less sedative. Metabolized by liver. No active metabolites, no accumulation in renal failure.
Alfentanil	20–50 µg/kg/h	Expensive. Shorter acting than fentanyl Good analgesic, less sedative. No active metabolites, no accumulation in renal failure. Rapid termination of effects after discontinuation
Remifentanil	0.1–0.25 µg/kg/min	More expensive still. Ultrashort-acting analgesic, very titratable Metabolized by plasma esterases Rapid clearance even after prolonged infusion Mostly used intraoperatively or for short-term ventilation Causes significant hypotension, avoid boluses

Ketamine is an anaesthetic agent that is also profoundly analgesic. Unlike other sedative agents it does not cause cardiovascular or respiratory depression at normal doses. Ketamine indirectly increases sympathetic activity, which in turn leads to increases in heart rate and blood pressure and produces bronchodilatation. These properties have made it a useful agent for anaesthesia in extreme environments outside hospital (e.g. for amputation at the scene of an accident) and would make it appear attractive as an agent for use in intensive care. Historically it has been used to provide short-term analgesia for painful procedures (e.g. burns dressings) and it is occasionally used as a sedative agent in severe asthma for its bronchodilator effects. Its general use is, however, limited by the incidence of unpleasant dreams, hallucinations and emergence phenomena.

TABLE 3.3 Common sedative agents (doses based on 70-kg adult)

Drug	Dose	Notes
Diazepam	5–10 mg bolus i.v.	Cheap, long-acting benzodiazepine. Reasonable cardiovascular stability, sedative, amnesic, anticonvulsant. Given by intermittent boluses. Metabolized in liver. Long elimination half-life. Parent drug and active metabolites can accumulate in sicker patients, therefore avoid continuous infusions
Midazolam	2–5 mg bolus i.v. 2–10 mg/h	Shorter-acting benzodiazepine. Similar properties to diazepam. Metabolized by the liver, no active metabolites. Can be given by continuous infusion
Etomidate	0.2 mg/kg bolus i.v.	Short-acting cardiovascular stable anaesthetic induction agent. Single dose used for induction of anaesthesia, e.g. prior to intubation. Associated with adrenal suppression. Not to be used by infusion
Propofol*	1–3 mg/kg bolus 2–5 mg/kg/h	Short-acting intravenous anaesthetic agent. Sedative anticonvulsant and amnesic properties. Used for induction of anaesthesia and intubation. May cause significant hypotension. Concerns about use in children

*Propofol 1–3 mg/kg is sufficient to induce anaesthesia (e.g. prior to intubation). Smaller doses 10–20 mg repeated to effect may be sufficient for increasing the depth of sedation, e.g. prior to suction or painful procedure. (See also Practical procedures: Intubation, p. 337.)

Problems of oversedation

Ideally patients should be awake, pain-free, able to move about as much as possible and be able to co-operate with physiotherapy and nursing care. Excessive sedation should be avoided. The potential problems associated with oversedation are:

- prolonged need for IPPV/intubation
- haemodynamic instability

- gastrointestinal tract stasis
- potential immune suppression
- potential organ toxicity
- difficulty in assessing neurological state.

Titration to effect

In order to avoid excessive sedation, agents should be titrated according to the balance of the patient's needs. In practice this can be difficult. The requirement for sedation differs markedly between patients. Younger, fitter patients generally require more sedative and analgesic drugs. Patients who abuse alcohol and other centrally acting drugs may be very difficult to sedate owing to cross-tolerance between the abused substance and the sedative or analgesic agents prescribed. Relatives and patients often deny such usage. Acute tolerance to drugs used for sedation in ICU may also occur.

In addition, the elimination of drugs by critically ill patients is very variable. There is only limited information on drug metabolism and excretion in the critically ill. Drug trials performed in rats, healthy 'volunteers', ASA I patients, compensated cirrhosis and uraemia bear little resemblance to the typical ICU patient. Therefore repeated assessment of sedation and analgesia is required. Where drugs are given by continuous infusion, consideration should be given to stopping them daily to avoid accumulation and oversedation. Studies have repeatedly shown that patients tend to be oversedated and that if sedation is reassessed regularly the duration of tracheal intubation and ventilatory support can be reduced.

Sedation scoring

Sedation scoring systems may be useful in helping titrate levels of sedation. A typical score, with the appropriate response to the hourly sedation score, is shown in Table 3.4. In this system levels −1 to +1 are ideal.

COMMON PROBLEMS RELATED TO SEDATION

Patient difficult to sedate

Check that sedative infusions are running correctly and at the prescribed dose. In addition:

- Exclude possible causes of agitation, including: full bladder, painful wound, hypoxia, hypercarbia, and endotracheal tube touching carina.
- Review other drug therapy and stop where appropriate. Many drugs (for example H_2 blockers) have the potential to induce confusional states.

TABLE 3.4 Typical sedation score

Description	Score	Comment
Agitated and restless	+3	Levels 3 to 2: inadequate sedation
Awake and uncomfortable	+2	Give bolus and increase infusion rates
Awake but comfortable	+1	Levels 1 to 0: appropriate levels of sedation
Roused by voice	0	Reassess regularly
Roused by touch	−1	Levels −1 to −3: excess levels of sedation
Roused by painful stimuli	−2	Reduce or stop infusion
Unrousable	−3	Restart when desired level attained
Natural sleep	A	Ideal
Paralysed	P	Difficult to assess level of sedation. Consider physiological response to stimulation

- Consider the value of tracheostomy over conventional intubation. This is often better tolerated and allows sedative and analgesic drugs to be significantly reduced.
- Consider alternative sedative agents.

Eventually all patients will need to be weaned off drugs and there is often a difficult phase when the patient is partially sedated but unable to cooperate due to residual drug effects. Real problem patients, for example, those post head injury or suffering from withdrawal of drugs or alcohol, may be best nursed on a mattress on the floor. This reduces risk of harm should the patient fall out of bed. (See Withdrawal phenomena below.)

Patient who will not wake up

If a patient fails to regain full consciousness after sedative and analgesic drugs have been stopped for a period of time, the question 'why?' invariably arises. This may be due to the accumulation of drugs or their active metabolites, which will resolve with time, but other causes of coma should be excluded. Consider:

- effects of sepsis (for example as part of multiple organ failure)
- metabolic derangement/encephalopathy
- structural brain damage (including CVA, hypoxic brain injury)
- awake patients who cannot respond ('locked-in syndrome')
- residual paralysis. (See Muscle relaxants, p. 37.)

TABLE 3.5 Naloxone and flumazenil

Drug	Dose	Notes
Naloxone	0.4–2 mg bolus i.v.	Competitive antagonist of opioid receptors* Used to reverse sedation and respiratory depression caused by opioids
Flumazenil	0.2–0.5 mg bolus i.v.	Competitive antagonist of benzodiazepine receptors* Used to reverse sedation and respiratory depression caused by benzodiazepines

*Both have short half-life (20 min) leading to recurrence of respiratory depression and sedation. Risk of fits, hypertension and arrhythmias (especially in patients who have taken mixed overdoses). Do not infuse over long periods of time. Ventilate the patient and await resolution as redistribution and metabolism of drugs occurs!

An EEG and CT scan may be helpful. If no other cause of coma can be established and failure to wake up is considered to result from the accumulation of sedative agents, a trial of naloxone or flumazenil may occasionally be diagnostic (Table 3.5).

Withdrawal phenomena following ICU sedation

When drugs used before admission, or sedative drugs given in ICU, are stopped, drug withdrawal states may develop. This may result in seizures, hallucinations, delirium tremens, confusional states, agitation and aggression. These phenomena are difficult to control without further heavy sedation, but usually settle over time. You should look for and treat any reversible causes of confusion (Table 3.6).

Drugs that can be useful for the control of acute confusional states, including those induced by the withdrawal of mixed sedative agents, are shown in Table 3.7. You should generally seek senior advice before resorting to these agents.

TABLE 3.6 Causes of acute confusional states

Side effects of prescribed drugs
Withdrawal of alcohol or other centrally acting drugs
Effects of sepsis
Renal and hepatic encephalopathy
Electrolyte disturbance
Hypoxia/hypercarbia
Brain injury
Sleep deprivation (especially REM sleep)
Elderly patients particularly susceptible

TABLE 3.7 Drugs for the treatment of acute confusional states

Drug	Dose	Notes
Lorazepam	1–3 mg bolus i.v.	Long-acting benzodiazepine Useful for controlling seizures and withdrawal phenomenon
Clonidine	50–150 µg bolus i.v.	α_2 agonist Useful for controlling withdrawal phenomenon See previous notes
Chlorpromazine	5–10 mg bolus i.v. Repeat as necessary	Major tranquillizer* Useful in acute confusional states
Haloperidol	5–10 mg bolus Repeat as necessary	Major tranquillizer* Useful in acute confusional states

*Large number of actions and side effects. Particularly beware of α blockade and hypotension.

MUSCLE RELAXANTS

The routine use of muscle relaxants in ICU is to be discouraged. The problems associated with muscle relaxants include:

- 'Awareness', when paralysed patients are inadequately sedated during unpleasant procedures. Beware, as increasing numbers of surgical procedures, such as tracheostomy, are performed in ICU!
- Accidental unnoticed disconnection of the ventilator may result in hypoxia because the paralysed patient cannot make any respiratory effort.
- Neuropathies and myopathies are common in patients with multiple organ failure and may be associated with the prolonged use of muscle relaxants.

Therefore use should be restricted to the following:

- To facilitate endotracheal intubation.
- The management of patients with acute brain injury or cerebral oedema (to prevent rises in ICP on coughing).
- The management of patients with critical cardiovascular or respiratory insufficiency where the balance between oxygen delivery and oxygen consumption may be improved by preventing muscle activity.

The choice of drugs depends upon the requirement and the patient's general condition.

Suxamethonium

(Only used for endotracheal intubation: 1 mg/kg i.v. bolus)

This is a short-acting depolarizing muscle relaxant, which gives good intubating conditions in less than a minute. It is useful for rapidly intubating patients in an emergency and has the advantage for the inexperienced that it has a short duration of action (2–4 minutes), so that if intubation is difficult, spontaneous respiratory effort is rapidly re-established. In a small number of patients, however, the effects are prolonged because of a genetic abnormality in the cholinesterase enzyme, which breaks down suxamethonium.

Side effects associated with the use of suxamethonium include bradycardia, hypotension, and increased salivation and bronchial secretions. These can be blocked by the use of atropine. Intraocular pressure and intracranial pressure are transiently increased. All patients suffer a small increase (0.5–1 mmol/1) in serum potassium following suxamethonium. It should be avoided, therefore, in patients with hyperkalaemia. In some groups of patients, this increase in potassium may be much greater and may result in a cardiac arrest.

> ⚠ **In some patient groups, suxamethonium is associated with serious, life-threatening side effects. This is one of the reasons why some people believe that suxamethonium should not be used in the ICU. Seek local advice. Make sure you know the contraindications to its use.**

TABLE 3.8 Contraindications to suxamethonium

Absolute	Relative
Recent burns or crush injuries	Severe overwhelming sepsis
Spinal injury	Prolonged immobility
Renal failure and raised K$^+$	Neuromyopathies
Myasthenia gravis	
Dystrophia myotonica	
History of malignant hyperpyrexia	

NON-DEPOLARIZING MUSCLE RELAXANTS

Currently available non-depolarizing muscle relaxants are slower in onset and of longer duration than suxamethonium. They can be used for intubation as an alternative to suxamethonium (when this is contraindicated) or when the risk of airway contamination with gastric contents is low. Non-depolarizing muscle relaxants can be used either by intermittent bolus or infusion to provide continuous muscle relaxation when this is required. Table 3.9 provides a guide to commonly used agents.

Monitoring neuromuscular blockade

The use of muscle relaxants should be regularly reviewed and consideration given to stopping them intermittently to assess the

TABLE 3.9 Common non-depolarizing muscle relaxants

Drug	Dose	Notes
Atracurium	0.5 mg/kg i.v. bolus 0.5–1.0 mg/kg/h infusion	Onset 1–2 minutes, duration 30 minutes Undergoes spontaneous degradation, no accumulation in hepatorenal failure. Ideal for use by infusion Localized histamine release common May cause bronchospasm
Cisatracurium	150 µg/kg i.v. bolus 1–3 µg/kg/min infusion	Onset 1–2 minutes, duration 45 minutes Similar to atracurium, less histamine release
Vecuronium	0.1 mg/kg i.v. bolus 0.05–0.2 mg/kg/h infusion	Onset 1–2 minutes, duration 40 minutes Can be associated with bradycardia Parent drug and active metabolites can accumulate in hepatorenal failure
Rocuronium	600 µg/kg i.v. bolus 300–600 µg/kg/h infusion	Faster onset of action than vecuronium More prolonged block Similar in other aspects to vecuronium
Pancuronium	0.1 mg/kg i.v. bolus	Onset 2 minutes, duration 1 hour Produces tachycardia and increased blood pressure Relatively long-acting, usually given by intermittent bolus Can accumulate in renal failure

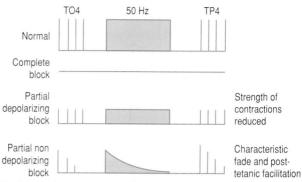

Fig. 3.1 Monitoring neuromuscular function: typical patterns. TO4, train of four.

adequacy of sedation. Neuromuscular blockade can be monitored if required using nerve stimulators. On the ICU this is most commonly required to exclude residual muscle paralysis, for example prior to performing brainstem death tests. An electric current is passed through a peripheral nerve and the response of the muscle supplied by that nerve observed. A common method of assessment is to produce four impulses, 0.5 s apart, known as a train of four (TO4), followed by a period of continuous tetanic stimulation at 50 Hz and then another train of four. Typical responses are shown in Figure 3.1.

Other than for intubation purposes, it is usually unnecessary to completely abolish all muscle response. When using non-depolarizing muscle relaxants by infusion, 75–90% block is usually adequate. This equates to 1 or 2 twitches present on a train of four.

PSYCHOLOGICAL CARE

Despite the provision of analgesic and sedative agents to patients on intensive care it is important to realize that they are not anaesthetized and may be aware of their surroundings during their stay. Even the sickest patients, who may be heavily sedated during critical phases of their illness, will hopefully go on to a period of convalescence, when they will be fully aware of their surroundings. This can be very stressful for patients. A number of factors may contribute to patients' distress.

Environment

The ICU is a very noisy place and often the only lighting is artificial. Patients may spend long periods in the same room with little knowledge of the outside world. Even the appreciation of day and night may be lost, resulting in disturbed sleep patterns. In addition, sedative drugs abolish rapid eye movement (dream) sleep and this can cause marked psychological disturbance, particularly during the convalescent stage.

Communication difficulties

Communication difficulties following tracheal intubation have not been adequately resolved. Written messages and letter boards are cumbersome, and lip reading is often difficult. Speaking aids for ventilated patients are available in the form of an artificial larynx to produce tones, but none is satisfactory for acute use as they take time and practice to work well. Speaking tracheostomy tubes are helpful in the recovery phase of illness.

Dependency

Patients in intensive care are totally dependent both on the nursing staff for their personal needs and on machines and drugs. In addition, they may be repeatedly visited by large groups of doctors and other staff. This may be humiliating and depersonalizing.

Pain, fear and anxiety

Many patients in intensive care will have painful surgical wounds and many will also have stiff painful limbs and joints as a result of immobility and critical illness neuropathy (see p. 254.) Almost all will be subjected to repeated, potentially painful, procedures. Patients may be aware how sick they are, or even that they are dying. The overall experience is very frightening.

To reduce the impact of these problems, think about the psychological care of your patient. In particular:

- Take time to get to know patients. Acknowledge their fears and anxieties. Give appropriate explanations and reassurance.
- Respect patient privacy as much as possible.
- Avoid unnecessarily large ward rounds and talking over the patient.
- Always explain procedures to patients and provide adequate analgesia or anaesthesia.
- Avoid disturbing the patient at night if possible. Encourage daytime stimulation in the form of visits from relatives and children. television and radio, all of which improve morale.

Despite every effort many patients on ICU will suffer distressing, vivid nightmares and dreams during their stay. Some will develop apparent psychoses, which require treatment. Others (particularly long-stay patients) may become markedly depressed and withdrawn. Consideration should be given to appropriate antidepressant therapy, although there are arguments against its use in so-called reactive depression. Amitriptyline at night may aid nocturnal sleep and help to elevate mood and motivation. One role of the intensive care follow-up clinic is to allow the late psychological sequelae of intensive care to be recognized and managed appropriately. (See ICU follow-up clinics, p. 13.)

FLUIDS AND ELECTROLYTES

The management of fluid and electrolyte balance in critically ill patients is fundamental to intensive care. In health, daily input and output are in balance and the figures (in ml) are approximately as shown in Figure 3.2. This translates to daily water and electrolyte requirements as shown in Table 3.10.

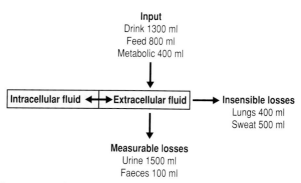

Input
Drink 1300 ml
Feed 800 ml
Metabolic 400 ml

Intracellular fluid ←→ Extracellular fluid → Insensible losses
Lungs 400 ml
Sweat 500 ml

Measurable losses
Urine 1500 ml
Faeces 100 ml

Fig. 3.2 Typical fluid balance for a healthy 70 kg adult under normal environmental conditions.

TABLE 3.10 Typical daily water and electrolyte requirements	
Water	30–35 ml/kg/day
Na^+	1–1.5 mmol/kg/day
K^+	1 mmol/kg/day

Simplistically therefore, fluid management is a matter of selecting an appropriate fluid and volume to provide the required amount of water and electrolytes. The constituents of commonly available fluids are shown in Table 3.11. Daily requirements could, for example, be provided by 2–3 litres of 4% dextrose and 0.18% saline, with 20 mmol of potassium added to each litre. For the critically ill patient on the intensive care unit, however, the situation is more complex than this. A number of factors need to be considered.

Reduced fluid requirement

- Stress response to critical illness. Increased activity of the renin–angiotensin–aldosterone axis results in reduced sodium excretion, while at the same time increased secretion of antidiuretic hormone (ADH) reduces secretion of free water. (See Stress response to critical illness, p. 298, and SIADH, p. 169.)
- Oliguric renal failure.

Increased fluid requirement

- Widespread capillary leak associated with sepsis and inflammatory conditions may result in redistribution of body water out of the vascular compartment, and the development of pulmonary and peripheral oedema.
- Gastrointestinal tract dysfunction, fluid sequestration and diarrhoea.
- Increased fluid losses associated with burns, skin loss, wounds and fistulae.
- Insensible losses are increased by pyrexia and poor humidification of inspired ventilator gases. (Fluid requirements may increase by as much as 150 ml/day for each 1°C rise in temperature.)
- Non-oliguric (high-output) renal failure and the recovery phase of acute tubular necrosis.
- Neurogenic diabetes insipidus may accompany brain injury.
- The effects of the underlying condition, multiple procedures and venesections may result in increased requirements for fluid or repeated blood transfusions. Significant coagulopathy may require use of other blood products such as fresh frozen plasma (FFP) and platelet concentrates. All these additional volumes of fluid influence overall fluid balance.

Altered electrolyte requirements

- At cellular level: hypoxia, acidosis, toxins and the effects of drugs can interfere with ionic pump mechanisms and lead to alterations in normal electrolyte balances and requirements.
- Fluid shifts and increased fluid losses can be associated with altered electrolyte balance.
- Altered renal function further impairs electrolyte homeostasis.

TABLE 3.11 Composition of commonly available intravenous fluids

	Na⁺ (mmol/l)	Cl⁻ (mmol/l)	K⁺ (mmol/l)	Ca²⁺ (mmol/l)	HCO₃⁻ (mmol/l)	Dextrose (mmol/l)	Osmolality* (mosmol/kg)
Hartman's/Ringer lactate	131	112	5.0	2.0	29		279
0.9% Saline	154	154					308
0.45% Saline	77	77					154
0.18% Saline 4% Dextrose	31	31				222	284
5% Dextrose						278	278

*Calculated osmolality. Measured osmolality may be less.

Practical fluid management

The aim is to keep the patient hydrated, with an adequate circulating volume and normal electrolytes. Exact fluid regimens will depend on the patient's clinical state of hydration (look at tongue, mucous membranes, tissue turgor, urine output), cumulative fluid balance on the daily charts, and electrolyte investigations.

- Measure 24-hour fluid balance accurately. The nurses will chart the totals of all fluids, in and out, hourly. This will include all intravenous and nasogastric fluids, all drugs and all measurable losses. It does not include unmeasurable insensible losses or shifts between intra- and extravascular spaces.
- Measure serum electrolytes frequently. Sodium (Na^+) and potassium (K^+) at least every 4–6 hours in sicker patients. Magnesium (Mg^{2+}), calcium (Ca^{2+}) and phosphate (PO_4^{3-}) daily or as required. Increasing Na^+ and urea suggest dehydration.
- Additional measurements such as plasma and urinary osmolality and urinary electrolytes are useful in difficult cases.
  (See Oliguria, p. 155.)

A typical fluid regimen for a 70 kg adult patient not receiving nutritional support, and with normal renal function, might be:

- Maintenance: dextrose 4% and saline 0.18% at 80–100 ml/h plus 20–60 mmol K^+ per litre.
- Additional NG/drain losses: replace ml for ml with normal saline (0.9%) with 20 mmol K^+/l.
- Additional K^+, Ca^{2+}, Mg^{2+} and phosphate as required.
- Colloids as additionally required to maintain adequate central venous filling pressures.
- Blood products as required.

Despite careful fluid management patients frequently become significantly fluid-overloaded, as measured by positive fluid balance and generalized oedema. This usually reflects the severity of the underlying clinical condition and resolves as the patient's condition improves. However, you should review the fluid balance and regimen regularly and adjust it as seems necessary. If in doubt, consider a fluid challenge or trial of diuretics. Low-dose diuretics (for example 10–20 mg furosemide (frusemide)) will often produce a good diuresis in the overloaded patient but have little effect in those who are not. (See Oliguria, p. 155.)

Disturbances of fluid and electrolyte balance are discussed further in Chapter 8.

NUTRITION

During the acute phase of illness, intensive care patients are generally catabolic. Muscle is broken down to provide amino acids for energy requirements and for synthesis of acute phase proteins. Nitrogen from protein breakdown is lost in the urine and patients develop a negative nitrogen balance. This may result in severe muscle wasting and weakness, greatly prolonging recovery. The aim of feeding patients is therefore to provide adequate amino acids and energy to minimize this process.

When examining patients in the ICU it is worth noting their nutritional status in terms of muscle bulk. Note that wasting may often be hidden by oedema fluid and it is only on recovery, when oedema fluids shift, that the true extent of wasting is visible. All critically ill patients should be assumed to have established or impending nutritional deficiency.

Nutrition can be provided by the enteral or parenteral route depending upon the circumstances, although the enteral route is preferred (see below). Whichever route is chosen, the aim is to provide all the patient's nutritional requirements. Typical daily requirements are given in Table 3.12. (See also Fluids and electrolytes, p. 42.)

Estimation of energy requirements

Energy requirements depend on body mass and metabolic rate. They are normally 30–40 kcal/kg/day, this may be increased in critical illness.

In most instances when starting nutritional support it is not necessary to calculate exact energy requirements. Standard feeds can be used and the energy content can be adjusted subsequently if necessary. If required, energy requirements can be estimated using formulae such as the one below. Seek advice from a dietician.

TABLE 3.12 Typical daily requirements

Item	Requirement	Typical daily requirement (70 kg adult)
Maintenance fluid	30–35 ml/kg/day	2500 ml
Na$^+$	1–1.5 mmol/kg/day	100 mmol
K$^+$	1 mmol/kg/day	60–80 mmol
Phosphate	0.5 mmol/kg/day	<50 mmol
Energy	30–40 kcal/kg/day*	

*Increased in critical illness (see below).

1. Estimate the resting energy requirements or basal metabolic rate (BMR) from nomograms (Table 3.13).
2. Adjust the basal metabolic rate according to the patient's individual circumstances (Table 3.14).
3. Add a factor for the level activity and metabolic effect of feed:

- Add 10% for bed-bound immobile.
- Add 15–20% if bed-bound mobile/sitting.
- Add 25% if mobile on ward.

An alternative method of estimating energy requirements is indirect calorimetry. Metabolic computers are available which sample the patient's inspired and expired gases and, using an assumed value for the respiratory quotient, can estimate total energy expenditure.

TABLE 3.13 Estimation of basal metabolic rate

Age (years)	Male	Female
15–18	BMR = $17.6 \times$ weight (kg) + 656	BMR = $13.3 \times$ weight (kg) + 690
18–30	BMR = $15.0 \times$ weight (kg) + 690	BMR = $14.8 \times$ weight (kg) + 485
30–60	BMR = $11.4 \times$ weight (kg) + 870	BMR = $8.1 \times$ weight (kg) + 842
>60	BMR = $11.7 \times$ weight (kg) + 585	BMR = $9.0 \times$ weight (kg) + 656

TABLE 3.14 Metabolic rate adjustment for stress

Burns 25–90% (1st month)	Add	20–70%
Severe sepsis/multiple trauma	Add	20–50%
Persistent increase temperature 2°C	Add	25%
Burns 10–25% (1st month) Multiple long bone fractures (1st week)	Add	10–30%
Persistent increase temperature 1°C	Add	12%
Burns 10% (1st month) Single fracture (1st week) Postoperative patient (1st 4 days) Inflammatory bowel disease Mild infection	Add	0–10%
Partial starvation (>10% loss body weight)	Subtract	0–10%

> ⚠ **While adequate calorie intake might prevent
> negative nitrogen balance (muscle breakdown) in a
> critically ill patient, excess feeding will not produce a positive
> nitrogen balance in a catabolic patient. This will only be
> achieved in the recovery phase of illness. Avoid excessive
> feeding. Seek specialist advice from a dietician.**

Energy requirements are generally provided as a mixture of
carbohydrate and fats.

Nitrogen (protein)

To prevent muscle breakdown adequate amounts of nitrogen must be
provided. This is generally of the order of 9–14 g nitrogen a day,
equivalent to 1–2 g protein/kg/day. Proteins should be provided in a
form that ensures that all the essential amino acids are provided.
There is increasing interest in the role of individual amino acids. For
example, glutamine has a specific role as a substrate for metabolism
within the gastrointestinal tract where it is important in maintaining
integrity and function.

Vitamins, minerals and trace elements

Vitamins, minerals and trace elements are essential for health
and many have important roles in enzyme pathways. Not much
is known, however, about the requirements during critical illness.
Both water- and fat-soluble vitamins can be provided by commercially
available preparations. Folic acid and vitamin B12 should be
prescribed separately. Trace elements and minerals, including
calcium, magnesium, iron, zinc, copper, selenium, molybdenum,
manganese and chromium, are available. Replacement is guided by
the reference values for daily recommended intake and signs of
deficiency.

Immunonutrition

There has been a lot of interest over the last 10 years in the role of
several specific nutrients in modulating the immune response.
Arginine, glutamine, nucleotides and omega-3 fatty acids have been
studied, either alone or in combination, in a variety of patient groups.
Although studies have shown conflicting results, there is a suggestion
that the addition of some supplements, particularly glutamine, may
improve outcome in critically ill patients. More research is needed in
this area.

ENTERAL FEEDING

Enteral feeding is the preferred means of nutritional support. Advice should be sought from the dietician for exact nutritional requirements; however, ready-to-use off-the-shelf enteral feeding formulae are available and are suitable for most patients. Therefore do not wait for specialist dietetic advice before starting enteral feeding. Start empirical feeds out of hours and seek a tailored approach on the next working day. It is unnecessary in intubated patients to stop feeds for repeated surgical procedures like daily pack changes or tracheostomy.

Indications

Unless there is a specific surgical contraindication, all patients should receive enteral feeding as soon as possible, preferably within 24 hours. This provides nutrition and helps to maintain gastrointestinal tract integrity and function. Potential benefits include:

- Reduced gut atrophy.
- Reduced bacterial and endotoxin translocation.
- Reduced incidence of septic complications and SIRS.
- Reduced length of hospital stay.

(See Stress ulcer prophylaxis, p. 53 and Gastrointestinal tract, p. 140)

Contraindications

Contraindications include paralytic ileus, intestinal obstruction and surgical conditions of the oesophagus or abdomen.

> The absence of bowel sounds alone in a ventilated patient without other evidence of ileus should not prevent attempts to commence enteral feeding.

Route of administration

The majority of patients in the ICU will already have a large-bore nasogastric tube in situ for gastric aspiration. This can be used for short-term feeding. In patients who require longer term feeding and who are convalescing, fine-bore nasogastric feeding tubes are more comfortable and less likely to cause mucosal erosions. (See Practical procedures, p. 357.)

Delayed gastric emptying is a major factor limiting the success of enteral feeding. There is increasing use of feeding tubes placed through the pylorus, which deliver enteral feed directly into the duodenum or jejunum. Although it is possible to place these tubes 'blindly', more commonly placement is guided by X-ray screening, ultrasound or endoscopy.

The use of percutaneous endoscopic gastrostomy (PEG) is increasing. This has the advantage that it can be performed on the ICU and allows all nasogastric tubes to be removed, reducing the risks of nosocomial infection.

Feeding regimen

Enteral feeds are given by continuous infusion. Typically, feed is given for 20 hours and then stopped for 4 hours. This rest period is to allow the gastric pH to return to normal (acid) levels. This helps to prevent colonization of the stomach with gastrointestinal tract flora, which is associated with an increased incidence of nosocomial pneumonia.

Many units have policies for the commencement of enteral feeding. For example:

- Commence enteral feed at 30 ml/h.
- Give feed for 4 hours.
- Aspirate NG tube to assess gastric residual volume.
- If feed absorbed, increase in 25 ml increments every 4 hours up to 100 ml/h.

Complications

The complications of enteral feeding are shown in Table 3.15. Misplacement or dislodgement of the NG tube can allow accidental delivery of, or aspiration of, feed into the lungs. The position of the tube must always be verified before feed or drugs are administered. (See Passing a nasogastric tube, p. 357) Blocked NG tubes can occasionally be 'rescued' by flushing with normal saline using a Luer–Lok syringe. Small syringes are more effective then large ones for this purpose.

TABLE 3.15 Complications of enteral feeding

Tube malposition or displacement
Tube occlusion
Abdominal cramps and bloating
Regurgitation and pulmonary aspiration
Diarrhoea
Increased risk of nosocomial infection associated with NG tubes
Metabolic derangement

COMMON PROBLEMS ASSOCIATED WITH ENTERAL FEEDING

Feed not absorbed

High gastric residual volume suggests enteral feed is not being absorbed. If after 4 hours' feed the gastric residual volume is more than 200 ml, return the aspirated feed to the stomach and rest for 1 hour. Then reassess.

Consider the need for further investigation such as plain abdominal X-ray to exclude obstruction. If possible, stop or reduce opioid analgesics that may delay gastric emptying. Ensure that the electrolyte balance is normal. Disturbances of potassium and magnesium in particular can contribute to gastrointestinal tract dysfunction. Consider the use of prokinetic drugs to promote gastric emptying. Choice will depend upon local protocol. Available agents include:

- metoclopramide
- erythromycin.

Unless there is a contraindication to feeding, do not stop enteral feeds purely because of 'failure to absorb'. Continue at a low rate, for example 10–20 ml/hour. Consider the use of a nasoduodenal/ nasojejunal tube.

Diarrhoea

Diarrhoea commonly complicates enteral feeding in the ICU. The causes of this are multifactorial. Diarrhoea is generally a nuisance rather than a serious problem; however, it may result in the need to abandon enteral feeding.

- Do not immediately stop enteral feed. Discuss, with the dietician changing the feed, reduction in the osmolality and increase in the fibre content.
- Perform a rectal examination to exclude faecal impaction (common in the elderly), which may be a cause of overflow diarrhoea. Consider suppositories or manual evacuation.
- Confirm diarrhoea is not infective in nature: send stool specimens for microscopy and culture (*Salmonella*, *Shigella* and *Campylobacter* species) and for *Clostridium difficile* toxin.
- Treat any infective process appropriately. For *Clostridium difficile* use oral or nasogastric metronidazole or vancomycin.
- Review the drug chart. Stop any prokinetic drugs such as metoclopramide. If the diarrhoea is non-infective consider the use of loperamide.

- If the diarrhoea is bloody or if the nature is unclear consider the need for surgical investigation, e.g. sigmoidoscopy or colonoscopy.

TOTAL PARENTERAL NUTRITION

If enteral feeding is contraindicated or cannot be established then total parenteral nutrition (TPN) may be required. It is generally not necessary if the patient is likely to be able to recommence enteral feeding within a few days, unless the patient is already severely wasted or malnourished. If in doubt seek senior advice.

Practical TPN

Most units now use one or two standard mixture feeds, prepared under sterile conditions in the pharmacy or bought in from an outside supplier. The typical composition of a standard feed in shown in Table 3.16.

Some patients need regimens specifically tailored to their needs. For example, patients in renal failure, who are not on renal support, require a reduced volume and restricted nitrogen intake to avoid rises in plasma urea. For most patients, however, a standard feed can be started and advice subsequently sought from dieticians, pharmacists or a parenteral nutrition team.

In practice, decide what volume of feed the patient will tolerate. Standard adult feeds are usually 2.5 litres a day, but smaller volume feeds are available for fluid-restricted patients.

Parenteral feeds are hypertonic and cause thrombophlebitis. They should normally only be given via central venous lines, although high-volume lower-osmolality feeds may be given via peripherally inserted feeding lines. When inserting multiple lumen central lines, it is a good idea to keep one lumen clean and dedicated for TPN. Parenteral nutrition mixtures make good culture mediums for bacteria, so do not break the line to give anything else. TPN is given by constant infusion over 24 hours and delivered by volumetric infusion pumps.

TABLE 3.16 Typical composition of standard TPN mixture	
Volume	2.5 litres
Nitrogen source (9–14 g nitrogen)	L-amino acid solution
Energy source (1500–2000 kcal)	Glucose and lipid emulsion
Additives	Electrolytes, trace elements, vitamins
Other additives	Insulin and H_2 blockers may be added if required

Monitoring TPN

Advice should be sought from the nutrition team and dietician. The following should be assessed daily:

- Fluid balance.
- Urea, electrolytes, phosphate.
- Glucose. Blood sugar will often rise and require the addition of an insulin infusion. Recent evidence suggests that close control of blood sugar levels may improve outcome of critically ill patients (see p. 179).
- Adequate energy requirements. Judged by degree of catabolism clinically. Nitrogen balance can be calculated but in practice rarely is.
- Liver function (albumin, transferrin and enzymes) indicate adequate protein synthesis and give an early indication of TPN-related complications.

Complications

The complications of TPN include all complications of central venous access. Metabolic derangement, particularly hyper- or hypoglycaemia, hypophosphataemia and hypercalcaemia, are not uncommon and require appropriate adjustment of the feed. Hepatobiliary dysfunction, including elevation of hepatic enzymes, jaundice and fatty infiltration of the liver may occur. This is usually caused by a combination of the patient's underlying disease processes and overfeeding. Reduce the volume of TPN and/or energy content. If the serum becomes very lipaemic it may be necessary to reduce the fat content. (See Complications of central venous cannulation, p. 324.)

STRESS ULCER PROPHYLAXIS

Early enteral feeding helps to maintain gastrointestinal mucosal blood flow, and provides essential nutrients to the mucosa. Early feeding is therefore important in reducing the incidence of both septic complications and stress ulceration. (See Gastrointestinal tract, p. 140.)

If enteral feeding cannot be established, patients should receive alternative prophylactic measures to prevent stress ulceration. For example:

- sucralfate 1 g NG 6-hourly
- ranitidine 50 mg i.v. 8-hourly.

Histamine (H_2 receptor) blocking drugs such as ranitidine raise intragastric pH. This is associated with an increased colonization of the upper gastrointestinal tract with lower gastrointestinal tract bacteria and a subsequent increase in the incidence of nosocomial infection. Therefore sucralfate, which acts as a protective barrier to the gastric mucosa without altering intragastric pH, may be the preferred agent for stress ulcer prophylaxis.

DEEP VENOUS THROMBOSIS PROPHYLAXIS

Patients requiring intensive care are at risk for the development of deep venous thrombosis (DVT) and pulmonary embolism (PE). Risk factors include immobility, venous stasis, poor circulation, major surgery, malignancy and pre-existing illness. Over and above these well-known factors, intensive care itself is an independent risk factor. Upper limb venous thrombosis is more common in ITU than in other settings, usually due to thrombosis following subclavian vein catheterization.

Despite all these risk factors there has been surprisingly little research performed to document either the true incidence of DVT or PE in such a population or what constitutes the best form of prophylaxis. The use of compression stockings and early mobilization of patients may help to reduce the risk. Once coagulation profiles are within normal ranges low-dose subcutaneous heparin should be given. For example:

- heparin 5000 units s.c. b.d.
- enoxaparin 20 mg s.c. daily.

Low molecular weight heparins (e.g. enoxaparin) may be associated with a lower incidence of haemorrhage than conventional heparin. APTT cannot, however, be used to monitor their effect. Specific assays of factor X activity are required, although these are time consuming. Fortunately it is not considered necessary to perform routine clinical monitoring of low molecular weight heparin therapy.

Suspected DVT can be confirmed by ultrasound or venography. If confirmed, the patient should be fully anticoagulated either with heparin or with high-dose low molecular weight heparin. This can be followed by warfarin when conditions allow. (See Pulmonary embolism, p. 89.)

CARDIOVASCULAR SYSTEM

SHOCK

The primary function of the cardiovascular system is to maintain the perfusion of organs and tissues with oxygenated blood. Complex homeostatic mechanisms exist to ensure that an adequate cardiac output and blood pressure are maintained to meet the needs of the individual. When these mechanisms fail, 'shock' ensues, which uncorrected can result in organ failure, prolonged ICU stay and death.

Definition

Shock is a syndrome of cardiovascular system failure resulting in inadequate tissue perfusion. Hypotension is a common but not universal feature.

Clinical features

The clinical features vary depending on the cause and the physiological response. Two patterns are typically recognized, although there is a continuum from one to the other:

- Warm pink vasodilated, hyperdynamic patient with high cardiac output and hypotension.
- Cold, grey, sweaty, vasoconstricted, peripherally shut down patient with low cardiac output. Blood pressure may be maintained in the early stages.

Other features of shock may include increased or decreased core temperature, hypoventilation or hyperventilation, renal and hepatic dysfunction, disseminated intravascular coagulation, and altered mental status. (See Systemic inflammatory response syndrome, p. 277 and Multiorgan dysfunction syndrome, p. 277.)

Aetiology

The aetiology of shock is frequently multifactorial. Typical causes are listed in Table 4.1. Although all causes of shock are seen on the ICU, the commonest in practice is septic shock (see p. 277).

Management

Apart from the mechanical causes of shock, in which relief of the mechanical obstruction may take priority, the principles of managing shock states are similar in all patients regardless of aetiology. They include:

- optimization of oxygen delivery
- optimization of cardiac output
- optimization of blood pressure

TABLE 4.1 Typical causes of shock	
Classification	*Underlying cause*
Hypovolaemia	Dehydration
	Haemorrhage
	Burns
	Sepsis
Cardiogenic	Myocardial infarction/ischaemia
	Valve disruption
	Myocardial rupture (e.g. VSD)
Mechanical/obstructive	Pulmonary embolism
	Cardiac tamponade
	Tension pneumothorax
Altered systemic vascular resistance	Sepsis
	Anaemia
	Anaphylaxis
	Addisonian crisis

● treatment of the underlying pathology
● support for any organ failure.

You should therefore understand the factors that influence oxygen delivery, oxygen consumption and cardiac output.

OXYGEN DELIVERY AND OXYGEN CONSUMPTION

Oxygen delivery (DO_2)

Oxygen delivery is defined as the total amount of oxygen delivered to the tissues per minute. It depends on the cardiac output (CO) and the oxygen content of arterial blood, as shown:

$$DO_2 = CO \times [\text{arterial oxygen content}]$$
$$DO_2 = CO \times [(SaO_2 \times Hb^* \times 1.34) + (\text{dissolved oxygen})]$$

Ignoring dissolved oxygen, which is insignificant at atmospheric pressure, typical figures are:

$$1000 \text{ ml/min} = 5000 \text{ ml} \times [(99/100 \times 15/100 \times 1.34)]$$

Hb^* = haemoglobin g/dl (divide by 100 for g/ml)
1.34 = amount of oxygen (ml) bound to 1 g of fully saturated haemoglobin.

Oxygen consumption (VO_2)

Oxygen consumption is the total amount of oxygen consumed by the tissues per minute. It can be calculated from the difference in oxygen

TABLE 4.2 Normal values: oxygen delivery and oxygen consumption

Oxygen delivery (DO_2)	1000 ml/min
Oxygen delivery index (DO_2I)	550 ml/min/m^2
Oxygen consumption (VO_2)	250 ml/min
Oxygen consumption index (VO_2I)	150 ml/min/m^2

content of arterial and mixed venous blood ($S\bar{v}O_2$) drawn from the pulmonary artery via a pulmonary artery catheter:

$$VO_2 = CO \times [(\text{arterial oxygen content}) - (\text{mixed venous oxygen content})]$$
$$VO_2 = CO \times [(SaO_2 \times Hb \times 1.34) - (S\bar{v}O_2 \times Hb \times 1.34)]$$

If cardiac index is used in the above calculations (see below), then oxygen delivery and oxygen consumption can also be expressed as an index. Typical normal values are shown in Table 4.2.

Under normal circumstances, oxygen consumption by the tissues is only about 25% of the oxygen delivered. This provides a large margin for safety, so that if oxygen requirements increase, for example in exercise, more oxygen can be extracted and utilized.

In disease states, however, while oxygen requirements may be raised, the ability of the tissues to extract and utilize oxygen may be impaired. Under these circumstances, tissue utilization of oxygen may become limited by the available supply. To prevent tissue hypoxia and organ dysfunction, optimal oxygen delivery must be ensured.

Optimizing oxygen delivery

● Ensure adequate arterial oxygen saturation.
● Optimize haemoglobin (see below).
● Optimize cardiac output. (See Optimizing haemodynamic status, p. 61).
● If oxygen delivery remains critical, consider muscle relaxants to reduce the muscle utilization of oxygen and reduce oxygen requirements.

Since haemoglobin (Hb) carries oxygen to the tissues one might assume that raising a patient's Hb to 15 g/dl might provide optimal oxygen delivery. However, this is associated with an increase in blood viscosity, which may actually result in worsening tissue perfusion. The ideal Hb for critically ill patients has therefore been a matter of debate. Recent work suggests that restrictive transfusion strategies produce the best outcome in critically ill patients and that the optimal level in most cases is an Hb of 8–10 g/dl. (See Indications for blood transfusion, p. 207.)

Mixed venous oxygen saturation (S$\bar{v}$O$_2$)

A guide to the balance between oxygen delivery and oxygen consumption can be obtained by the measurement of mixed venous oxygen saturation. This may either be intermittent, by measurement of blood gases on a sample drawn from the distal port of a pulmonary artery catheter, or continuous using a fibreoptic pulmonary artery catheter.

> If the patient does not have a pulmonary artery catheter in situ, use oxygen saturation of blood drawn from a central venous catheter with the tip in the superior vena cava. This provides close correlation.

Resuscitation guided by S$\bar{v}$O$_2$ has been shown to improve outcome by reducing the severity of organ failure and the duration of intensive care. Normal S$\bar{v}$O$_2$ is 55–75%. Levels below this imply inadequate oxygen delivery. Levels above this imply either adequate oxygen delivery or reduced oxygen consumption. Conditions which may result in impaired oxygen consumption include sepsis, metabolic poisoning and widespread cellular death.

> ⚠ **Despite adequate global oxygen delivery as described above, differences in regional perfusion may still result in some tissues receiving an inadequate oxygen delivery. The splanchnic circulation, for example, is at particular risk of hypoperfusion.**

(See GIT failure, p. 140, Sepsis, p. 277.)

CARDIAC OUTPUT

Assuming that oxygen saturation and haemoglobin are adequate, then the main determinant of oxygen delivery is cardiac output (CO). This is defined as the volume of blood ejected by the heart per minute. It is the product of heart rate (HR) and stroke volume (SV), as shown:

cardiac output (CO) = heart rate (HR) × stroke volume (SV)

In order to take account of patient size, cardiac output is usually expressed as cardiac index (CI), which is the CO divided by the

TABLE 4.3 Typical values of cardiac output	
Cardiac output (CO)	4–6 l/min
Cardiac index (CI)	2.5–3.5 l/min/m²

patient's body surface area (BSA). BSA can be derived from a patient's height and weight using nomograms. In practice, however, height and weight are entered directly into monitoring systems and all necessary calculations performed automatically. Typical values are shown in Table 4.3.

The factors that affect cardiac output are discussed below.

Heart rate

In a healthy heart there is little change in stroke volume with fluctuations in heart rate occurring within the physiological range (70–160 beats/min). Therefore, as heart rate increases, CO increases. The elderly, those with pre-existing heart disease, and critically ill patients, however, tolerate a much narrower range of heart rates, and values outside 100–120 beats/min may significantly compromise CO.

At low heart rates, SV may be maintained but CO falls as a function of heart rate. At high rates, inadequate filling leads to a fall in SV and a subsequent reduction in CO. Tachycardias associated with abnormalities of cardiac rhythm (e.g. atrial fibrillation) further reduce ventricular filling and CO. Tachycardias also lead to increased myocardial oxygen consumption, while simultaneously reducing the time for diastolic perfusion of the ventricles. In patients with ischaemic heart disease, this may produce significant myocardial ischaemia, which may further compromise CO.

Stroke volume (SV)

SV is determined by preload, contractility and afterload.

Preload

This is defined as the ventricular wall tension at the end of diastole. In simple terms preload refers to the degree of ventricular filling. According to the Frank–Starling law of the heart, the greater the degree of ventricular filling, the greater the force of myocardial contraction and thus SV. Above a certain point, however, the ventricle becomes overstretched and further filling may result in a fall in SV. Heart failure and pulmonary oedema may then develop (Fig. 4.1).

Preload is therefore a function of the volume status of the patient. It also depends, however, upon adequate ventricular relaxation in order to allow ventricular filling to take place. Ventricular relaxation is

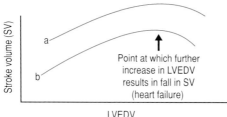

Fig. 4.1 Frank–Starling curves. (a) Increasing LVEDV leads to increased SV. (b) Effect of increased contractility, e.g. as a result of inotropes.

an active process. In critically ill patients, failure of ventricular relaxation (diastolic failure) may result in the ventricle becoming stiff and non-compliant. When this occurs, the ventricle cannot fill normally, regardless of the patient's volume status, and cardiac output is reduced.

Contractility

This represents the ability of the heart to work independently of the preload and afterload. Increased contractility, as for example produced by inotropes, results in increased SV for the same preload (Fig. 4.1). Decreased contractility may result from intrinsic heart disease, or from the myocardial depressant effects of acidosis, hypoxia and disease processes, e.g. sepsis.

Afterload

This is defined as the ventricular wall tension at the end of systole. In simple terms this is a measure of the load against which the heart is working. It is increased by ventricular dilatation, outflow resistance (for example, aortic valve stenosis) and increases in peripheral vascular resistance.

OPTIMIZING HAEMODYNAMIC STATUS

Optimization of haemodynamic status may be of benefit both to the critically ill patient and the high-risk patient undergoing major surgery. This encompasses both optimization of CO and oxygen

delivery and also maintenance of adequate organ perfusion pressure or
blood pressure.

Although considerable information on the cardiovascular status of
a patient can be obtained from simple clinical examination (peripheral
temperature, pulse, blood pressure, urine output, etc.), additional
information obtained from invasive monitoring is useful, particularly
when assessing the response to changes in therapy.

Invasive arterial pressure monitoring

Arterial cannulation allows beat-to-beat measurement of arterial blood
pressure and easy serial blood gas sampling. Significant respiratory
variation in the amplitude of the arterial pressure wave ('respiratory
swing') is characteristic of hypovolaemia. (See Arterial cannulation,
p. 312.)

Central venous pressure

Central venous catheterization provides a route of delivery for drugs
and fluids and enables measurement of right heart filling pressures
(CVP). Central venous access can be achieved via the jugular,
subclavian, brachial or femoral routes. (See Central venous
cannulation, p. 316, and Optimizing filling status, p. 65.)

Pulmonary artery catheterization

Pulmonary artery (PA) catheterization has for a number of years been
the gold standard cardiovascular monitoring tool in ICU (see p. 327).
This technique enables the measurement of pulmonary artery pressure,
pulmonary artery occlusion pressure (PAOP) and CO, and also allows
many other haemodynamic variables to be calculated or derived.
Typical values are given in Table 4.4.

The value of pulmonary artery catheters has recently been questioned
and the technique is currently the subject of a major multicentre trial. This
is likely to lead to a critical re-evaluation of the role of PA catheterization.
It has been suggested that the use of PA catheters is associated with an
increased mortality in critically ill patients and that this may be the result
of inappropriate interventions based on the information obtained.
Although PA catheterization remains in widespread use, there has been a
move towards alternative forms of monitoring. Relatively non-invasive
systems for continuous cardiac output monitoring are available based
on transthoracic bioimpedance, Doppler and pulse contour analysis.

Pulse contour analysis

Currently, systems based on pulse contour analysis are perhaps the
most likely to enter widespread use. In general terms these require
venous access (peripheral or central) and an arterial line with a sensor

TABLE 4.4 Normal values of common haemodynamic variables derived from PA catheterization

Central venous pressure (CVP)	4–10 mmHg
Pulmonary artery occlusion pressure (PAOP)	5–15 mmHg
Cardiac output (CO)	4–6 l/min
Cardiac index (CI)	2.5–3.5 l/min/m^2
Stroke volume (SV)	60–90 ml/beat
Stroke volume index (SVI)	33–47 ml/beat/m^2
Systemic vascular resistance (SVR)	900–1200 dyne.s/cm^5
Systemic vascular resistance index (SVRI)	1700–2400 dyne.s/cm^5/m^2
Pulmonary vascular resistance (PVR)	<250 dyne.s/cm^5
Pulmonary vascular resistance index (PVRI)	255–285 dyne.s/cm^5/m^2

These 'normal values' provide a guide only. They may not be achievable or appropriate for all critically ill patients. (See Goal directed therapy below).

either built in or attached. To calibrate the system an indicator is injected into the venous catheter and is detected by the arterial line producing a standard dilutional CO measurement. From this the systems are able to provide continuous CO, SV and systemic vascular resistance by analysis of the pulse waveform. To maintain accuracy they must be calibrated every 8–12 hours or whenever there is a significant change in cardiovascular status. If these systems are in use in your unit you should seek instruction on their use. (See also Volumetric haemodynamic monitoring, p. 66.)

Oesophageal Doppler

A Doppler ultrasound probe is placed in the oesophagus and directed to obtain a signal from the descending aorta. The signal obtained is displayed on the screen and indicates peak velocity and flow time. By making a number of assumptions about the nature of flow in the aorta, the cross-sectional area of the aorta (estimated from body surface area and age) and the percentage of CO passing down the aorta, SV and CO can be estimated. Trends in values and response to changes in therapy are more useful than absolute values. It is particularly useful for assessing response to fluid challenges.

Goal-directed therapy

There has been great interest in the manipulation of haemodynamic variables in an attempt to improve the outcome of critically ill patients. Shoemaker, for example, compared measured variables in survivors and non-survivors and suggested that we should aim to achieve supranormal values of cardiac index (4.5 l/min/m^2), oxygen delivery index (650 ml/min/m^2) and oxygen consumption index (165 ml/min/m^2). There is little evidence that this approach improves outcome in critically ill patients.

Rational approach to optimization of haemodynamic status

Avoid aiming to achieve absolute numbers for CO, etc. Use normal values only as a guide and think in terms of achieving adequate haemodynamic performance for the individual patient. A rational approach is to optimize fluid (filling) status first and then to add an inotrope or vasoconstrictor as required. This is summarized in Figure 4.2.

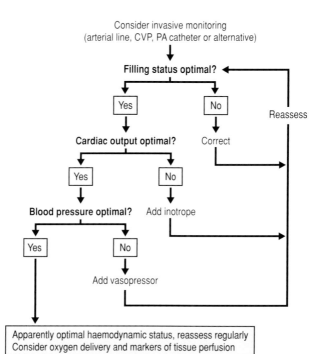

Fig. 4.2 Optimization of the haemodynamic system.

TABLE 4.5 Effects of agonists on vasoactive receptors

Receptor	Effects
α_1	Vasoconstriction
β_1	Increase myocardial contractility and heart rate
β_2	Vasodilatation (and bronchodilatation)
DA	Splanchnic and renal vasodilatation

The algorithm for optimizing haemodynamic (Fig. 4.2) provides a common approach to the management of shock regardless of the underlying cause. For many patients in the ICU the primary problem will be sepsis, which typically produces a high CO, low pressure state. Following the algorithm, if CO is adequate, attention moves directly to perfusion pressure.

There is a tendency to refer to all vasoactive drugs as inotropes. This is not only incorrect but can lead to confusion when deciding which agent to choose in any given circumstance. By classifying the available agents according to their receptor pharmacology and actions, a rational approach to their use can be achieved. Table 4.5 shows the effects of agonists at various receptors.

On the basis of activity at these receptors, drugs can be classified as inotropes (directly increase cardiac contractility), vasodilators, vasopressors, or a combination of these, e.g. inodilator or inopressor. Classifying agents in this way enables rational choices to be made in selecting agents for use. (See Optimizing cardiac output and Optimizing perfusion pressure below.)

OPTIMIZING FILLING STATUS

The optimal filling status for a patient is that which achieves the maximal CO while at the same time avoiding any deterioration in gas exchange due to the development of pulmonary oedema. If this cannot be achieved, then assisted ventilation may be required.

Use of CVP/PAOP

The use of right atrial pressure (CVP) and left atrial pressure (PAOP) to guide fluid therapy is commonplace. Fluids are typically given to achieve a predetermined CVP or PAOP. This approach should be avoided.

The relationship between filling pressure and volume status (ventricular end-diastolic volume) is complex and depends on the compliance of the ventricle. This compliance varies both between individuals and in different disease states. It may also change acutely in a single individual in response to pathophysiological changes such as myocardial ischaemia or acidosis.

Any predetermined figure for CVP/PAOP is bound, therefore, to be somewhat arbitrary and may not be optimal for an individual patient. Rather than aiming for a specific CVP or PAOP, try and determine the filling pressure which produces the best haemodynamic response from an individual patient.

● Give fluid to increase the CVP or PAOP in small increments and measure the increase in CO or SV. Continue until there is no further improvement or until there is deterioration in arterial blood gases or evidence of pulmonary oedema. (Note: stroke volume index of 50 ml/m² represents a full ventricle.)
● Remember also that optimal filling may actually mean use of fluid restriction, diuretics and vasodilators to reduce preload in patients with heart failure.

Volumetric haemodynamic monitoring

Increasing recognition that the concept of using 'filling pressure' (CVP or PAOP) as a measure of ventricular filling status is flawed has led to the development of monitoring systems capable of directly measuring (estimating) volume status. Detailed description is beyond the scope of this book. If volumetric monitoring is available in your unit you should seek instruction on its use. A guide to normal values for volume indices is given in Table 4.6.

There is currently no consensus as to which of these variables is the most useful in assessing volume status. As with other haemodynamic variables, it is the trend and response to therapy which is more important than the absolute values obtained. If volumetric monitoring is not available echocardiography can also be used to provide useful information about filling status.

OPTIMIZING CARDIAC OUTPUT

In all but the simplest cases of circulatory failure, where CO is inadequate consider an echocardiogram to establish diagnosis and

TABLE 4.6 Typical values of volumetric haemodynamic variables

Right ventricular ejection fraction (RVEF)	35–45%
Right ventricular end-diastolic volume (RVEDV)	100–160 ml
Right ventricular end-diastolic volume index (RVEDVI)	60–100 ml/m²
Intrathoracic blood volume index (ITBVI)	850–1000 ml/m²
Extravascular lung water index (EVLWI)	3–7 ml/kg

exclude treatable mechanical causes. Transthoracic and transoesophageal echocardiography give useful information on structural and functional cardiac abnormalities, including pericardial collections, valvular lesions and contractility. Filling, regional wall motion abnormalities and an estimate of flows/pressures can also be made. Many critically ill patients will have small pericardial effusions. These do not normally require drainage unless CO is impaired. (See Pericardiocentesis, p. 332)

Inotropes

If despite optimal filling CO remains inadequate, inotropes may be added to improve cardiac performance (Fig. 4.2.). The rational use of inotropes requires an understanding of the receptor pharmacology of the commonly used agents. These are summarized in Table 4.7.

Dobutamine (1–20 µg/kg/min)

Increases CO and causes a variable degree of peripheral vasodilatation. It is useful in low CO states when vasomotor tone and mean arterial pressure are reasonably well maintained.

Dopexamine (1–5 µg/kg/min)

At doses up to 1 µg/kg/min dopexamine has little inotropic activity and increases in CO are mediated primarily by peripheral vasodilatation (reduced afterload) and reflex tachycardia. This results in improved blood flow primarily in the splanchnic and renal circulation. At doses above these, there is some intrinsic inotropic activity. Dopexamine may be useful in low CO states when there is increased peripheral vasomotor tone and mean arterial blood pressure

---

TABLE 4.7 Actions of commonly used inotropic agents

Drug	Receptor	Actions*	Classification
Dobutamine	β_1 β_2	↑ Heart rate and stroke volume Peripheral vasodilatation	Inodilator
Dopexamine	β_2 DA	Peripheral and splanchnic vasodilatation ↑ Heart rate	Inodilator
Adrenaline (epinephrine)	α_1 β_1 β_2	↑ Heart rate and stroke volume Peripheral vasoconstriction	Inopressor
Dopamine	DA α_1 β_1	Actions varied depending on dose (see below)	Variable

*See notes on individual drugs (above and below).

is maintained. In addition it may be used to promote renal–splanchnic blood flow. (See Oliguria, p. 155, and GIT failure, p. 140.)

Adrenaline (epinephrine) (0.1–0.5 µg/kg/min)

At low doses the primary effect is increased CO; at higher doses there is additional potent vasoconstriction. It is useful in low output states associated with low peripheral vasomotor tone and low mean arterial pressure. Adrenaline (epinephrine) is the drug of choice in an emergency and in hypotensive states when the overall haemodynamic status is not clear. Its prolonged use is associated with impaired splanchnic perfusion, hyperglycaemia and increased serum lactate.

Dopamine (2.5–5 µg/kg/min)

Dopamine acts on α_1 and β_1 adrenoceptors and DA receptors and releases noradrenaline (norepinephrine) from adrenergic nerves. The actions of dopamine therefore vary depending on the dose. At low doses, up to 5 µg/kg/min, the primary action is said to be on DA receptors, resulting in increased splanchnic and renal perfusion. Dopamine may therefore be useful to help maintain renal blood flow and promote urine output, although the evidence for this is poor (see Oliguria, p. 155). At doses above 5 µg/kg/min vasoconstrictor and cardiac effects predominate.

Choice of inotrope

From the table and notes above, select the most appropriate inotrope for the patient's clinical condition. Generally:

- If despite low CO mean arterial blood pressure is well maintained use dobutamine or dopexamine to increase CO and improve perfusion.
- If low CO is associated with low blood pressure use adrenaline (epinephrine).
- If you are uncertain, the mixed actions of dopamine make it a reasonable choice in most settings. It is commonly used as a first-line agent in Europe; however, in the UK it has lost favour and has tended to be used primarily for its supposed renal effects.

Start infusions at the lowest infusion rate possible to achieve the desired effect and continually reassess the response. Potential adverse effects include tachycardia, arrhythmias and increased myocardial oxygen consumption. Hyperglycaemia and lactic acidosis may also occur.

OPTIMIZING PERFUSION PRESSURE

If, despite adequate filling and best achievable CO, the mean arterial pressure remains low, then vasoconstrictors should be used. The commonly available agents are shown in Table 4.8.

TABLE 4.8 Actions of commonly used vasopressor agents

Drug	Receptor	Actions	Classification
Noradrenaline (norepinephrine)	α_1	Peripheral vasoconstriction	Vasopressor
Phenylephrine	α_1	Peripheral vasoconstriction	Vasopressor

- Phenylephrine (1–5 µg/kg/min).
- Noradrenaline (norepinephrine) (0.1–0.5 µg/kg/min).

Both drugs have direct action on α_1 receptors and increase blood pressure by causing vasoconstriction. There is no appreciable direct effect on CO. They are used to generate an adequate perfusion pressure for vital organs, in particular the brain, liver and kidneys.

Excessive use of vasoconstrictors may, however, be associated with a number of adverse effects. These include increased afterload and reduced CO, reduced renal blood flow, reduced splanchnic blood flow and impaired peripheral perfusion. Vasoconstrictors should, therefore, be used only in the lowest possible doses required to achieve the desired effect. In particular, vasoconstrictors should only be titrated against the mean arterial blood pressure and not other derived variables such as systemic vascular resistance.

⚠ **Vasoconstrictors should be titrated against blood pressure and not against the SVR. Systemic vascular resistance is mathematically derived from CO and perfusion pressure, and is not a directly measured, independent variable:**

systemic vascular resistance = perfusion pressure × constant/cardiac output

SVR = (MAP – CVP) × 80/CO

Vasopressin

There is increasing evidence that in profound shock states vasopressin or antidiuretic hormone (ADH), which is normally secreted by the posterior pituitary, becomes depleted. Replacement at physiological rather than pharmacological doses, by infusion of vasopressin at 0.1–0.4 µg/kg/min, can help restore vascular reactivity and tone. Usually used in combination with other vasopressor agents.

RATIONAL USE OF INOTROPES AND VASOPRESSORS

Except in emergency, do not start inotropes or vasopressors until adequate fluid loading has been achieved. Give only into central veins, using dedicated lines.

Following each change in therapy you should reassess the patient's haemodynamic status. In particular, check filling status is still optimal and whether therapies have had the desired effect. When optimal haemodynamic status is apparently achieved, ensure oxygen delivery is adequate and consider markers of regional perfusion such as renal output.

No response to inotropes/vasoconstrictors

- Check that arterial and other monitoring lines are functioning correctly (check blood pressure manually) and that transducers are appropriately zeroed and at the correct level.
- Ensure that filling status is optimal. Inotropes and vasoconstrictors are of little value if the circulation is empty!
- Exclude mechanical causes of low CO and hypotension such as tension pneumothorax, pulmonary embolus and cardiac tamponade.
- Ensure that the appropriate inotrope or vasoconstrictor agent has been started. Check that the infusion is running at the correct rate. Note that if an infusion is started at a low rate it may take some time for the active drug to reach the end of the dead space in the infusion line.
- The myocardium responds poorly to inotropes in the presence of acidosis. Therefore, if a significant acidosis is present (pH < 7.2) consider correcting this with sodium bicarbonate. (See Metabolic acidosis, p. 146.)
- Check the ionized calcium and consider giving additional calcium. (Never give calcium and sodium bicarbonate together down the same line!)
- If there is no improvement in haemodynamic status increase the infusion rate until an appropriate response is obtained. If there is still no response, and particularly if the inotropes or vasoconstrictors have been in use for some time, consider the possibility of tachyphylaxis and receptor downregulation. Start an alternative or additional agent.
- Consider the possibility of adrenocortical failure (rare) or functional adrenal insufficiency. Consider corticosteroid replacement. (See Adrenal insufficiency, p. 183.)

Weaning inotropes and vasoconstrictors

As the patient's condition improves, inotropes and vasoconstrictor agents can be gradually reduced. Ensure optimal filling at all times and reduce drugs according to the results of haemodynamic monitoring.

HYPOTENSION

(See Optimizing haemodynamic status, p. 61.)

Assess the patient
- Is the blood pressure adequate for the patient? A MAP of 60 mmHg is generally adequate but this will depend on the patient's normal blood pressure, which will vary with age and premorbid state.
- Is there evidence of inadequate tissue oxygenation or organ perfusion (acidosis, oliguria or altered conscious level)? If not, further treatment may not be necessary.
- Is there an obvious cause for hypotension, e.g. hypovolaemia (bleeding), myocardial failure, sepsis? This will guide specific treatment.

Optimize filling status
- Unless there is evidence of fluid overload or myocardial failure, give a fluid challenge to optimize cardiac filling, even if measured CVP is apparently adequate (e.g. 100–500 ml colloid). If there is no response (particularly if there is no rise in measured filling pressures) consider a further fluid bolus.
- If there is still no response, establish invasive monitoring with a pulmonary artery catheter in order to measure PAOP and CO. (See Practical procedures, p. 327.)

> Faced with significant hypotension in the absence of invasive haemodynamic monitoring, start an adrenaline (epinephrine) infusion. This has both inotrope and vasoconstrictor actions and is the agent of choice in the first instance. It can be continued or replaced once invasive monitoring is established.

Optimize cardiac output
- Give further fluid bolus if appropriate to increase PAOP and observe the change in CO. Titrate fluids to determine PAOP that gives optimum cardiac output.
- If CO remains low, add an inotrope. The choice will depend on the clinical condition of the patient. If the peripheral resistance is low adrenaline (epinephrine) is useful as a first-line agent.

Optimize perfusion pressure

● If mean arterial blood pressure remains low despite adequate filling pressure and CO, add a vasoconstrictor to maintain diastolic blood pressure, e.g. noradrenaline (norepinephrine).

HYPERTENSION

Although hypotension is more of a problem in intensive care, hypertension can also occur. This may be a manifestation of pre-existing essential hypertension, but is frequently secondary to other factors. Typical causes are shown in Table 4.9.

Management

In intensive care short periods of hypertension, for example during weaning from ventilation, are not uncommon and do not generally result in any harm unless there is associated myocardial, cerebral or vascular disease. Therefore:

● Do not over treat hypertension.
● If using an arterial line check the blood pressure reading using a blood pressure cuff. The readings sometimes disagree, in which case the non-invasive measurement may be the more accurate. (See Arterial cannulation, p. 312.)
● Ensure adequate analgesia and sedation.
● Ensure normal fluid status and blood gases.
● Correct hypothermia.
● Reduce or stop inotropes and vasoconstrictors as appropriate.

Treatment will depend upon the absolute blood pressure, age and condition of the patient. The typical hypertensive patient is the elderly postoperative arteriopath with ischaemic heart disease. Treatment is generally only required if there is sustained diastolic blood pressure > 110 mmHg, systolic > 200 mmHg or associated myocardial ischaemia. If treatment is required consider:

TABLE 4.9 Causes of hypertension in ICU

Pre-existing hypertension/vascular disease
Pain and anxiety
Effects of exogenous catecholamines
Intracranial lesion
Hypervolaemia
Hypoxia
Hypercarbia
Hypothermia

- Nifedepine 10–20 mg s.l. (Nifedepine capsules can be punctured with a needle and the contents given sublingually. This produces a gentle reduction in blood pressure within 20 minutes and can be repeated 6–8-hourly.)
- Hydralazine 10 mg i.v. repeated as necessary.
- GTN infusion. Particularly if hypertensive episodes are associated with myocardial ischaemia or failure.
- Labetalol is used in small incremental boluses (5–10 mg) and by infusion.

Young hypertensive patients

The young patient with unexplained sustained hypertension, particularly if associated with end organ damage, for example left ventricular hypertrophy, warrants further investigation. Consider other causes such as renal artery stenosis and phaeochromocytoma (see Phaeochromocytoma, p. 184.)

DISTURBANCES OF CARDIAC RHYTHM

Disturbances in cardiac rhythm are common in the ICU and this highlights the need for careful monitoring of all patients. Dysrhythmias may result from underlying heart disease, e.g. ischaemic heart disease, cardiomyopathy or valve lesions. Other predisposing factors are listed in Table 4.10.

TABLE 4.10 Factors predisposing to dysrhythmias

Pain and anxiety (inadequate analgesia and sedation)
Increased catecholamine levels (endogenous or from inotrope infusions)
Hypoxia
Hypercarbia
Endocrine abnormalities
Electrolyte disturbance (hypokalaemia, hyperkalaemia, hypomagnesaemia)
Hypovolaemia
Pyrexia and myocardial effects of sepsis
Drugs

Initially, ensure adequate oxygenation and ventilation together with correction of predisposing factors. Where there is no improvement or there is haemodynamic disturbance, definitive treatment is required.

Sinus tachycardia

This is a common problem and generally represents an appropriate response. Management is, therefore, correction of the underlying cause(s).

⚠ **Do not give β blockers to control sinus tachycardia. This may result in decompensation. Sinus tachycardia will usually resolve when the underlying condition improves.**

Bradycardia

Bradycardia frequently reflects intrinsic disease of pacemaker tissue or the conducting system. It may be precipitated by increased vagal tone, hypoxia (particularly in children) and the myocardial depressant effect of drugs. Initially, as heart rate falls, CO is maintained by increases in SV. Thereafter, as heart rate falls further, CO and blood pressure will fall. Junctional or ventricular escape rhythms may appear.

The algorithm for the management of bradycardia is shown in Figure 4.3. In the intensive care unit, if bradycardia occurs in association with significant hypotension then consider adrenaline (epinephrine). Give 50–100 μg (0.5–1 ml of 1:10 000 adrenaline) boluses and titrate to effect.

Supraventricular tachycardia (SVT) (Figs 4.4, 4.5)

SVT encompasses all forms of tachydysrhythmia originating above the ventricles. In practice it is useful to distinguish atrial fibrillation and atrial flutter from other forms of SVT. In SVT the QRS complexes are always narrow (narrow complex tachycardia) unless there is an associated conduction defect (Fig. 4.5).

The management depends on the degree of haemodynamic disturbance and likely origin. Atrial fibrillation is considered separately (see p. 76). Amiodarone may be the drug of choice for the treatment of SVT that is not associated with haemodynamic compromise (Fig. 4.4).

There is increasing use of magnesium sulphate to treat supraventricular dysrhythmias. This is as effective as amiodarone. The typical dose is 10–20 mmol over 10 minutes followed by 50–100 mmol over 24 hours.

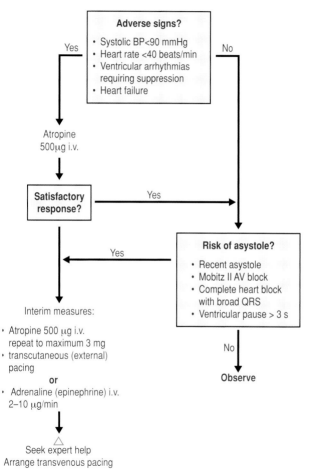

Bradycardia
(includes rates inappropriately slow for haemodynamic state)

If appropriate, give oxygen and establish i.v. access

Adverse signs?
- Systolic BP<90 mmHg
- Heart rate <40 beats/min
- Ventricular arrhythmias requiring suppression
- Heart failure

Yes

No

Atropine
500µg i.v.

Satisfactory response?

Yes

Risk of asystole?
- Recent asystole
- Mobitz II AV block
- Complete heart block with broad QRS
- Ventricular pause > 3 s

Yes

No

Interim measures:

- Atropine 500 µg i.v. repeat to maximum 3 mg
- transcutaneous (external) pacing

or

- Adrenaline (epinephrine) i.v. 2–10 µg/min

Observe

△
Seek expert help
Arrange transvenous pacing

Fig. 4.3 Algorithm: bradycardia. Resuscitation Council UK Guidelines 2000.

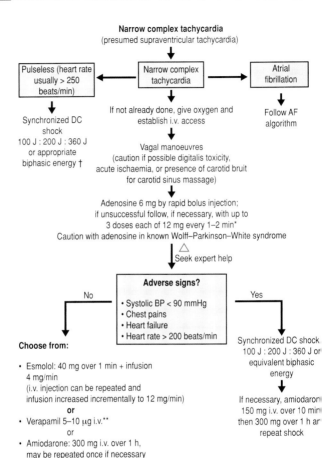

Narrow complex tachycardia
(presumed supraventricular tachycardia)

| Pulseless (heart rate usually > 250 beats/min) | ← | Narrow complex tachycardia | → | Atrial fibrillation |

Synchronized DC shock
100 J : 200 J : 360 J
or appropriate biphasic energy †

If not already done, give oxygen and establish i.v. access

Follow AF algorithm

Vagal manoeuvres
(caution if possible digitalis toxicity, acute ischaemia, or presence of carotid bruit for carotid sinus massage)

Adenosine 6 mg by rapid bolus injection; if unsuccessful follow, if necessary, with up to 3 doses each of 12 mg every 1–2 min*
Caution with adenosine in known Wolff–Parkinson–White syndrome

△ Seek expert help

Adverse signs?
- Systolic BP < 90 mmHg
- Chest pains
- Heart failure
- Heart rate > 200 beats/min

No

Yes

Choose from:

Synchronized DC shock 100 J : 200 J : 360 J or equivalent biphasic energy

- Esmolol: 40 mg over 1 min + infusion 4 mg/min
  (i.v. injection can be repeated and infusion increased incrementally to 12 mg/min)
  or
- Verapamil 5–10 μg i.v.**
  or
- Amiodarone: 300 mg i.v. over 1 h, may be repeated once if necessary
  or
- Digoxin: maximum dose 500 μg i.v. over 30 min x 2

If necessary, amiodarone 150 mg i.v. over 10 min then 300 mg over 1 h and repeat shock

Doses throughout are based on an adult of average body weight
A starting dose of 6 mg adenosine is currently outside the UK licence for this agent.

* Note 1: Theophylline and related compounds block the effect of adenosine. Patients on dipyridamole, carbamazepine, or with denervated hearts have a markedly exaggerated effect which may be hazardous.
† Note 2: DC shock is always given under sedation/general anaesthesia.
** Note 3: Not to be used in patients receiving beta-blockers.

Fig. 4.4 Algorithm: narrow complex tachycardia. Resuscitation Council UK Guidelines 2000.

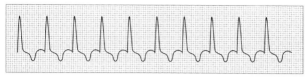

Fig. 4.5 Narrow complex tachycardia (SVT).

Atrial fibrillation (AF)

This is the commonest dysrhythmia seen in the ICU (Fig. 4.6), particularly in the elderly patient with postoperative sepsis and inotrope dependency. Consider the underlying causes of dysrhythmia above.

When sudden in onset, restoration of sinus rhythm (where possible) should be attempted. Treatment depends on the ventricular rate and the degree of associated haemodynamic disturbance. (Fig. 4.7).

Chronic AF may be associated with ischaemic heart disease or mitral valve disease. Restoration of sinus rhythm is unlikely and control of the ventricular rate is the main aim. Digoxin may be the drug of choice:

● Digoxin is infused 0.5 mg i.v. over 30 minutes, followed by 0.25–0.5 mg after 2 hours if necessary. Once daily dose, thereafter, depending on response and levels.

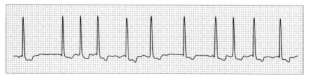

Fig. 4.6 Atrial fibrillation.

Atrial flutter

In atrial flutter the atrial rate is about 300 beats per minute and the P waves have a saw tooth appearance (Fig. 4.8). The AV node cannot conduct all the P waves to the ventricle and there is often associated 2:1 AV block. Therefore, suspect if the ventricular rate is 150. At this rate use a 12-lead ECG to identify flutter waves:

● Treatment: synchronized DC cardioversion (50 J: 100 J: 200 J).

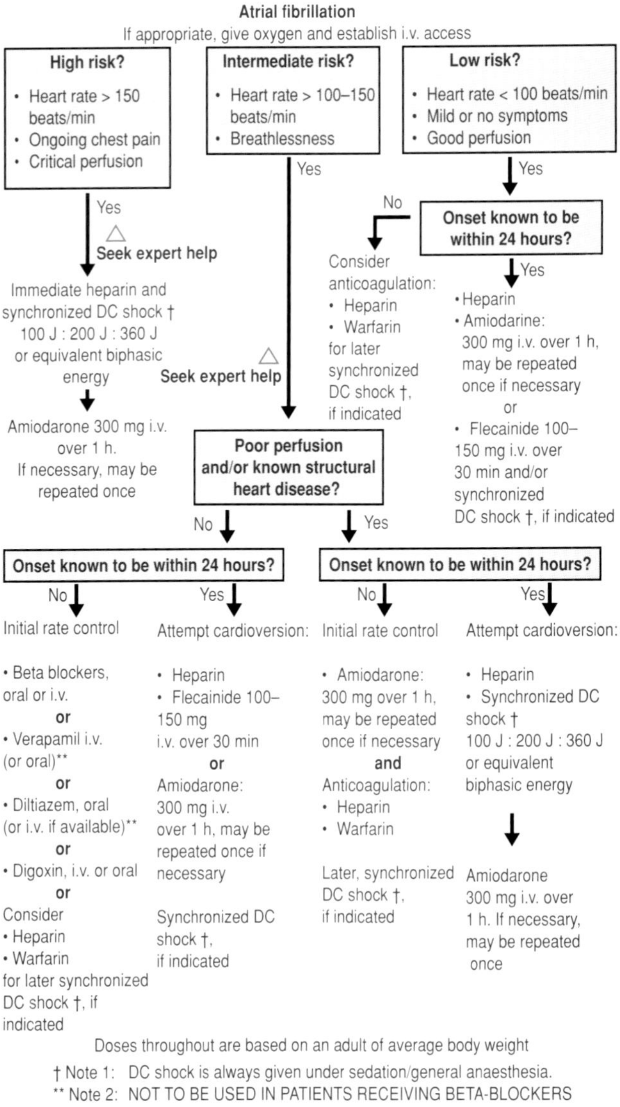

Atrial fibrillation

If appropriate, give oxygen and establish i.v. access

High risk?
- Heart rate > 150 beats/min
- Ongoing chest pain
- Critical perfusion

Intermediate risk?
- Heart rate > 100–150 beats/min
- Breathlessness

Low risk?
- Heart rate < 100 beats/min
- Mild or no symptoms
- Good perfusion

Yes

△
Seek expert help

Immediate heparin and synchronized DC shock †
100 J : 200 J : 360 J or equivalent biphasic energy

Amiodarone 300 mg i.v. over 1 h.
If necessary, may be repeated once

Yes

No → Consider anticoagulation:
- Heparin
- Warfarin
for later synchronized DC shock †, if indicated

△
Seek expert help

Poor perfusion and/or known structural heart disease?

Yes

Onset known to be within 24 hours?

Yes

- Heparin
- Amiodarone: 300 mg i.v. over 1 h, may be repeated once if necessary
  or
- Flecainide 100–150 mg i.v. over 30 min and/or synchronized DC shock †, if indicated

No

Onset known to be within 24 hours?

No
Initial rate control

- Beta blockers, oral or i.v.
  or
- Verapamil i.v. (or oral)**
  or
- Diltiazem, oral (or i.v. if available)**
  or
- Digoxin, i.v. or oral
  or
Consider
- Heparin
- Warfarin
for later synchronized DC shock †, if indicated

Yes
Attempt cardioversion:

- Heparin
- Flecainide 100–150 mg i.v. over 30 min
  or
Amiodarone: 300 mg i.v. over 1 h, may be repeated once if necessary

Synchronized DC shock †, if indicated

No
Initial rate control

- Amiodarone: 300 mg over 1 h, may be repeated once if necessary
  and
Anticoagulation:
- Heparin
- Warfarin

Later, synchronized DC shock †, if indicated

Yes
Attempt cardioversion:

- Heparin
- Synchronized DC shock †
  100 J : 200 J : 360 J or equivalent biphasic energy

↓

Amiodarone 300 mg i.v. over 1 h. If necessary, may be repeated once

Doses throughout are based on an adult of average body weight

† Note 1: DC shock is always given under sedation/general anaesthesia.
** Note 2: NOT TO BE USED IN PATIENTS RECEIVING BETA-BLOCKERS

Fig. 4.7 Algorithm: atrial fibrillation. Resuscitation Council UK Guidelines 2000.

Ventricular premature beats (VPBs)

VPBs occur normally in the general population and their significance
is uncertain. They are more common in the presence of heart disease
and may be increased by the effects of digoxin toxicity,
catecholamines and hypokalaemia. Asymptomatic unifocal VPBs
occurring less than 5 per minute are considered to be benign.
Treatment may be indicated if associated with poor haemodynamic
state, if multifocal, or if occurring in runs of two or more.

- Correct hypoxia, hypercarbia, acidosis and hypokalaemia.
- Consider lidocaine (lignocaine) 1 mg/kg followed by infusion
  2 mg/min.
- Consider magnesium.

Broad complex tachycardia

Broad complex tachycardia (Fig. 4.9) is usually ventricular in origin,
but may occasionally be supraventricular if there is an associated
conduction defect, e.g. bundle branch block. Haemodynamic status is
a poor guide to the underlying rhythm. An ECG may help to
distinguish between the two (Table 4.11, p. 81). If in doubt, broad
complex tachycardia should be assumed to be ventricular in origin
until proved otherwise. Management of broad complex tachycardia is
shown in Figure 4.10.

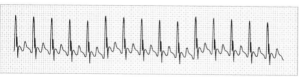

Fig. 4.8 Atrial flutter (with 2:1 block).

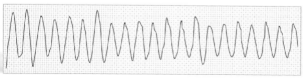

Fig. 4.9 Broad complex tachycardia.

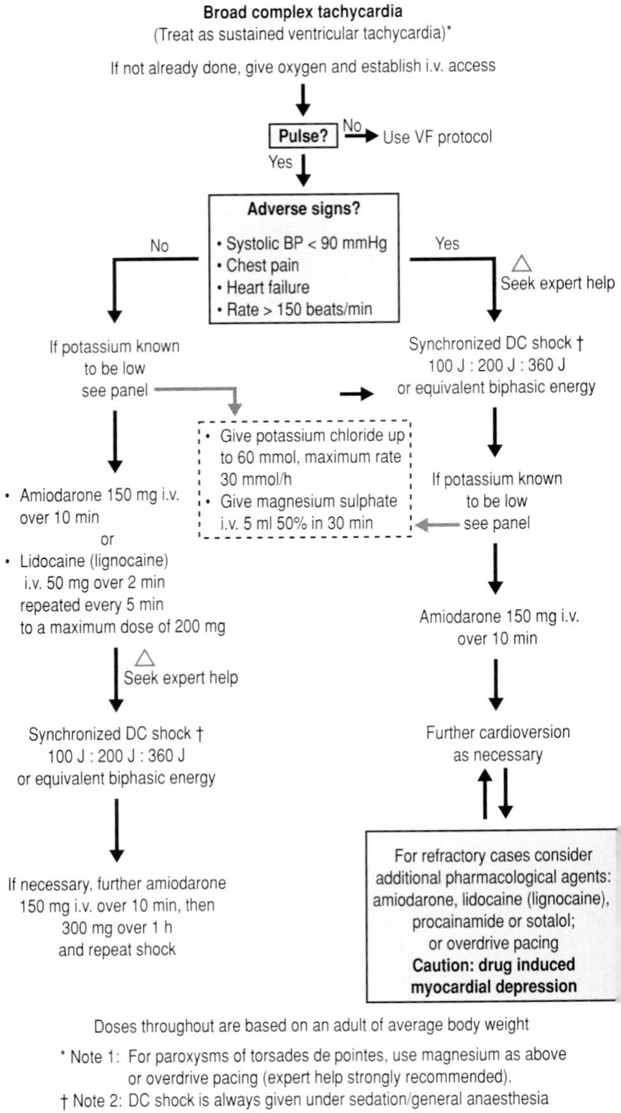

Broad complex tachycardia
(Treat as sustained ventricular tachycardia)*

If not already done, give oxygen and establish i.v. access

Pulse? → No → Use VF protocol

Yes

Adverse signs?
• Systolic BP < 90 mmHg
• Chest pain
• Heart failure
• Rate > 150 beats/min

No

Yes

△ Seek expert help

If potassium known
to be low
see panel →

→ Synchronized DC shock †
100 J : 200 J : 360 J
or equivalent biphasic energy

• Give potassium chloride up
to 60 mmol, maximum rate
30 mmol/h
• Give magnesium sulphate
i.v. 5 ml 50% in 30 min

• Amiodarone 150 mg i.v.
over 10 min
or
• Lidocaine (lignocaine)
i.v. 50 mg over 2 min
repeated every 5 min
to a maximum dose of 200 mg

△ Seek expert help

If potassium known
to be low
see panel ←

Amiodarone 150 mg i.v.
over 10 min

Synchronized DC shock †
100 J : 200 J : 360 J
or equivalent biphasic energy

Further cardioversion
as necessary

If necessary, further amiodarone
150 mg i.v. over 10 min, then
300 mg over 1 h
and repeat shock

For refractory cases consider
additional pharmacological agents:
amiodarone, lidocaine (lignocaine),
procainamide or sotalol;
or overdrive pacing
**Caution: drug induced
myocardial depression**

Doses throughout are based on an adult of average body weight

* Note 1: For paroxysms of torsades de pointes, use magnesium as above
or overdrive pacing (expert help strongly recommended).
† Note 2: DC shock is always given under sedation/general anaesthesia

Fig. 4.10 Algorithm: broad complex tachycardia. Resuscitation Council UK
Guidelines 2000.

TABLE 4.11 ECG features of broad complex tachycardia

VT more likely if:
QRS very broad >0.14 s
Evidence of AV dissociation (capture beats or fusion beats)
Dominant first R wave in VI
Deep S wave V6
QRS direction same all V leads

Polymorphic ventricular tachycardia (torsade de pointes)

Torsade de pointes is a form of VT in which the complexes have a pointed shape, vary from beat to beat and the axis of the rhythm constantly changes. It is usually self-limiting but may give rise to VF. Hypokalaemia, prolonged QT interval, bradycardia and antidysrhythmic drugs may be causes. Seek expert help.

- Give magnesium 10 mmol i.v. stat followed by 50 mmol infusion over 12 hours.
- Consider β blockers.
- Consider overdrive pacing and DC cardioversion.

(See Defibrillation and DC cardioversion, p. 335.)

CONDUCTION DEFECTS

In addition to the dysrhythmias discussed above, AV conduction defects can result in haemodynamic compromise.

1st degree heart block

PR interval > 0.2 seconds (1 large square on standard ECG trace). This does not require treatment but is indicative of underlying heart disease, electrolyte disturbance or drug toxicity, e.g. digoxin.

2nd degree heart block

This may be of two types:

- Mobitz type 1 (Wenkebach phenomenon). There is progressive lengthening of the PR interval followed by a P wave which is not conducted to the ventricle and then repetition of the cycle. This is usually self-limiting.
- Mobitz type 2. The PR interval is constant but occasional P waves are not conducted to the ventricle. If high levels of block are present, e.g. 2:1 or 3:1 block, there is a significant risk that this will progress to complete heart block.

Complete heart block

No atrial electrical activity is conducted to the ventricle. This may result in ventricular standstill (no CO!) or there may be an idioventricular escape rhythm. In this case there is no discernible relationship between visible P waves and QRS complexes on the ECG.

Treatment of heart block

Asymptomatic 1st or 2nd degree heart block does not require treatment. Any symptomatic episodes of heart block do require treatment:

- See bradycardia algorithm above.
- Consider pacing: external or temporary pacing wire.

Indications for temporary cardiac pacing are given in Table 4.12.

Pacemakers

Patients with permanent indwelling pacemakers are normally seen in pacemaker clinic regularly and should carry a card indicating the type of pacemaker that has been fitted. These are described using a coding system (Table 4.13).

TABLE 4.12 Indications for temporary pacing

Symptomatic bradycardia unresponsive to treatment (Fig. 4.3)
Mobitz type 2 heart block
Complete heart block
RBBB + left anterior or posterior hemiblock in association with prolonged PR interval*

*Relative indication.

TABLE 4.13 Pacemaker coding system

Chamber paced	V = ventricle, A = atrium, D = dual
Chamber sensed	V = ventricle, A = atrium, D = dual
Mode of response	T = triggered, I = inhibited, D = dual, O = none
Programmable functions	P = simple, M = multiple, C = communicating, O = none
Antitachydysrhythmia functions	B = bursts, N = normal rate competition, S = scanning, E = externally activated

The commonest pacemaker is still the ventricular demand pacemaker (VVI). While the pacemaker senses normal ventricular activity the function of the pacemaker is inhibited. If ventricular activity is not sensed the pacemaker stimulates the ventricle.

Pacemaker technology has advanced dramatically over recent years and many pacemakers are now complicated programmable microprocessors. For this reason advice should always be sought from a cardiologist regarding any patient with a pacemaker.

> ⚠ **Traditional VVI pacemakers could be switched from demand to fixed rate with a magnet. Do not attempt to alter the function of a pacemaker with a magnet unless advised to do so. Programmable pacemakers may be damaged.**

MYOCARDIAL ISCHAEMIA

Ischaemic heart disease (IHD) is extremely common and ranges from the asymptomatic, through stable angina to crescendo angina and myocardial infarction. The understanding of acute coronary syndromes has increased in recent years. (See Troponin, p. 86.)

Many patients admitted to intensive care will already be on a number of cardiovascular medications and these should be reviewed in the light of the patient's condition. Where appropriate, existing drug therapy should be continued; however, many oral cardiac drugs have no parenteral preparation. In practice it is common to stop such medication in the acute phase of a critical illness and reintroduce it as the patient's condition improves.

- Oral nitrates can be replaced with GTN patches (5–10 mg every 24 hours) or GTN infusion.
- Warfarin (for prosthetic valves or chronic AF) should be replaced by heparin infusion and the APTT monitored. The required level will depend upon the indication for coagulation.
- Diuretics may be continued in equivalent doses i.v.
- Ca^{2+} channel blockers, β blockers and angiotensin converting enzyme (ACE) inhibitors are usually withheld.

Many patients in the ICU are unable to indicate the onset of ischaemic chest pain because of the effects of sedation and ventilation. However, changes in ECG monitoring, such as ST depression, and deteriorating myocardial performance, such as reduced CO, may indicate ischaemia. The management will depend upon the apparent degree of ischaemia and associated haemodynamic disturbance.

Simple angina/ST depression

- Give oxygen.
- Correct precipitating factors such as tachycardia, hypertension or hypotension.
- Administer GTN either sublingually or as oral spray. Consider GTN infusion.
- Give analgesia if required. Usually a bolus of morphine or diamorphine i.v.

Unstable angina/increasing ST depression (crescendo angina)

If angina or ST depression do not settle or become more severe, myocardial infarction may be imminent. The commonest mechanism of infarction is rupture of a soft atheromatous plaque and subsequent occlusive thrombus formation within the coronary artery. Management is based at preventing this. In addition to the above:

- Give aspirin 300 mg oral followed by 75 mg daily (beware contraindications).
- Consider clopidogrel 300 mg oral followed by 75 mg daily.
- Start enoxaparin 1 mg/kg s.c. twice a day.
- Consider β blocker (e.g. atenolol 100 mg daily) if there are no contraindications (bradycardia, hypotension, heart failure, asthma).
- Consider GTN infusion to reduce preload and reduce myocardial work. 1–2 mg/h and titrate to response.

ACUTE MYOCARDIAL INFARCTION

Patients may be admitted to intensive care following a myocardial infarct or may suffer an infarction during their stay on intensive care.

The diagnosis of myocardial infarction is usually made on the basis of a characteristic history of chest pain, ECG changes, elevation of cardiac troponin and the interpretation of cardiac enzymes. Patients in the ICU may not be able to give a history of classic chest pain and great reliance has to be placed on the clinical picture, ECG changes and confirmatory tests.

The clinical picture of myocardial infarction may include the sudden development of hypotension, cardiac failure (3rd or 4th heart sound), pericardial rub and pyrexia. If myocardial infarction is suspected, appropriate management should be instituted. Measure cardiac troponin and perform serial ECG and cardiac enzyme studies for 3 days.

ECG changes

The typical ECG changes accompanying acute myocardial infarction are:

- ST segment elevation > 1 mm in precordial leads or > 2 mm in limb leads which persists for more than 24 hours. Usually returns to normal within 2 weeks. (Persistent ST elevation at 1 month suggests development of left ventricular aneurysm.)
- Reciprocal ST segment depression in the opposite leads.
- Development of new Q waves greater than 25% of the 'R' wave and 0.04 s duration.
- T wave inversion. (This is not diagnostic by itself.)

The location of these changes on the ECG identify the region of the infarction (Table 4.14).

Enzyme changes

Patterns of enzyme changes following myocardial infarction are shown in Table 4.15.

Creatinine phosphokinase (CK) is released from all damaged muscle cells, whereas CK–MB is specific to heart muscle. If the total CK is raised and the ratio of CK–MB to CK is greater than 6–8%, myocardial infarction is highly likely.

TABLE 4.14 Myocardial infarction and ECG patterns

Area of infarction	ECG leads
Inferior	aVF, II & III
Anteroseptal	VI–V4
Anterior	V3–V4
Anterolateral	V3–V6
Posterior	V1

TABLE 4.15 Patterns of enzyme change following myocardial infarction

Enzyme	Peak (hours)	Duration (days)
Creatinine kinase (CK–MB)	12–24	1–3
Total creatinine kinase	18–30	2–5
Aspartate transaminase	20–30	2–6
Lactate dehydrogenase	30–48	5–14

Cardiac troponin

Cardiac troponin (troponin I) is a protein released by damaged myocardial cells. The availability of troponin assays has led to an increased understanding of the relationship between myocardial ischaemia and myocardial damage. Changes range from mild damage common after anaesthesia, major surgery and during critical illness, to massive irreversible damage, which accompanies myocardial infarction.

The measured level in fit and healthy people is normally less than 0.1 µg/l. Values above this usually indicate an acute myocardial ischaemic event or infarction. In critically ill patients, however, myocardial damage may arise from causes other than ischaemia and minor rises in cardiac troponin may occur. The diagnostic threshold for an acute ischaemic event or myocardial infarction in intensive care patients is therefore a little higher. Levels above 0.5 µg/l are strongly suggestive of myocardial infarction.

Management

Management is similar to crescendo angina above:

- Oxygen.
- Analgesia.
- Give aspirin 300 mg oral followed by 75 mg daily (contraindications GI bleed, asthma, renal impairment).
- Consider thrombolysis. Streptokinase 1.5 million units in 100–200 ml 0.9% saline i.v. over 1 hour or tissue plasminogen activator (TPA) 100 mg over 90 minutes. (Follow local protocol.)
- Consider β blocker (e.g. atenolol 100 mg daily), if there are no contraindications (bradycardia, hypotension, heart failure, asthma).
- Consider GTN infusion to reduce preload and reduce myocardial work; 1–2 mg/h. Titrate to response.

Thrombolysis aims to limit the size of myocardial infarction by dissolving coronary artery thrombus and allowing reperfusion of the myocardium. This is only indicated if there is irrefutable ECG evidence of acute infarction. It should be started as soon as possible and preferably within 6 hours of the onset of chest pain unless there are contraindications (Table 4.16).

TABLE 4.16 Contraindications to thrombolysis

Recent surgery
Intracranial pathology, e.g. previous CVA
Previous GI haemorrhage
Bleeding from any site
Allergy to streptokinase
Prolonged external cardiac massage

If thrombolysis is contraindicated, consider anticoagulation as for crescendo angina above. There may be a role for emergency angiography, and either acute angioplasty or acute coronary artery bypass grafts. Seek advice from a cardiologist.

CARDIAC FAILURE

Heart failure is common and represents an inability of the heart to maintain sufficient CO despite adequate filling. The clinical picture may range from mild peripheral oedema and shortness of breath to florid pulmonary oedema and hypotension. The principles of management are the same:

- Give oxygen.
- Consider CPAP by face mask or non-invasive ventilation.
- Institute invasive monitoring as necessary. Arterial line, central venous or pulmonary artery catheter or equivalent.
- Optimize preload. Consider the use of diuretics and GTN infusion to reduce both preload and afterload.
- Add inotropes if required.
- ACE inhibitors have been shown to improve long-term survival and should be considered as soon as possible. These agents may cause profound hypotension (especially first dose) and should be introduced gradually. They should also be used cautiously in renal impairment. Seek advice.

Right heart failure and pulmonary hypertension

Both mitral valve disease and chronic pulmonary disease may result in pulmonary hypertension and subsequent right heart failure. This is a very difficult condition to manage. When pulmonary artery and right ventricular pressures are high, systemic pressure falls and perfusion of the right ventricle is impaired. This results in worsening right ventricular performance and rapid deterioration.

- Maintain systemic arterial blood pressure. Avoid drugs that lower systemic arterial pressure. Vasoconstrictors may be necessary to maintain systemic blood pressure and right ventricular perfusion. Consider intra-aortic balloon counter pulsation pumps to maintain systemic diastolic pressure. (See Cardiogenic shock below.)
- Optimal filling of the right ventricle is vital. Use volumetric haemodynamic monitoring or right heart ejection fraction pulmonary artery catheters if available to directly estimate right ventricular end-diastolic volume.
- Consider inotropes to improve right ventricular contractility.

- Consider measures to reduce pulmonary vascular pressures and right ventricular afterload. Epoprostenol (prostacyclin) is effective but is not selective and may also reduce systemic blood pressure. Nitric oxide is more selective and may be useful particularly when pulmonary hypertension is secondary to hypoxic pulmonary vasoconstriction associated with primary lung disease. (See ARDS, p. 128.)

CARDIOGENIC SHOCK

This is the failure to adequately perfuse tissue as a result of poor cardiac function. It is characterized by high cardiac filling pressures, low cardiac output and increased systemic vascular resistance. This is associated with a very high mortality. The main aim is to restore oxygen delivery to tissues by increasing CO:

- Ventilate with high inspired oxygen concentration and correct any dysrhythmias (non-invasive ventilation may be appropriate).
- Establish invasive monitoring with arterial pressure and central venous or pulmonary artery catheter or equivalent.
- Optimize filling pressure. Cardiogenic shock is generally associated with a high PAOP and pulmonary oedema. Consider diuretics to remove fluid. Vasodilators such as GTN may reduce preload if the blood pressure is adequate.
- Rationalize inotropes. In the first instance adrenaline (epinephrine) infusion may be a reasonable choice. This will increase CO and maintain some degree of peripheral vasoconstriction. Once invasive monitoring is established, inodilator drugs such as dopexamine and dobutamine may be more appropriate.
- Obtain an ECG to assess myocardial function and exclude surgically correctable problems such as cardiac tamponade and acute valvular dysfunction.
- If CO fails to improve, consider enoximone. This is a phosphodiesterase inhibitor (PDE-III), which acts at an intracellular level, effectively bypassing the β receptors. It is an inodilator, and causes both an increase in CO and peripheral vasodilatation. It may be associated with a marked fall in blood pressure. Do not give loading doses: start infusion at a low level and increase according to response. Hypotension may require concomitant use of a vasoconstrictor such as noradrenaline (norepinephrine) to maintain adequate diastolic pressure.
- Where there is no improvement with these measures, consider intra-aortic balloon counterpulsation. The balloon is inserted via a femoral artery and inflates in the aorta during diastole to maintain diastolic perfusion of the myocardium.

- Occasionally younger patients may be suitable for acute heart transplantation. Seek senior advice.

PULMONARY EMBOLISM

Pulmonary thromboembolism is common in immobile, critically ill, traumatized and postoperative patients. The effects range from mild discomfort and shortness of breath to sudden profound collapse and cardiac arrest. Typical clinical features are shown in Table 4.17.

Investigations
- CXR: reduced vascular markings (oligaemia).
- ECG tachycardia, right ventricular strain pattern, right axis deviation, right bundle branch block and P pulmonale.
- Plasma D-dimer raised.
- Traditional V/Q scans (ventilation/perfusion scans) are often not practical in ICU patients and may be difficult to interpret if there is a significant pre-existing lung problem.
- Spiral CT scans may demonstrate blood clot in the pulmonary artery and are usually the most useful investigation for ICU patients.
- Pulmonary angiography.

Management
- Give high inspired oxygen; intubate/ventilate as necessary.
- Optimize cardiovascular status.
- For major embolism consider thrombolysis, e.g. streptokinase 0.5 million units over 30 minutes followed by 0.1 million units per hour/24 hours. Then anticoagulate. Seek senior advice.
- For smaller embolism consider anticoagulation, either heparin infusion, e.g. 20–40 000 units/24 hours (monitor APTT and aim to keep $2-3 \times$ normal) or high-dose low molecular weight heparin.

TABLE 4.17 Typical clinical features of pulmonary embolism

Pleuritic chest pain
Dyspnoea
Haemoptysis
Severe hypoxia
Right ventricular failure
Cardiogenic shock/hypotension

PERICARDIAL EFFUSION AND CARDIAC TAMPONADE

Pericardial effusions may be caused by a variety of medical conditions. In the ICU small pericardial effusions are common in patients with widespread capillary leak and generalized tissue oedema. Significant effusions are less common but should be considered in patients with haemodynamic compromise or who fail to respond to resuscitation, particularly if there is evidence of recent chest trauma, cardiothoracic surgery or central venous access procedures.

The haemodynamic consequences of a pericardial effusion depend on the size and speed of accumulation. Large, rapidly formed collections typically compress the right atrium and ventricle, preventing filling and impairing CO. The clinical signs include tachycardia, elevated central venous pressures, hypotension, pulsus paradoxus, and muffled heart sounds. This may progress to profound collapse and PEA (pulseless electrical activity) arrest.

None of these signs is specific. Except in emergency circumstances a confirmatory 'echo' should be obtained before attempting pericardial drainage. The typical findings in cardiac tamponade are a large pericardial effusion with right atrial and right ventricular diastolic collapse. Urgent pericardiocentesis is required. Seek senior help. (See Pericardial aspiration, p. 332.)

CARDIAC ARREST

Most deaths in the ICU are expected and sudden unexpected cardiac arrest is actually infrequent. If patients arrest despite optimal intensive care management, unless the problem is one of transient ventricular dysrhythmia, it is unlikely that the outcome will be favourable. Follow the advanced life support algorithm for the management of cardiac arrest in adults (Fig. 4.11).

Ventricular fibrillation

The chances of a successful outcome from VF are thought to be best if defibrillation is achieved within 90 seconds of onset and decrease with time thereafter. In a witnessed arrest a single precordial thump may terminate fibrillation, after which the application of defibrillating DC shock should not be delayed.

Asystole

Chances of recovery from asystolic arrest are poor. Be sure that the diagnosis is correct. Check that the ECG leads are correctly attached

Advanced life support algorithm for the management of arrest in adults

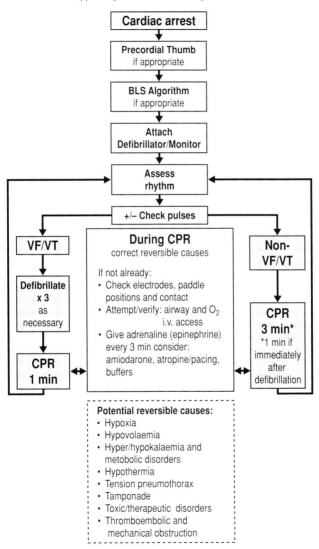

Fig. 4.11 Algorithm: cardiac arrest. Resuscitation Council UK Guidelines 2000.

and that the gain on the monitor is maximal. If VF cannot be excluded, then management commences as for VF.

Pulseless electrical activity (PEA)

Previously referred to as electromechanical dissociation. This term is used to describe the situation where electrical activity is present on the ECG but there is no discernable cardiac output. Hypovolaemia and mechanical obstruction of the cardiac output (e.g. tension pneumothorax and cardiac tamponade) should be excluded.

Management of patients following cardiac arrest

Patients who are resuscitated from cardiac arrest outside the ICU frequently require admission to intensive care. This may be because of failure to regain adequate conscious level, or inadequate cardiac, respiratory or renal function. The management of these patients depends upon the underlying clinical condition, the type of arrest and the timing and adequacy of the initial resuscitation measures.

The commonest problem posed by these patients is difficulty determining the extent and nature of neurological injury resulting from the period of hypoxia. It is very difficult to make any assessment of this in the first 24–48 hours and most patients, therefore, will require a period of stabilization and assessment:

- Institute positive pressure ventilation according to arterial blood gases.
- Optimize haemodynamic status.
- Correct acidosis and electrolyte abnormalities.
- Treat any underlying conditions appropriately.
- If required, use short-acting drugs for sedation.

If the patient's neurological condition fails to improve over 48 hours then the outcome is likely to be poor. Seek advice. (See Hypoxic brain injury, p. 243.)

CHAPTER 5

RESPIRATORY SYSTEM

INTERPRETATION OF BLOOD GASES

The interpretation of blood gases is fundamental to the management of all patients requiring intensive care, not just those with respiratory failure. When drawing an arterial blood sample into a heparinized syringe, ensure that any liquid heparin is completely expelled from the syringe before use, as this will contaminate the sample and influence the results. Arterial blood is obtained either by direct puncture of an artery or from an indwelling arterial line. (See Practical procedures: Arterial cannulation, p. 312.)

Most ICUs now have a blood gas analyser for 'near patient testing'. These are expensive to maintain and repair. You will be unpopular if you damage it by, for example, blocking the sample channels with clotted blood. If you do not know how to use it, ask for help. Normal blood gas values are as shown in Table 5.1.

When interpreting blood gases from a patient use the following system:

- What is the inspired oxygen concentration? Look at the PaO_2. Is the patient hypoxaemic? What is the A–a gradient? (See APACHE scoring: calculating A–a gradient, p. 8.)
- Look at the $PaCO_2$. Is it low, normal or high?
- Look at the pH. Is the patient acidotic (pH < 7.34) or alkalotic (pH > 7.45)?

If the patient has a disturbance of acid–base balance then it is necessary to examine the blood gas further to determine the cause:

- Look again at the $PaCO_2$. Is the $PaCO_2$ consistent with the change in pH, i.e. if the patient is acidotic, is the $PaCO_2$ raised? If the patient is alkalotic, is the $PaCO_2$ low? If so the primary abnormality is likely to be respiratory.
- If the $PaCO_2$ is normal or does not explain the abnormality in pH, look at the base deficit/base excess.

The base deficit/base excess is a calculation of how much base (e.g. bicarbonate) would need to be added to or taken away (by titration) to

TABLE 5.1 'Normal' blood gas values	
pH	7.35–7.45
PaO_2	13 kPa
$PaCO_2$	5.3 kPa
HCO_3	22–25 mmol/l
Base deficit or excess	−2 to +2 mmol/l

normalize the pH of the sample. For example, in a metabolic acidosis, bicarbonate would need to be added to correct the pH because there is insufficient buffering capacity present, i.e. there is a base deficit. In metabolic alkalosis, bicarbonate would need to be taken away to correct the pH, because there is too much base (or insufficient hydrogen ions) present, i.e. there is a base excess.

- If the base deficit/base excess is consistent with the abnormality in pH then the primary abnormality is metabolic.
- If both the $PaCO_2$ and the base excess/base deficit are altered in a way that is consistent with the abnormality in pH then a mixed picture is present.

This simple scheme for the interpretation of blood gases is practical and will suffice for most situations. More complex systems, which take account of other plasma constituents, such as that described by Stewart, are beyond the scope of this book. If in doubt always seek senior help.

A number of patterns of disturbance of acid–base balance can be recognized.

Respiratory acidosis
Hypoventilation from any cause results in accumulation of CO_2 and respiratory acidosis. Over time, the bicarbonate concentration may rise (base excess) in an attempt to balance this and a compensated respiratory acidosis may develop in which the pH is nearly normal.

Respiratory alkalosis
Hyperventilation from any cause results in a lowering of the $PaCO_2$ and a respiratory alkalosis. Bicarbonate concentration may fall (base deficit) in an attempt to compensate.

Metabolic acidosis
There are a number of causes of metabolic acidosis resulting from the accumulation of organic acids or the loss of bicarbonate buffer. Bicarbonate concentration is low (base deficit). If the patient is breathing spontaneously, compensatory hyperventilation may result in a low $PaCO_2$. (See Metabolic acidosis, p. 176.)

Metabolic alkalosis
This is relatively uncommon and may result from the loss of acid, for example from excessive vomiting or nasogastric drainage, or from excessive administration of alkali. Other causes include hypokalaemia, diuretics and liver failure. The bicarbonate concentration is raised (base excess) and the patient may hypoventilate in an attempt to

compensate, resulting in a raised $PaCO_2$. (See Metabolic alkalosis, p. 178.)

> Neither respiratory compensation nor metabolic compensation for an acid/base disturbance is ever complete. The pH will always distinguish the underlying abnormality.

DEFINITIONS OF RESPIRATORY FAILURE

Respiratory failure occurs when pulmonary gas exchange becomes impaired such that normal arterial blood gas tensions are no longer maintained, and hypoxaemia is present with or without hypercapnia. Two patterns are described: types 1 and 2.

Type 1 (hypoxic) respiratory failure

$PaO_2 < 8$ kPa with normal or low $PaCO_2$
(Breathing air at sea level)

Type 1 respiratory failure is caused by disease processes that directly impair alveolar function, e.g. pneumonia, pulmonary oedema, adult respiratory distress syndrome (ARDS) and fibrosing alveolitis.

Type 2 (hypercapnic) respiratory failure

$PaO_2 < 8$ kPa and $PaCO_2 > 8$ kPa
(In absence of metabolic alkalosis)

Type 2 respiratory failure is caused by failure of alveolar ventilation. It occurs most commonly in association with chronic obstructive pulmonary disease (COPD) but may be caused by reduced respiratory drive, airway impairment, neuromuscular conditions and chest wall deformity.

> ⚠ **These definitions are somewhat theoretical, as patients with severe type 1 hypoxic respiratory failure will eventually become exhausted, develop alveolar hypoventilation and then retain carbon dioxide.**

These definitions relate to patients breathing air at normal atmospheric pressure. When interpreting blood gases the inspired oxygen concentration (FiO_2) must be known. Clearly a patient who is already receiving significant oxygen therapy and still has poor PaO_2 is considerably worse than a patient with the same PaO_2 on air. For this reason, PaO_2/FiO_2 ratio, alveolar–arterial (A–a) gradient, and shunt fraction have all been used to describe the severity of hypoxia.

Shunt occurs when blood from the right ventricle reaches the left-sided circulation without being exposed to a functioning (oxygenating) alveolar unit. Shunt may be anatomical (e.g. bronchial venous drainage, ventricular septal defect) or 'physiological' (e.g. atelectasis). Shunt fraction is an estimate of how much mixed venous blood would need to be reaching the left side of the heart without oxygenation to produce an observed arterial PaO_2 and can be used to describe the degree of hypoxaemia.

> Ventilation–perfusion mismatch can be thought of as comprising two elements: dead space ventilation and shunt. Dead space ventilation describes those areas of the lung that are ventilated but not perfused, while shunt describes those areas of the lung that are perfused but not ventilated.

Normal and abnormal values for PaO_2/FiO_2 ratio, A–a gradient and shunt fraction are shown in Table 5.2.

ASSESSMENT OF RESPIRATORY FAILURE

Common causes of respiratory failure are listed in Table 5.3.

Blood gases are only one indicator of respiratory function. The primary assessment of a patient with respiratory failure is clinical:

- Look at the patient.
- Is the patient conscious? Is he or she able to talk and lucid?
- Is the patient using accessory muscles of respiration and making adequate respiratory effort, or is he or she exhausted and respiratory effort minimal? Is there an adequate cough?
- If possible, take a history. If the patient is too short of breath to talk, the history may be obtained from the notes, staff or relatives. Try to obtain some idea of the patient's normal respiratory reserve. How far can the patient walk? Is he or she oxygen dependent?

TABLE 5.2 Measures of hypoxia in respiratory failure

	Normal	Severe hypoxia
PaO_2/FiO_2 ratio	>300 mmHg	<200 mmHg
A–a gradient*	<26	>45
Shunt fraction	0–8 %	>30%

*Calculation of A–a gradient, see p. 8.

TABLE 5.3 Common causes of respiratory failure	
Loss of respiratory drive	CVA/brain injury
	Metabolic encephalopathy
	Effects of drugs
Neuropathy and neuromuscular disease	Spinal cord injury
	Phrenic nerve injury
	Guillain–Barré syndrome
	Myasthenia gravis
Chest wall abnormality	Trauma
	Scoliosis
Airway obstruction	Foreign body
	Tumour
	Infection
	Sleep apnoea
Lung pathology	Asthma
	Pneumonia
	COPD
	Acute and chronic fibrosing conditions
	ALI/ARDS

- Examine the patient, particularly the cardiovascular and respiratory systems, bearing in mind the causes of respiratory failure. Note:
  — Pulse, BP, JVP, heart sounds, peripheral oedema. Is there any evidence of cardiac failure or of dehydration?
  — Increased or decreased respiratory rate, tracheal shift, percussion, bilateral air entry. Presence of crackles or wheeze. Is there any evidence of obstruction, collapse or consolidation, bronchospasm, pleural effusion?
- If there is wheeze, peak flow measurement may help to document severity but is often unrecordable in the critically ill.
- Look at the CXR, blood gases and other available investigations.

MANAGEMENT OF RESPIRATORY FAILURE

> ⚠ If the patient is in extremis due to respiratory failure then immediate action is required. Support respiration with a bag and mask using 100% oxygen. Intubate and continue positive pressure ventilation. Beware of cardiovascular collapse.
> (See Practical procedures: Intubation, p. 337.)

Management is based around treatment of the underlying condition, correction of hypoxia and ventilatory support if required.

Treatment of the underlying condition

● Bronchodilators. If there is wheeze, nebulized bronchodilators may help. In more severe cases consider intravenous bronchodilators and steroids. (See Asthma, p. 123)

● Physiotherapy may help clear secretions and re-expand areas of collapse.

● Antibiotic therapy is best directed on the basis of Gram stains of sputum and on subsequent culture results. Seek microbiological advice. In the first instance broad-spectrum cover, e.g. with a cephalosporin, is probably appropriate. Erythromycin may be added if there is a possibility of an atypical chest infection. (See Pneumonia, p. 115.)

● Diuretics. If there is evidence of congestive cardiac failure and pulmonary oedema, then diuretics may help. Furosemide (frusemide) 40 mg or bumetanide 1–2 mg i.v.

● Continually reassess response to treatment. If there is no improvement or if the patient's condition worsens, tracheal intubation and assisted ventilation may become necessary.

Hypoxaemia

Hypoxaemia is the primary concern and should be corrected:

● If there is evidence of chronic CO_2 retention, give controlled oxygen therapy via a Venturi system. (See COPD, p. 125.)

● In all other cases give high flow oxygen via a face mask, preferably via a humidified system.

● Consider facial CPAP or non-invasive ventilation. (See Non-invasive ventilation, p. 101.)

Hypercapnia

Exhausted patients with minimal respiratory effort will require immediate intubation and ventilation. In those patents that are not in extremis, non-invasive ventilation together with treatment of the underlying condition may lead to improvement. (See Non-invasive ventilation, p. 101.)

Continually reassess the response to treatment. If there is no improvement or if the patient's condition worsens, intubation and ventilation may become necessary. Possible indications for intervention are shown in Table 5.4.

TABLE 5.4 Indications for ventilatory support in respiratory failure

Reduced conscious level
Exhaustion
Tachycardia/bradycardia
Hypotension
Increasing respiratory rate
Falling PaO_2 despite oxygen therapy
Rising $PacO_2$ despite therapy
Worsening acidosis

CONTINUOUS POSITIVE AIRWAY PRESSURE

Continuous positive airway pressure (CPAP) is a system (Fig. 5.1) for spontaneously breathing patients which is analogous to PEEP in ventilated patients. (See p. 104.) It may be provided either through a tight-fitting face mask or via connection to an endotracheal/tracheostomy tube. A high gas flow (which must be greater than the patient's peak inspiratory flow rate) is generated in the breathing system. A valve on the expiratory port ensures that pressure in the system, and the patient's airways, never falls below the set level. This is usually +5 to +10 cmH$_2$O.

The application of CPAP has a number of effects:

● Airways are splinted open, reducing alveolar collapse.
● Alveolar recruitment leads to improved oxygenation.
● Increased functional residual capacity (FRC) allows the lung to function on a more favourable part of the compliance curve and may therefore reduce the work of breathing.

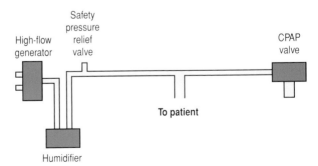

Fig. 5.1 Typical CPAP system.

CPAP is well tolerated by patients even via a tight fitting face mask. Relative disadvantages include noise, difficulties with humidification, distension of the stomach and increased risks of reflux and aspiration.

NON-INVASIVE POSITIVE PRESSURE VENTILATION

Over recent years there has been increased use of non-invasive ventilation to manage acute respiratory failure. It may avoid the need for endotracheal intubation and conventional ventilation, so avoiding many of the associated complications. Patients with acute exacerbations of COPD have been demonstrated to have a better outcome where non-invasive positive pressure ventilation (NIPPV) has been used in place of conventional ventilation. Non-invasive ventilation techniques are also increasingly being used in the management of pulmonary oedema in congestive cardiac failure and to aid weaning from conventional ventilation.

(See COPD, p. 125, and Weaning from artificial ventilation, p. 111.)

Biphasic positive airways pressure (BIPAP)

The most commonly used form of NIPPV is biphasic positive airway pressure (BIPAP). A high flow of gas is delivered to the airway via a tight fitting face or nasal mask, to create a positive pressure. (See CPAP above.) The ventilator alternates between higher inspiratory and lower expiratory pressures. The higher inspiratory pressure augments the patient's own respiratory effort and increases tidal volume, while the lower expiratory pressure is analogous to CPAP/PEEP. Typical initial settings are shown in Table 5.5. Once established, the inspiratory pressure and inspiratory time can be adjusted to create the optimal ventilatory pattern for the patient.

BIPAP is generally well tolerated by patients. The face or nasal mask can be removed intermittently for short periods to enable eating and drinking and oral medication. Regular arterial blood gas measurement should be performed to assess response to treatment. If the patient's condition deteriorates, conventional ventilation may still be required.

TABLE 5.5 Typical initial settings for BIPAP non-invasive ventilation

Inspiratory pressure (IPAP)	10–12 cmH$_2$O
Expiratory pressure (EPAP)	4–5 cmH$_2$O
Inspiratory time (It)	1.2 s
FiO$_2$	As required to maintain oxygen saturation

BASICS OF ARTIFICIAL VENTILATION

Most intensive care ventilators are now highly sophisticated, computer-controlled machines with complicated interfaces, a large number of different ventilatory modes, and inbuilt monitoring and alarm systems. Detailed descriptions and discussion are beyond the scope of this book.

One problem is that there is no uniformly agreed terminology in relation to ventilator modes and different manufacturers use different terms for similar functions. The following terms and modes are in common use but are by no means universal. Before using a ventilator you should familiarize yourself with it. If you have any difficulties seek advice.

Volume controlled ventilation

The simplest form of volume controlled ventilation is controlled mandatory ventilation (CMV; Fig. 5.2). The patient is ventilated at a preset tidal volume and rate (for example, tidal volume 500 ml and rate 12 breaths/min).

This is suitable for patients who are heavily sedated and/or paralysed and who are making no respiratory effort. It is not suitable for patients who are attempting spontaneous breaths. There is no pressure support for spontaneous breaths and ventilator valves may be closed during attempted inspiration or expiration. The ventilator may also deliver a breath immediately after the patient's own inspiration, or as the patient tries to breathe out. This is uncomfortable and distressing, and may result in trauma to the lungs (see below).

Pressure controlled ventilation

CMV and SIMV (see below) are both traditionally volume controlled modes of ventilation. This means that the tidal volume delivered is

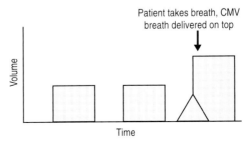

Fig. 5.2 Controlled mandatory ventilation.

predetermined and the peak pressure required to deliver this volume varies depending upon other ventilator settings and the patient's pulmonary compliance. One disadvantage, therefore, of volume controlled modes of ventilation is that high peak airway pressures may result and this can lead to lung damage or barotrauma.

To reduce this risk, pressure controlled modes of ventilation are preferred in patients with poor pulmonary compliance. Instead of setting a predetermined tidal volume, a peak inspiratory pressure is set. The tidal volume delivered is a function of the peak pressure, the inspiratory time and the patient's compliance. By using lower peak pressures and slightly longer inspiratory times the risks of barotrauma can be reduced. As the patient's condition improves and lung compliance increases, the tidal volume achieved for the same settings will increase and the inspiratory pressure can therefore be reduced. (See ARDS, p. 128.)

It is important when using pressure controlled ventilation to understand the relationship between rate, inspiratory time and the I:E ratio (ratio of inspiratory time:expiratory time). Rate determines the total time period for each breath (60 seconds divided by rate = duration in seconds for each breath). The I:E ratio then determines how time is apportioned between inspiration and expiration. For example:

If respiratory rate is 10/minute,
total time for breath 60/10 seconds = 6 seconds.
If I:E ratio 1:2, then
inspiratory time = 2 seconds and expiratory time = 4 seconds.

If the rate is reduced while the I:E ratio is fixed, inspiratory time becomes progressively longer, effectively holding the patient in sustained inspiration. To avoid this, the inspiratory time should be fixed whenever pressure controlled ventilation is used (e.g. 1.5–2 seconds), so that, as the respiratory rate is changed, it is only the length of expiration which alters.

Synchronized intermittent mandatory ventilation (SIMV)

Although historically a volume controlled mode of ventilation, the equivalent of SIMV is now available in both volume controlled and pressure controlled modes (Fig. 5.3). Immediately before each breath there is a small time window during which the ventilator can recognize a spontaneous breath and respond by delivering the set (SIMV) breath early.

SIMV modes improve patient synchrony with the ventilator and reduce the problems described with CMV above. SIMV modes are therefore potentially more comfortable for the patient.

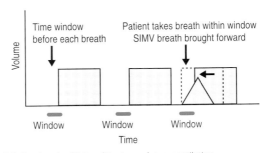

Fig. 5.3 Synchronized intermittent mandatory ventilation.

Pressure support/assisted spontaneous breathing (ASB)

Breathing through a ventilator can be difficult because respiratory muscles may be weak and ventilator circuits provide significant resistance to breathing. These problems can be minimized by the provision of pressure support. The ventilator senses a spontaneous breath and augments it by addition of positive pressure. This reduces the patient's work of breathing and helps to augment the tidal volume. Pressure support modes are available on all modern ventilators and can be used in conjunction with both volume and pressure controlled modes of ventilation.

Pressure support is usually set at 15–20 cmH$_2$O in the first instance and can be reduced as the patient's condition improves. It is best not to remove pressure support completely, however, because of the resistance of the ventilator. (See Weaning from artificial ventilation, p. 111.)

Positive end expiratory pressure (PEEP)

Intubation, artificial ventilation and the effects of lung disease lead to reduction in functional residual capacity (FRC) of the lung. This results in the collapse of small airways, particularly in dependent lung zones, increasing ventilation–perfusion mismatch and worsening blood gases. To prevent this +5 to +10 cmH$_2$O of PEEP can be used to help maintain FRC and alveolar recruitment. Disadvantages of PEEP include reduced venous return to the heart and a subsequent reduction in CO and blood pressure. Unnecessarily high levels of PEEP are therefore best avoided.

Patients with severe expiratory airflow limitation, e.g. due to asthma or obstruction, may develop high levels of *intrinsic* PEEP, with the risk of progressive air trapping. Most modern ventilators include functions for displaying dynamic compliance curves and calculating intrinsic PEEP. If you are unsure how to use or interpret these functions seek advice.

If a patient has high levels of intrinsic PEEP, evidence suggests that applying external PEEP up to, but not exceeding, the level of intrinsic PEEP, causes little cardiovascular compromise, does not increase air trapping and may improve gas exchange by facilitating recruitment in non-flow limited parts of the lung. Increasing external PEEP above the level of intrinsic PEEP may worsen hyperinflation and should be avoided. Seek advice.

PEEP is relatively contraindicated in asthmatics and in chronic emphysema.

VENTILATOR SETTINGS AND VENTILATION STRATEGY

Volume controlled ventilation

In most patients an SIMV volume controlled mode of ventilation with added pressure support will be adequate. Typical initial ventilator settings for an average adult are as shown in Table 5.6.

Pressure controlled ventilation

Pressure controlled ventilation can be used for all patients, although it is frequently reserved for those with poor pulmonary compliance. Typical initial settings are as shown in Table 5.7.

Ventilation strategy

Over the past few years the role that mechanical ventilation plays in producing lung damage has been increasingly recognized. There is evidence that the ventilation strategy used can adversely affect outcome. (See Complications of IPPV below.) Current trends in ventilation strategy are therefore based on the following:

TABLE 5.6 Typical ventilator settings (SIMV, volume control and pressure support)	
Tidal volume	6–10 ml/kg*
Rate	8–14 breaths/min
I:E ratio	1:2
PEEP	5–10 cmH$_2$O
Pressure support	15–20 cmH$_2$O
FiO$_2$	As required to maintain oxygenation
*See Ventilation strategy below.	

TABLE 5.7 Typical ventilator settings (SIMV, pressure control and pressure support)

Peak inspiratory pressure	20–35 cmH$_2$O
Rate	8–14 breaths/min
Inspiratory time	1.5–2 s
PEEP	5–10 cmH$_2$O
Pressure support	15–20 cmH$_2$O
FiO$_2$	As required to maintain oxygenation

- Limit tidal volume to 6 ml/kg.
- Limit peak pressure to 35 cmH$_2$O.
- Accept higher than normal $PaCO_2$ levels (6–8 kPa), so-called 'permissive hypercapnia'.
- Accept PaO_2 7–8 kPa, SaO$_2$ ≥ 90%.
- Use higher levels of PEEP to improve alveolar recruitment.
- Use longer inspiratory times.
- Use ventilation modes which allow and support spontaneous respiratory effort.

See ARDS, p. 128.

CARE OF THE VENTILATED PATIENT

Care of the ventilated patient encompasses many elements discussed earlier, including provision of adequate analgesia, sedation and psychological support. In addition, a number of other factors are important.

Humidification

Some form of humidification is essential in every case. Adequate humidification prevents drying and thickening of secretions that can accumulate in the airways and endotracheal tube. Humidification is generally provided by a heated water bath on the inspiratory limb of the ventilator circuit.

Physiotherapy and tracheal suction

The presence of an endotracheal tube and the effects of analgesia and sedation impair the ability to cough and clear secretions. Regular physiotherapy and suction of the airway is essential to prevent accumulation of secretions.

Monitoring

In addition to the clinical progress of the patient, continuous SaO_2 monitoring and regular blood gases measurement, ventilator function should be continuously monitored. Modern intensive care ventilators have a large number of built-in monitors and alarms which do this, although you may have to set values or limits for some of these. In particular you should note:

- Inspired oxygen concentration.
- Tidal volume and minute volume delivered and expired. A discrepancy between the two indicates a leak in the circuit.
- Peak airway pressure. If the peak airway pressure does not reach a predetermined value, the breathing circuit may have become disconnected. If the peak pressure is too high this may indicate obstruction of the airway or breathing circuit, or poor compliance. The patient may be at risk of barotrauma.
- Spontaneous effort. Many ventilators are able to record and measure any spontaneous contribution the patient makes to the minute volume.

COMPLICATIONS OF ARTIFICIAL VENTILATION

There are many complications of artificial ventilation. These include the following:

- Risks associated with endotracheal intubation, including inability to intubate and dislodgement or blockage of the endotracheal tube, for example with secretions.
- Prolonged tracheal intubation may be associated with damage to the larynx (particularly the vocal cords) and trachea. Traditionally tracheostomy was performed at about 14 days but many units now perform percutaneous tracheostomy earlier. (See Practical procedures: Tracheostomy, p. 342.)
- The drying effect of gases and impaired cough lead to retention of secretions and increases the likelihood of chest infection. (See Nosocomial pneumonia, p. 118.)
- Problems associated with the need for anaesthesia and/or sedation. Include cardiovascular depressant effects of drugs, delayed gastric emptying reduced mobility and delayed recovery. (See Sedation and analgesia, p. 30.)
- Haemodynamic effects of IPPV and PEEP include reduced venous return, reduced CO and reduced blood pressure. In turn this reduces gut/renal blood flow and function.
- Barotrauma. The effects of high pressures applied to the airway can result in damage to the delicate tissues of the lung. This may be

manifest as pneumothorax, pneumopericardium, subcutaneous surgical emphysema, interstitial emphysema and even air embolism. Where possible peak pressure should not be allowed to exceed 35–40 cmH$_2$O. If pressures above this are required, consider the underlying cause and the need for pressure controlled ventilation and 'permissive hypercapnia'. (See ARDS, p. 128.)

- Volume trauma. Even at low pressures excessively large tidal volumes or unequal distribution of the tidal volume through the lung, so that some segments become over distended, can result in volume trauma. The clinical manifestations of this are similar to barotrauma above and include air leaks and cystic and emphysematous changes in the lung parenchyma.

COMMON PROBLEMS DURING ARTIFICIAL VENTILATION

Poor oxygenation

Gradual deterioration in oxygenation may represent continuing development of the pathophysiological process, while more sudden deterioration may represent the onset of a new problem or complication.

- Check the ventilator settings, FiO$_2$ and PEEP.
- Are both sides of the chest being ventilated equally? Check the position of the endotracheal tube. Is the tube too long or the tip abutting the carina on CXR.
- Is there any evidence of new collapse, pulmonary oedema, effusions or pneumothorax. Obtain a CXR. (Effusions/ pneumothoraces may be better demonstrated on erect or semi-erect films.) Treat any findings as appropriate.
- Increase FiO$_2$. Consider increasing PEEP, tidal volume and altering the I:E ratio (increase the inspiratory time). Consider pressure control ventilation, and alveolar recruitment manoeuvres.
- Ensure that the cardiac output and haemodynamic status are optimal.
- Consider permissive hypoxaemia where aggressive ventilation is more likely to result in harm than poor oxygenation. PaO_2 above 8 kPa and SaO$_2$ above 90% are considered safe. (See Ventilation strategy, p. 108, and ARDS, p. 128.)

Hypercapnia

Hypercapnia generally results from inadequate ventilator settings and is simple to resolve. It may be associated with complications of ventilation which result in reduced compliance, particularly pneumothorax. Occasionally it may result from hypermetabolic states in which there is increased CO_2 production.

- Check ventilator settings, tidal volume and rate. Ensure that dead space in the ventilator circuit is minimal.
- Check the endotracheal tube. Is there any evidence of obstruction (e.g. tube kinked or blocked with secretions)? Are both sides of the chest being ventilated equally? Are there any new clinical signs? Particularly, evidence of pneumothorax? Obtain a CXR if there is any doubt. Treat findings as appropriate.
- Is there any evidence of bronchospasm? Consider bronchodilators.
- Increase tidal volume and/or rate.
- Consider permissive hypercapnia: sometimes an elevated $PaCO_2$ is appropriate, either because lung pathophysiology makes reduction difficult/hazardous, or because the patient's habitual $PaCO_2$ is elevated. Remember head-injured patients and those at risk of raised intracranial pressure may be harmed by an elevated $PaCO_2$.

Increased airway pressures

Increases in airway pressure generally indicate a significant problem and should be dealt with promptly, both to resolve the underlying cause and to prevent injury from barotrauma. Common causes of increased airway pressure are shown in Table 5.8.

- Disconnect the patient from the ventilator and attempt to ventilate with 100% oxygen via a bag and mask.

TABLE 5.8 Common causes of increased airway pressure

Endotracheal or tracheostomy tube	Kinked
	Patient biting endotracheal tube
	Obstructed with blood, secretions, etc.
	Too long (endobronchial)
	Misplaced outside trachea
Major airway	Obstructed with blood, secretions, etc.
Reduced compliance	Pulmonary collapse/consolidation
	Pneumothorax
	Pleural effusion
	Bronchospasm
Poor synchrony with ventilator	Inadequate sedation
	Inappropriate ventilator settings

- Check the patient. Is there partial or complete obstruction of the endotracheal tube or major airway? Suction may clear this. Consider bronchoscopy to clear major airways.
- If there is any doubt about the patency of the endotracheal or tracheostomy tube, remove/change it. Use a bougie or airway exchange catheter if any difficulty is anticipated.
- Are there any new clinical signs? Is there evidence of bronchospasm or pneumothorax? Treat any findings as appropriate. This may require physiotherapy and suction, improved humidification, nebulized bronchodilators.
- Check ventilator settings. Are tidal volume, I:E ratio and inspiratory flow rate appropriate?
- If there is no evidence of an acute problem and airway pressures are rising due to reduced lung compliance or underlying pathophysiology, consider pressure control or alternative modes of ventilation.

HIGH FREQUENCY MODES OF VENTILATION

In patients with low pulmonary compliance, conventional IPPV can result in high airway pressures, barotrauma and haemodynamic disturbance. High frequency ventilation has been tried as a means of reducing transpulmonary pressure, while providing adequate gas exchange. In most cases the tidal volume generated is less than anatomical dead space, and the exact mechanisms by which gas exchange is maintained are poorly understood. If you are considering these alternative modes of ventilation seek senior advice.

High frequency oscillation
A piston oscillates a diaphragm across the open airway resulting in a sinusoidal flow pattern with I:E ratio 1:1 (variable). This is unique in that both inspiration and expiration are active. Airway pressure oscillates around a slightly increased mean but the peak airway pressure is reduced. Increasing the mean airway pressure recruits more alveoli and improves oxygenation. CO_2 clearance is controlled by altering the rate and amplitude of oscillation. Clearance of secretions is improved. This type of ventilation is well established in neonatal and paediatric intensive care. Oscillators capable of use in adults have recently become available and are currently being evaluated.

Jet ventilation
Pulses of gas are delivered at high pressure either through an attachment to the endotracheal tube or via a special endotracheal tube.

TABLE 5.9 Typical settings for jet ventilator	
Driving pressure	1.5–2.5 atmospheres (150–250 kPa)
Frequency	60–200/min
I:E ratio	1:1 – 1:1.5

The driving pressure and frequency can be varied. The jet of gas produced entrains air/oxygen from an open circuit (e.g. T-piece) and the tidal volume generated is generally of the order of 70–170 ml. Expiration is passive. Gas trapping may occur. The technique can be noisy and cumbersome. Humidification can be problematic. Typical settings are shown in Table 5.9.

There are two main roles for jet ventilation:

- Management of bronchopleural fistulae. During conventional ventilation most of the tidal volume may be lost through the fistula, making effective ventilation of the patient impossible. Jet ventilation is claimed to reduce transpulmonary pressures, thus reducing the leak.
- As an aid to weaning. Patients can comfortably breathe over jet ventilation. As the patient's condition improves, driving pressure is reduced and frequency increased. The use of non-invasive ventilation as an aid to weaning has reduced the use of jet ventilation for this indication.

WEANING FROM ARTIFICIAL VENTILATION

As the patient's condition improves, artificial ventilation can gradually be reduced until the patient is able to breathe unassisted. The decision to start weaning is largely one of clinical judgement, based on improving respiratory function and resolving underlying pathology. Typical criteria for successful weaning are shown in Table 5.10. Studies have shown, however, that weaning is often delayed unnecessarily and there is evidence that the use of weaning protocols may reduce the time to extubation and reduce ICU stay.

Some patients, particularly postoperative elective surgical cases, will tolerate weaning well and can be rapidly extubated. Others, particularly those who have been ventilated for some time, or who have significant lung damage or muscle wasting, may take longer and benefit from tracheostomy. There is no widely agreed policy on the best way to wean patients from ventilation. A typical approach is described below:

TABLE 5.10 Typical criteria for successful weaning

Neuromuscular	Awake and co-operative
	Good muscle tone and function
	Intact bulbar function
Haemodynamic	No dysrhythmias
	Minimal inotrope requirements
	Optimal fluid balance
Respiratory	FiO_2 <0.5
	(A–a) DO_2 <40–45 kPa
	Vital capacity >10 ml/kg
	Tidal volume >5 ml/kg
	Can generate negative inspiratory pressure >20 cmH$_2$O
	Good cough
Metabolic	Normal pH
	Normal electrolyte balance
	Adequate nutritional status
	Normal CO_2 production
	Normal oxygen demands

- Ensure patient's general condition is optimal.
- Reduce/stop sedative drugs.
- Ensure adequate but not excessive analgesia for surgical wounds, etc.
- Where possible sit the patient up or out in a chair, and mobilize as much as possible.
- Gradually reduce the ventilator rate to allow the patient to take more breaths. Ensure adequate pressure support and PEEP to reduce the work of breathing.
- When the patient is taking an adequate number of breaths with a good and sustained respiratory pattern, switch to CPAP with pressure support.
- If the patient manages well, gradually reduce the level of pressure support further. When the pressure support is down to 10 cmH$_2$O do not reduce it any further.
- Either extubate directly from CPAP and pressure support if the patient is likely to manage or switch to separate flow generator CPAP system.
- Extubate at any stage when it is clear that the patient will manage.

Different patients will progress through weaning at different rates depending on their underlying problems. Some patients may be so agitated that there is no choice but to rapidly wean and extubate. Others may manage only brief periods of CPAP and pressure support before getting tired, as indicated by sweating, increasing pulse and respiratory rate (rapid shallow breaths). These patients will need rest periods on the ventilator between periods of CPAP and pressure support and weaning is often protracted.

Following weaning some patients will extubate without difficulty, others will rapidly deteriorate. This is often due to inability to clear secretions. These patients will require reintubation, ventilation and another period of optimization. Consider tracheostomy to aid clearance of secretions and weaning. (See Percutaneous tracheostomy, p. 342.)

Role of 'non-invasive' ventilation in weaning

There has been increasing recognition over the past few years of the role of 'non-invasive' ventilation techniques as an aid to weaning. Patients with difficulty weaning from conventional ventilation can, for example, be extubated and managed on BIPAP delivered via face mask. This is more comfortable for the patient than prolonged intubation, may avoid the need for tracheostomy and, as the patient's condition improves, can be removed intermittently to allow eating and drinking. Patients who have required a tracheostomy can also be weaned using similar ventilators (via the tracheostomy). This has led to interest in the concept of regional weaning centres, where patients who no longer require intensive care but still need respiratory support might be managed.

AIRWAY OBSTRUCTION

Airway obstruction is common in the immediate postoperative period while patients are in the recovery room and the effects of anaesthetic drugs wear off. Occasionally airway obstruction may persist or may be a potential risk following a particular surgical procedure. These patients will frequently be admitted to the ICU. Causes of airway obstruction are shown in Table 5.11.

TABLE 5.11 Causes of airway obstruction

Facial trauma
Soft-tissue obstruction in upper airway
Bleeding/swelling/tumour/foreign body in upper airway
Vocal cord paralysis following damage to laryngeal
nerve/hypocalcaemia
Bleeding/swelling/tumour/foreign body in lower airway
External compression of trachea, e.g. from bleeding/swelling in the
neck
Collapse of trachea, e.g. tracheomalacia

It is crucial to recognize actual or impending airway obstruction before the patient suffers a hypoxic episode. In the spontaneously breathing patient, airway obstruction produces obvious respiratory distress. Tracheal tug, intercostal recession (mostly in children) and paradoxical respiratory movements all suggest significant obstruction. Stridor is typical, but indicates at least some airflow; the silent patient may be in much greater danger.

Management

The management of any patient with airway obstruction is essentially the same, i.e. secure the airway by endotracheal intubation or tracheostomy as soon and as safely as possible. There are, however, a few points to bear in mind, depending on the situation and your own experience:

- Do not leave the patient unattended.
- Do not delay management of the problem by sending the patient for investigations.
- Give oxygen by face mask. Support ventilation with a bag and mask if necessary and practicable.
- Simple manoeuvres such as extending the neck, jaw thrust and suctioning of the airway may improve the situation.
- Seek help from senior anaesthetist and ENT surgeon as appropriate. In these circumstances intubation/reintubation can often be difficult.

The definitive management is to secure the airway by tracheal intubation or tracheostomy. If time allows, this should be performed in theatre with surgeons scrubbed and prepared for emergency tracheostomy. Awake fibreoptic intubation, awake tracheostomy or gaseous anaesthetic induction with the patient breathing spontaneously may be appropriate, depending on the circumstances. It is beyond the scope of this text to cover these in detail. The usual problem at intubation is gross swelling and distortion of the tissues, which makes the laryngeal inlet difficult to visualize. Often the endotracheal tube has to be passed blindly through swollen tissues into the larynx. Occasionally obstruction proves to be lower down the airway and ventilation may be impossible even when the trachea is intubated.

Once the airway is secured the management is that of the underlying condition. Allow time for swelling to subside. Steroids may be of value. Elevate the head of the bed, and reassess over time.

Airway obstruction in the intubated patient

This is common in the ICU and may be due to kinking of the endotracheal or tracheostomy tube or the effects of thick secretions, blood clot or even occasionally a foreign body. Adequate humidification, regular suctioning and careful fixation of endotracheal tubes avoids most problems, but these may still arise, particularly in children where the endotracheal tube is smaller in diameter and blocks more easily.

It is important to recognize and act on these problems immediately. Typical clues are increased airway pressure, inability to inflate the chest manually with a bag, falling SaO_2 and absent $ETCO_2$ trace.

● Ventilate with 100% oxygen if possible. If not remove the endotracheal tube and manually ventilate the patient with a bag and mask before reintubation.

> ⚠ **Both misplacement and obstruction of endotracheal and tracheostomy tubes is common. If ever in doubt about tube placement or patency, remove immediately and use bag and mask ventilation until the tube can be replaced.**

● If able to ventilate satisfactorily, suction the endotracheal tube. Use 10–20 ml saline instilled down the endotracheal tube to loosen secretion.
● Bronchoscopy may be helpful.
● In 'ball valve' obstruction the chest can be inflated but exhaled gas is trapped by a plug of mucus or blood impinging on the end of the tracheal tube. Apply suction directly to the endotracheal tube and remove it, dragging the plug out at the same time. Ventilate the patient by bag and mask before reintubation.

Post extubation stridor

Airway obstruction and stridor may occur following extubation. This may be as a result of underlying pathology but frequently results from laryngeal oedema, particularly in children whose airways are narrower. This may occasionally require reintubation.

Two or three doses of dexamethasone (4 mg) given around the time of extubation may reduce laryngeal swelling.

COMMUNITY-ACQUIRED PNEUMONIA

Pneumonia is defined as infection occurring in terminal respiratory airways. The pattern of illness and pathogens responsible depend on whether the infection was acquired in the community or in hospital, and on the patient's immune status. Community-acquired pneumonias can be divided into those of 'typical' and 'atypical' presentation.

Table 5.12 Causes of typical community-acquired pneumonia	
Lobar pneumonia	*Streptococcus* sp.
Bronchopneumonia	*Streptococcus* sp.
	Staphylococcus sp.
	Haemophilus sp.
	Coliform bacilli (Gram-negative species)

TYPICAL PNEUMONIA

Features of a 'typical' pneumonia include the following:

- sudden onset of fever with rigors
- cough productive of mucopurulent sputum
- shortness of breath
- pleuritic chest pain.

Chest X-rays show the appearances of consolidation, which may affect a single lobe, a whole lung or both lungs. The diagnosis is confirmed by raised WCC (predominantly neutrophils), and by results of sputum and blood culture.

The usual causative organisms are shown in Table 5.12.

ATYPICAL PNEUMONIA

Atypical pneumonias are so called because their mode of presentation is different from that seen in classic pneumonia. In particular the following presentations occur:

- Present over a few days, compared to the 24–36 hours of classic pneumonia.
- Non-respiratory symptoms may predominate. Fever, malaise, myalgias and arthralgias are common. Some may be associated with severe systemic illness.
- Cough may only appear after a few days. Often non-productive. Sputum which is produced is clear and often negative on Gram stain and culture.
- Disparity between the clinical signs on chest examination and the CXR. Often minimal signs on examination of the chest, whereas CXR shows widespread patchy consolidation with interstitial and alveolar infiltrates.
- WCC may be normal or mildly elevated.

Causes of atypical community-acquired pneumonia are shown in Table 5.13. While the list of causes is not exhaustive it gives an

TABLE 5.13 Causes of atypical pneumonia	
Viral	Influenza A, B
	Parainfluenza
	Respiratory syncytial virus
	SARS*
Bacterial	*Legionella pneumophila*
	Coxiella burnetii
	Mycobacterium tuberculosis
Chlamydia	*Chlamydia psittaci*
Mycoplasma	*Mycoplasma pneumoniae*
*See below.	

indication of the range of pathogens that may be responsible. The
difficulty is often in making the diagnosis. You should seek advice
from local microbiologists regarding investigations and treatment. The
features of some atypical pneumonias are described below.

Mycoplasma pneumonia

Mycoplasma pneumonia is a community-acquired infection that tends
to affect young adults. It may progress to a multisystem disease with
the following features:

- haemolytic anaemia, thrombocytopenia
- pericarditis, myocarditis, rarely endocarditis
- meningitis, encephalitis, peripheral and central nerve palsies
- vomiting and diarrhoea, hepatitis
- rashes, myalgias and arthralgias.

The diagnosis is confirmed by rising antibody titre. Cold agglutinins
occur in up to 50% of patients, although this is non-specific and can
occur in other atypical pneumonias, notably *Legionella*.

Legionella pneumonia

Legionella may occur in outbreaks associated with infected showers
and water-cooling systems, but also occurs sporadically, particularly
among older patients. Typical features are:

- prodromal flu-like illness
- dry cough
- fever up to 40°C associated with rigors
- mental confusion
- nausea, vomiting, diarrhoea and abdominal pain, jaundice
- haematuria and renal failure may develop
- multilobar shadowing and small pleural effusions on CXR.

The diagnosis is confirmed by rising antibody titre. *Legionella* may be identified by immunofluorescence on sputum, bronchial washings and urine.

Severe adult respiratory syndrome (SARS)

At the time of writing a new atypical pneumonia thought to be due to a novel coronavirus has caused a number of deaths in various parts of the world. Symptoms include sudden onset of high fever, sore throat and severe respiratory distress. The mortality rate is high (estimated between 5 and 20%) and health care workers have been affected. Treatment is supportive and infection control measures are paramount due to the high infectivity of secretions. Although initial outbreaks have been controlled by public health measures, there is an unquantifiable risk of this disease emerging seasonally and becoming pandemic. Detailed advice is beyond the scope of this book. If faced with a possible SARS patient, follow all prevailing recommendations and policies.

NOSOCOMIAL PNEUMONIA

Nosocomial or hospital-acquired pneumonias are a common cause of morbidity in hospitalized patients. Up to 20% of all mechanically ventilated patients develop nosocomial pneumonia and the incidence is higher in the immunocompromised patient. Gram-negative organisms and *Staphylococcus aureus* are particularly common.

A number of factors may increase the risk of nosocomial pneumonia in critically ill patients, by impairing host defence mechanisms and increasing colonization of the upper airway. These are summarized in Table 5.14.

Since little can be done to improve host defence mechanisms in the critically ill ventilated patient, the best approach to reducing the incidence of nosocomial infection is to prevent contamination of the airway with pathogenic bacteria, in particular by reducing the incidence of colonization of the upper airway.

Hygiene measures

Ensure adequate hygiene procedures and aseptic technique at all times. Suction the oropharynx regularly to prevent secretions pooling above the larynx and nurse patients in a semirecumbent position to reduce the risk of passive aspiration. Ensure adequate humidification

TABLE 5.14 Factors predisposing to nosocomial pneumonia

Critical illness	Impaired host defences and immune systems
Sedation	Impaired mucus transport and cough mechanisms
Endotracheal and tracheostomy tubes	Bypass normal host defence mechanisms Increased colonization of upper airways Laryngeal incompetence increases risk of aspiration
Antacids	Reduce gastric acidity, allow increased colonization of stomach with lower GI flora
Nasogastric tubes	Provide route for increased colonization of upper airway with lower GI flora from stomach
Broad-spectrum antibiotics	Destroy normal commensal flora and promote colonization with pathogenic microorganisms

of inspired gases and regular physiotherapy and tracheal suction. Use closed suction devices or wear sterile gloves when suctioning the airway.

Maintenance of gastric acidity

The maintenance of a normal gastric pH is a major barrier to the colonization of the upper airway with gut flora, occurring via nasogastric tubes or the reflux of gastric contents. The use of H_2 blockers, such as ranitidine, to reduce gastric acidity and prevent stress ulceration is therefore potentially undesirable. Consider sucralfate as an alternative. Establish enteral feeding early but stop feed periodically to allow gastric acidity to return to normal. (See Stress ulcer prophylaxis, p. 53, and Enteral feeding, p. 49.)

Selective decontamination of the digestive tract (SDD)

SDD is a method of reducing colonization of the upper airways by using oral, non-absorbable antibiotics in an attempt to reduce the bacterial load in the GI tract. There is some evidence that this is effective at reducing nosocomial infection; however, at the current time SDD is not in widespread use.

PNEUMONIA IN IMMUNOCOMPROMISED PATIENTS

(See also Haematology: The immunocompromised patient, p. 219.)

Patients who are immunocompromised for any reason may present with pneumonia. In addition to the typical and atypical conditions

---

TABLE 5.15 Opportunistic infections

Pneumocystis carinii
Cytomegalovirus (CMV)
Herpes virus (simplex and zoster)
Candida sp.
Aspergillus sp.

---

already described, a number of other opportunistic pathogens typically infect these patients. These are shown in Table 5.15.

Pneumocystis carinii pneumonia (PCP)

Typical features are:

- fever
- dry cough
- breathlessness and severe hypoxaemia
- bilateral diffuse alveolar and interstitial shadowing.

Eighty per cent of PCP can be detected by bronchoalveolar lavage (BAL). Occasionally transbronchial biopsy may be necessary.

Fungal pneumonia

Colonization of the pharynx, GIT, perineum, wounds and skin folds is common and rarely requires treatment. Significant fungal infections may occur after prolonged treatment with antibiotics and particularly in immunocompromised patients. Infection is suggested by significant growth in sputum, tracheal aspirates, BAL fluids and blood cultures. In addition there may be rising serum antibody titres to *Candida* or the presence of *Aspergillus* antigens. Fungal infection, particularly fungal septicaemia, is associated with a high mortality.

Cytomegalovirus (CMV)

CMV pneumonitis in immunocompromised patients is generally part of a disseminated infection in which there is also encephalitis, retinitis and involvement of the gastrointestinal tract. Cytology (BAL washings or biopsy) may show characteristic inclusion bodies. Diagnosis may be made by polymerase chain reaction (PCR), fluorescent antibody tests and tissue culture.

MANAGEMENT OF PNEUMONIA

All patients with pneumonia requiring admission to intensive care should have full blood count, urea and electrolytes, liver function tests, C–reactive protein (CRP) and CXR performed. Possible microbiological investigations are summarized in Table 5.16. Not all

TABLE 5.16 Microbiological investigations for pneumonia

Sample	Investigation
Sputum/tracheal aspirate	Microscopy, culture and sensitivity
BAL	MC & S (including AAFB) *Legionella* immunofluorescence Viruses Fungi Pneumocystis
Nasopharyngeal aspirate	Viruses
Blood	Blood culture Serology (acute and convalescent samples) Viral titres Complement fixation (*Mycoplasma*, *Chlamydia*)
Urine	*Legionella* immunofluorescence

patients require the full spectrum of investigations: these should be guided by severity, risk factors and response to treatment.

The treatment of any pneumonia is twofold:

- Supportive therapy including humidified oxygen and ventilation as necessary. Regular physiotherapy and tracheal suction to aid clearance of secretions.
- Antibiotic therapy. Choice will depend upon the clinical picture and the nature of the infecting organism. Wherever possible microbiological specimens should be obtained prior to the commencement of antibiotics.

Recommended empirical antibiotic therapy for severe community-acquired pneumonia is either a broad-spectrum lactamase stable antibiotic (e.g. co-amoxiclav) or a second-generation cephalosporin (e.g. cefuroxime) *plus* a macrolide antibiotic (e.g. clarithromycin) to cover the common atypical agents.

Where specific infective agents are identified or suspected, treatment should be based on microbiological advice.

Nosocomial pneumonia

The management of nosocomial pneumonia is the same as for the management of any pneumonia (see above). Ideally antibiotics should be used only for microbiologically proven infection. If, however, the patient's condition dictates blind antibiotic therapy, ensure microbiological specimens are obtained before commencing treatment. Antibiotic therapy needs to be guided by the likely source of the pathogens and by the local pattern of microbial antibiotic resistance. (See Empirical antibiotic therapy, p. 282, MRSA, p. 284, and VRE, p. 284.)

Pneumonia in immunocompromised patients

The management of pneumonia in immunocompromised individuals is essentially the same as in non-immunocompromised, although the range of potential infective agents is greater. Always seek advice on the likely pathogens, appropriate investigations and initial treatment. Common first-line agents are as follows:

● Pneumocystis pneumonia. High-dose co-trimoxazole (Septrin) and steroids to reduce the inflammatory response.
● Fungal pneumonia. High-dose fluconazole or (liposomal) amphotericin.
● Cytomegalovirus (CMV). Ganciclovir. Beware of nephrotoxicity and bone marrow suppression.

ASPIRATION PNEUMONITIS

Patients with impaired conscious level, cough or gag reflexes are at risk of aspiration of gastric contents into the airway.

Aspiration may present with acute airway obstruction if the aspirated matter is solid. More commonly it presents as gradual onset of respiratory distress and respiratory failure, either due to bacterial infection of the lungs or due to the inflammatory effects of acid aspiration. Some patients will develop ARDS following aspiration. (See ARDS, p. 128.)

If a patient is known to have aspirated gastric contents, e.g. during an anaesthetic, management is as follows:

● Suction the trachea to remove debris. If possible suction should be applied before any form of positive pressure ventilation.
● Consider bronchoscopy and lavage if available.
● Monitor clinical condition and oxygen saturation. Give humidified oxygen as required.
● Avoid antibiotics unless there is evidence of infection. If necessary, antibiotic therapy should cover the normal respiratory pathogens plus Gram-negatives and anaerobes. A combination of broad-spectrum cephalosporin and metronidazole is appropriate initially. Further treatment should be guided by the results of microbiological investigation.
● There is no role for routine prophylactic steroids.

- Treat bronchospasm appropriately. If wheeze persists, consider possible foreign body aspiration and the need for rigid bronchoscopy.
- If the patient's condition deteriorates, ventilatory support may be necessary.

ASTHMA

Asthma occurs principally in young people and the incidence of this potentially life-threatening condition is increasing. Asthma involves increased airway reactivity, often triggered by an environmental stimulus, or following infection. An inflammatory process results in narrowing of small airways, mucus plugging, expiratory wheeze and air trapping. Severe asthma is a medical emergency. It may be rapidly progressive and clinical signs may be misleading. The clinical signs of severe asthma are shown in Table 5.17.

> ⚠ The usual response to asthma is hyperventilation and a low $PaCO_2$. If $PaCO_2$ starts to rise this is a grave sign indicating exhaustion of the patient and the imminent need for ventilation (see below).

Management
- Give high flow humidified oxygen and monitor oxygen saturation continually.
- Give nebulized β agonists (salbutamol 2.5–5 mg neb.) and anticholinergics (ipratropium bromide 0.5 mg neb.). Repeat as frequently as required. Ensure nebulizers are given in oxygen not air.

TABLE 5.17 Clinical signs of severe asthma	
Severe asthma	Life-threatening asthma
Inability to talk in sentences	Exhaustion, confusion, reduced conscious level
Peak flow <50% predicted/best	Peak flow <33% predicted/best
Respiratory rate >25/min	Feeble respiratory effort or 'silent' chest
Pulse rate >110/min	Bradycardia or hypotension
Pulsus paradoxus	SaO_2 <92% PaO_2 <8 kPa $PaCO_2$ >5 kPa pH <7.3

- Give i.v. corticosteroids to suppress the inflammatory response. Hydrocortisone 200 mg bolus then 100 mg 6-hourly.
- There is no role for antibiotics unless there is clear evidence of a precipitating bacterial infection.
- Commence i.v. fluid, e.g. dextrose 4% saline 0.18% to correct dehydration.
- If there is no improvement, commence i.v. β agonist, either salbutamol 4 μg/kg loading dose over 10 minutes followed by infusion 5 μg/min or aminophylline 5 mg/kg loading dose over 10 minutes followed by infusion 0.5 mg/kg/h.

 Do not give a loading dose of aminophylline to patients who are already taking oral theophyllines (risk of dysrhythmias). All patients receiving aminophylline require measurement of theophylline levels during treatment.

- Consider a single bolus dose of magnesium sulphate 1.2–2 g i.v. over 20 minutes.
- If there is no improvement or the patient's condition is life-threatening, consider need for ventilation. Seek senior advice. Indications for ventilation are shown in Table 5.18.

Ventilation in asthma can be extremely hazardous. Always seek senior help.

Patients with severe life-threatening asthma often have high levels of endogenous catecholamines. When anaesthesia is induced to facilitate intubation, the cardiovascular depressant effects of the drugs, the reduction in endogenous catecholamines and the effects of dehydration and acidosis can lead to profound cardiovascular collapse.

Following intubation ensure adequate analgesia and sedation. The presence of an endotracheal tube in the larynx of an inadequately

TABLE 5.18 Indications for ventilation in asthma

Exhaustion
PaO_2 <8 kPa
$PaCO_2$ >6.5 kPa
pH <7.3
Cardiorespiratory arrest

sedated asthmatic is a potent source of irritation and continued bronchoconstriction. Standard sedative regimens are generally sufficient. There may be a role for ketamine infusion both as a sedative agent and as a bronchodilator in refractory bronchospasm. Muscle relaxation may be required in severe cases.

During ventilation, severe bronchoconstriction may result in air trapping and hyperinflation. This may lead to difficulty in ventilating the patient adequately using conventional ventilator settings. High airway pressure may be required, with the risk of barotrauma and development of a pneumothorax.

> ⚠ **Sudden deterioration in a ventilated asthmatic should be assumed to be due to pneumothorax until proven otherwise.**

To minimize these problems, ventilator settings should be adjusted to allow adequate time for expiration. The optimal combination of ventilation settings in any individual patient is best determined by trial. In general, set a slow rate and prolonged expiratory time (I:E, 1:3–1:4) to allow adequate time for full expiration. The short inspiratory time may result in higher peak airway pressure. This is partly offset by the slower rate. In severe cases it may be necessary to accept a higher $PaCO_2$ rather than increase inspiratory pressures.

The role of PEEP in asthma is controversial. In theory, adding PEEP increases FRC and may worsen air trapping in patients who are hyperinflated. Judicious levels of PEEP have, however, been used to recruit airways and improve ventilation. In practice, try adding PEEP cautiously and observe the response. (See PEEP, p. 104.)

If severe hyperinflation becomes a problem it may be necessary to disconnect the patient from the ventilator and manually ventilate with a long expiratory time. Manual compression of the chest wall has been used to expel trapped air and improve respiratory mechanics. Volatile anaesthetic agents may be useful in severe bronchospasm.

CHRONIC OBSTRUCTIVE PULMONARY DISEASE

Chronic obstructive pulmonary disease (COPD) is a broad 'description' applied to patients with chronic bronchitis and emphysema. These conditions frequently coexist, and in severe cases result in respiratory failure, episodes of which may be precipitated by intercurrent viral or bacterial respiratory infection.

Acute exacerbation

Patients with so-called acute exacerbations of COPD are generally managed in A&E and on medical wards with a combination of antibiotics, bronchodilators, controlled oxygen therapy (usually 24–35% oxygen by a fixed performance, Venturi system) and non-invasive ventilation. There are increasing numbers of respiratory care units that provide high dependency care to this group of patients, who are, therefore, only likely to be admitted to an ICU when these measures have failed and tracheal intubation and full ventilatory support is required (See Non-invasive ventilation, p. 101.)

If you are asked to assess a patient with COPD you should consider the following:

- Due to the effects of long-term compensatory mechanisms, these patients often tolerate markedly deranged blood gases (hypoxia and hypercapnia) very well. Therefore, it is the clinical condition of the patient rather than blood gases that determines the need for ventilatory support. Assess the patient clinically. If able to talk, and not distressed, the patient is unlikely to need immediate ventilation, regardless of the blood gas picture.
- Correct hypoxia by incremental increase in FiO_2. Aim to achieve PaO_2 7–8 kPa, $SaO_2 \geq 90\%$ or that which is normal for the patient.
- In some patients with COPD and type 2 respiratory failure, chronic hypercapnia results in loss of the normal ventilatory responsiveness to CO_2. In these patients hypoxia is the main stimulus to respiration. High concentrations of inspired oxygen can result in the loss of the stimulus to respiration and precipitate respiratory arrest. Look at the bicarbonate concentration on the blood gas. If this is normal, or only slightly raised (< 30 mmol/l), chronic CO_2 retention is unlikely to exist and the patient should not be dependent on hypoxic drive. Increase the inspired oxygen concentration as necessary and repeat the blood gases after half an hour. In cases where the patient is dependent on hypoxic drive, the $PaCO_2$ may rise and the need for assisted ventilation may be precipitated earlier.
- Avoid respiratory stimulants such as doxapram. These generally do not help and can result in patients becoming exhausted and requiring ventilation. Only use as an interim measure to allow transport to an intensive care bed or when a decision has been made not to ventilate a patient (see below).
- Give nebulized β agonists (salbutamol 2.5–5 mg neb.) and anticholinergics (ipratropium bromide 0.5 mg neb.). Repeat as frequently as required. Ensure nebulizers are given in oxygen not air.

- Give i.v. corticosteroids (hydrocortisone 200 mg bolus then 100 mg 6-hourly) to suppress the inflammatory response.
- There is no role for antibiotics unless there is clear evidence of a precipitating infection.
- Commence i.v. fluid, e.g. dextrose 4% saline 0.18% to correct dehydration.
- If there is no improvement, commence i.v. β agonist, either salbutamol 4 μg/kg loading dose over 10 minutes followed by infusion 5 μg/min or aminophylline 5 mg/kg loading dose over 10 minutes followed by infusion 0.5 mg/kg/h.
- If the patient remains severely hypoxic, becomes increasingly hypercapnic, acidotic or clinically exhausted, urgent ventilation is likely to be necessary.
- Most patients with acute exacerbations of COPD who require a short period of ventilation do well and leave hospital. Patients in end-stage respiratory failure, however, particularly those that have been ventilated before and who have been difficult to wean from ventilators, may not be suitable for further admission to intensive care. This decision should be taken by a senior doctor in consultation, where possible, with the patient and/or the next of kin. Seek senior advice.

> ⚠️ **If the patient is in extremis there may not be time for a full assessment. In this case you should institute appropriate resuscitative measures, including ventilation, without delay. Considered decisions regarding further management can be made subsequently.**

Intensive care management

These patients are typically very distressed and have a high level of sympathetic catecholamine activity. Anaesthetic drugs used to intubate may abolish this and unmask relative hypovolaemia with subsequent cardiovascular collapse. In addition, there are frequently coexisting medical problems such as ischaemic heart disease. Therefore:

- Where possible transfer the patient directly to the ICU for intubation and ventilation rather than attempting this on the ward.
- If the patient's condition allows, site an arterial line and institute arterial pressure monitoring before induction.
- Consider giving a fluid bolus (e.g. 500 ml of colloid) prior to induction. Have adrenaline (epinephrine) available for resuscitation.
- After securing the airway, institute IPPV. SIMV mode is usually adequate. Avoid hyperventilation. Rapid lowering of the $PaCO_2$ may further reduce sympathetic drive and lower the blood pressure.

- Continue antibiotic therapy according to local protocol. (See Pneumonia, p. 115, and Empirical antibiotic therapy, p. 282.)
- Give nebulized bronchodilators. Salbutamol 2.5 mg and ipratropium bromide 500 µg.
- Consider intravenous bronchodilator therapy. Aminophylline 5 mg/kg loading dose (if not on long-term theophylline and not already loaded) followed by infusion aminophylline 0.5 mg/kg/h. Check levels.
- Corticosteroids. Hydrocortisone 200 mg initially then 100 mg 6-hourly.

Many of these patients require a relatively short period of ventilation and wean easily from the ventilator. Weaning can often be facilitated by the use of non-invasive ventilation techniques such as BIPAP. Some patients, however, particularly those with type 2 respiratory failure, may be more difficult to wean and early tracheostomy may be considered to facilitate tracheal toilet and improve patient comfort while allowing a reduction in sedative drugs. Once stable, patients on BIPAP via mask or tracheostomy may be transferred to medical wards or weaning units for further weaning. (See Weaning, p. 111.)

ADULT RESPIRATORY DISTRESS SYNDROME

The clinical signs of acute lung injury (ALI) and acute respiratory distress syndrome (ARDS) are those of increasing respiratory distress, with associated tachycardia, tachypnoea and onset of cyanosis. Blood gases indicate severe hypoxaemia. The CXR shows acute bilateral interstitial and alveolar shadowing. The non-cardiogenic nature of the alveolar oedema can be confirmed by pulmonary artery catheterization, (PAOP < 18 mmHg, CI > 2 l/min/m^3) and infective processes excluded by BAL.

The principal diagnostic criterion used to distinguish ALI and ARDS is the degree of hypoxaemia, as shown in Table 5.19.

TABLE 5.19 Criteria for diagnosis of ALI and ARDS

	Timing	Oxygenation (PaO_2/FiO_2)	Chest X-ray	PAOP
ALI	Acute onset	<300 mmHg (regardless of PEEP)	Bilateral infiltrates	<18 mmHg or no evidence of left atrial hypertension
ARDS	Acute onset	<200 mmHg (regardless of PEEP)	Bilateral infiltrates	<18 mmHg or no evidence of left atrial hypertension

TABLE 5.20 Conditions associated with ALI/ARDS		
Physical	*Infective*	*Inflammatory/immune*
Trauma	Pneumonia	Blood transfusion
Acid aspiration	Septicaemia	Cardiopulmonary bypass
Fat embolism	Pancreatitis	Anaphylaxis
Smoke inhalation		

Pathophysiology

A large number of conditions have been associated with the onset of
ALI/ARDS, as indicated in Table 5.20.

It is clear that an ALI can develop in response to a wide range of
insults. The exact processes by which this occurs are not fully
understood. It is characterized by proliferation of inflammatory cells,
increased permeability of the alveolar capillaries and leak of
proteinaceous fluid into the alveoli (so-called 'non-cardiogenic
pulmonary oedema'). This protein-rich material precipitates, forming
hyaline membranes. In survivors, the acute inflammatory process
gradually subsides and healing occurs. This may result in widespread
interstitial lung fibrosis. Not all patients who have ALI go on to
develop severe ARDS. There is a spectrum of disease ranging from
mild to severe.

Although used primarily as a research tool, a scoring system for
grading the severity of ALI/ARDS has been devised. This is shown in
Table 5.21.

Management

Severe ARDS is associated with a high mortality ranging from
approximately 25 to 80% in different series. The best outcomes have
been reported from centres using strict protocols for management. In
general:

- Treat the underlying cause, as appropriate.
- Institute invasive cardiovascular monitoring (arterial line and
  pulmonary artery catheter or equivalent) and use
  inotropes/vasopressors as appropriate to optimize CO, perfusion
  pressure and oxygen delivery.
- Artificial ventilation is usually necessary. Reduced pulmonary
  compliance results in high inflation pressures, which are associated
  with increased risks of barotrauma. Current ventilatory strategies
  are intended to limit ventilator-associated lung damage while
  providing for alveolar recruitment. Pressure control ventilation,
  with longer inspiratory times (reversed I:E ratio) may be used to
  limit peak airway pressure. Tidal volumes should not exceed

TABLE 5.21 Scoring system for acute lung injury

Component	Assign value
Chest X-ray appearance	
No alveolar consolidation	0
Alveolar consolidation in 1 quadrant	1
Alveolar consolidation in 2 quadrants	2
Alveolar consolidation in 3 quadrants	3
Alveolar consolidation all 4 quadrants	4
Hypoxaemia score (PaO_2/FiO_2 mmHg)	
>300	0
225–299	1
175–224	2
100–174	3
<100	4
Compliance (ml/cmH$_2$O)	
>80	0
>60	1
>40	2
>20	3
<20	4
PEEP (cmH$_2$O)	
<5	0
6–8	1
9–11	2
12–14	3
>15	4

Score generated by dividing sum of component values by number of components used.

Score 0	No lung injury
Score <2.5	Mild to moderate lung injury
Score >2.5	Severe lung injury (ARDS)

Source: Murray JF, Matthay MA, Luce JM, Flick MR 1989
American Review of Respiratory Disease 139: 1065.

6 ml/kg. Increased levels of PEEP are used to promote alveolar recruitment and improve oxygenation.

- The FiO$_2$ should be kept to the minimum necessary to maintain acceptable oxygenation (PaO_2 7–8 kPa, SaO$_2$ ≥ 90%) in order to reduce lung damage associated with oxygen toxicity. Moderate levels of hypercarbia may be tolerated (permissive hypercapnia) if excessive ventilatory pressures would otherwise be required.
- BAL should be performed to identify infection, and, if appropriate, antibiotics started.
- Although in ARDS pulmonary oedema is classically thought of as non-cardiogenic, these patients often have multiple organ failure. It is estimated that 25% may develop myocardial failure, and fluid

overload is common. Diuretics may be given to 'dry' the patient and may help to reduce the extent of pulmonary oedema.

(See Ventilation strategy, p. 105.)

Nitric oxide

Nitric oxide is a naturally occurring vasodilator produced by the endothelium of blood vessels. If added to the inspiratory gases in concentrations of 5–20 v.p.m. it results in pulmonary vasodilatation in those areas of the lung that are well ventilated. Blood is diverted away from poorly ventilated areas. Ventilation–perfusion mismatch is reduced and there is an improvement in oxygenation. At the same time pulmonary hypertension and the risk of right heart failure is reduced. Nitric oxide has a short half-life when inhaled and is generally safe for the patient. It is, however, a toxic gas and should only be used according to the protocols established in your unit. Although nitric oxide may produce an improvement in oxygenation and therefore allow reduced FiO_2 and airway pressures, there is little evidence that it improves outcome.

Prone positioning

Turning the patient prone may improve V/Q mismatch and blood gases. The response in individual patients is unpredictable. The benefit tends to be temporary (24–48 hours) and patients may need to be turned alternately prone and supine. The risks of turning large patients include injury to staff and the patient, accidental tracheal extubation, and loss of venous access, chest drains, etc. There is little evidence to show improved outcome. (See Practical procedures, p. 359.)

ECMO

Extracorporeal membrane oxygenation is a technique that allows oxygenation to be maintained while the lungs recover. The benefits are well recognized in neonatal and paediatric practice, but are less well established in adult practice. In the UK, ECMO is only provided in a limited number of centres. Transfer of patients with severe hypoxaemia is hazardous and there is a mortality of approximately 30% associated with commencing ECMO. The use of ECMO is not therefore widespread. Evidence suggests that to be of benefit it should be started within 5–7 days of artificial ventilation being commenced.

Steroids in ARDS

The traditional view was that steroids were of no benefit in ARDS. There is increasing evidence, however, that high-dose steroids are of value in reducing the inflammatory and fibroproliferative aspects of ARDS, particularly in the convalescent phase.

Outcome from ALI/ARDS

Mortality in patients with ARDS is high; however, many of these patients die from the effects of multiple organ failure rather than directly from hypoxaemia. Lung function in survivors of ALI/ARDS often slowly improves over weeks or months but in severe cases lasting lung damage may persist.

INTERPRETING CHEST X-RAYS

The combination of tracheal intubation or tracheostomy and IPPV makes interpretation of classic respiratory signs in the noisy environment of the ICU very difficult. The CXR therefore assumes additional importance when evaluating the patient's condition.

You must be able to recognize the typical abnormal appearances seen in intensive care, particularly those that relate to complications of procedures. It is best, therefore, to have a standard system for evaluating the chest X-ray:

● Check name, date and orientation of film. The normal CXR orientation is posteroanterior (PA). That is, the X-rays are passed through the patient from behind towards the film, which is in front. Films taken in intensive care are generally anteroposterior (AP). (This alters the magnification of structures.)
● Check penetration and rotation of film.
● Check mediastinal structures, including cardiac shadow, lung hilum and pulmonary vessels.
● Check lung fields. Note position of diaphragms.
● Check bones and soft tissues.

All tracheal tubes, central venous and pulmonary artery catheters, nasogastric tubes and any drains visible by CXR should be checked for both correct placement and evidence of complications. In particular, note the following:

● Endotracheal tube, correct position above the carina, not endobronchial.
● Central venous catheters. Check intravascular placement with the tip positioned in the superior vena cava, above the pericardial reflections (see Fig. 15.3, p. 323).
● Pulmonary artery catheter. Check tip lying in the pulmonary artery, preferably on the right side and not too distal (within 2 cm of edge of the spinal column).
● Nasogastric tube in the stomach.

A number of CXR patterns are common in intensive care.

Consolidation and collapse

These terms are often used incorrectly and even interchangeably. The X-ray appearances of consolidation and collapse are, however, quite distinct (Fig. 5.4).

Typical features of consolidation are:

- opacification of a lobe or segment (may be patchy)
- no loss of lung volume
- mediastinal and diaphragmatic borders partially preserved
- air bronchograms may be present.

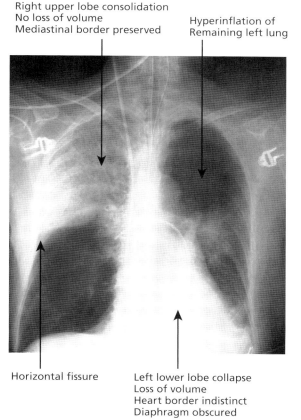

Right upper lobe consolidation
No loss of volume
Mediastinal border preserved

Hyperinflation of
Remaining left lung

Horizontal fissure

Left lower lobe collapse
Loss of volume
Heart border indistinct
Diaphragm obscured

Fig. 5.4 Chest X-ray features of collapse and consolidation.

Typical features of collapse include:

- loss of volume on side of collapse
- compensatory hyperinflation of remaining lobes
- shift of mediastinal structures towards side of collapse
- cardiac and diaphragmatic boarders obscured.

Collapse of the left lung

An extreme example of collapse is collapse of an entire lung. In intubated and ventilated patients this may occur as a result of

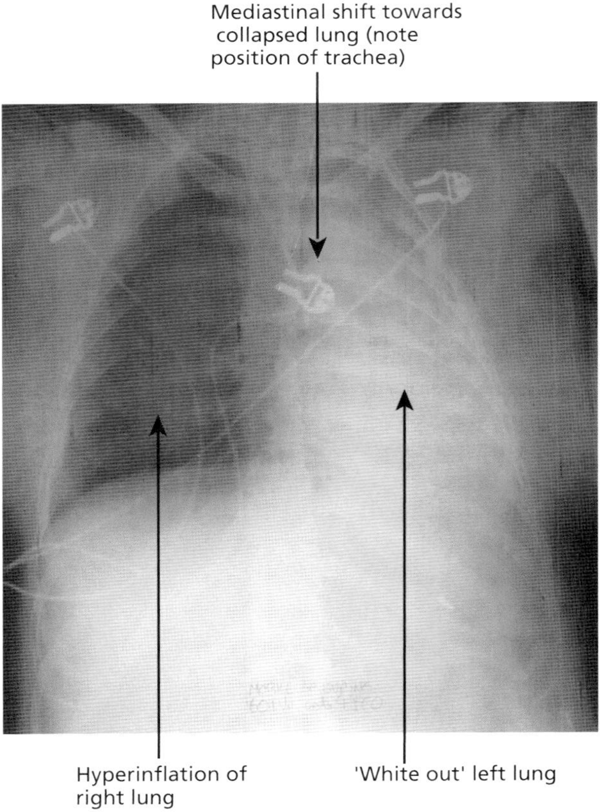

Mediastinal shift towards collapsed lung (note position of trachea)

Hyperinflation of right lung

'White out' left lung

Fig. 5.5 Collapse of left lung.

obstruction of the bronchus (e.g. by mucus plugging) or following endobronchial intubation. The anatomy of the bronchial tree is such that endotracheal tubes are more likely to pass down the right main bronchus than the left. This commonly leads to collapse of the left lung, the typical appearances of which are shown in Figure 5.5.

Pleural effusion/haemothorax

The classical feature of a pleural effusion in an upright patient is that of uniform opacification in the pleural space, typically obscuring the

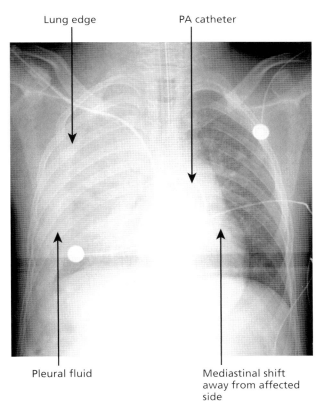

Lung edge

PA catheter

Pleural fluid

Mediastinal shift away from affected side

Fig. 5.6 Chest X-ray appearances of pleural effusion. Note general haze of right lung field. May be the only evidence of small effusion in a supine patient.

costodiaphragmatic recess. In critically ill patients, CXRs are generally taken with the patient supine, and therefore the classic appearance of pleural effusion may be missed. The only evidence of a small or moderate pleural effusion may be a general white haze to the whole lung field (imagine fluid lying posteriorly in the pleural space). Larger effusions usually have the classic features and may produce shift of mediastinal structures towards the other side (Fig. 5.6).

Pneumothorax

Pneumothorax should be suspected in any patient who deteriorates while on a ventilator, particularly if there is associated trauma or recent central line insertion. The typical appearances are that of a visible lung edge and translucent free air in the pleural space, as shown in Figure 5.7.

Air in
pleural
space

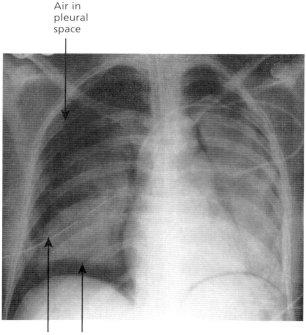

Chest drain   Lung edge

Fig. 5.7 Chest X-ray showing bilateral pneumothorax with lung edge. Right lung has not expanded despite chest drain. Check drain not blocked or kinked (presence of respiratory swing). Consider low suction. Similar changes on left but less marked.

The appearance may not, however, always be so obvious. In the critically ill supine patient with a small pneumothorax, free air may lie anteriorly over the lung and there may be no visible lung edge on CXR. (This is analogous to small pleural effusions lying posteriorly above.) The only evidence may be that of an increased translucency (blackness) anteriorly, as shown in Figure 5.8. If in doubt a lateral CXR or CT scan may help.

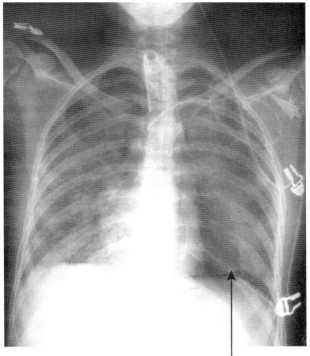

Appearance of free
air anteriorly in
pleural space

Fig. 5.8 Chest X-ray appearance of anterior pneumothorax.

Pulmonary oedema

Pulmonary oedema is common on the intensive care unit and may indicate heart failure, fluid overload or evidence of acute lung injury.

There is a spectrum from mild interstitial oedema to gross alveolar shadowing. Features include:

- interstitial shadowing (Kerley B lines)
- perihilar shadowing
- alveolar shadowing
- fluid in fissures (particularly horizontal fissure)
- pleural effusions.

Adult respiratory distress syndrome

The CXR appearances of ARDS are not specific. The common response to lung injury is leaking of capillaries, accumulation of alveolar fluid and subsequent development of areas of collapse and consolidation. The features are therefore a combination of those described above. A typical example is shown in Figure 5.9.

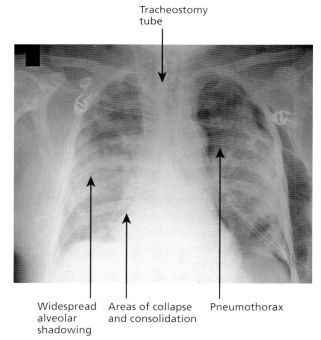

Tracheostomy
tube

Widespread alveolar shadowing   Areas of collapse and consolidation   Pneumothorax

Fig. 5.9 Chest X-ray showing typical features of severe ARDS.

CHAPTER 6

GASTROINTESTINAL SYSTEM

ROLE OF THE GASTROINTESTINAL TRACT IN CRITICAL ILLNESS

In addition to being a common site of surgical intervention and a common source of intra-abdominal sepsis, the gut plays a major role in the pathophysiology of critical illness. In particular, the gut is pivotal, as follows:

- as a large third space for fluid loss within the lumen of the gut
- as a reservoir for bacteria which may ascend the gastrointestinal tract and colonize/infect the respiratory tract
- as a site for altered blood flow (AV shunting) during shock states
- as a reservoir for bacteria and endotoxins which may translocate into the portal and systemic circulations, producing systemic inflammatory response syndrome, sepsis and multiorgan failure, particularly during periods of altered blood flow. (See Sepsis, p. 277.)

The maintenance of gastrointestinal integrity and function is therefore of major importance during critical illness. The key to this is preservation of adequate splanchnic blood flow. In this respect, early aggressive resuscitation is crucial. Several studies have shown that both volume resuscitation and the maintenance of adequate perfusion pressure using vasopressor agents are independently important. In those patients who are adequately resuscitated, early enteral nutrition may also be of value in helping to preserve mucosal integrity and gastrointestinal function.

GASTROINTESTINAL TRACT FAILURE

Failure of the gastrointestinal tract during critical illness may present in a number of ways (Table 6.1).

TABLE 6.1 Clinical features of GI tract failure

Delayed gastric emptying
Failure to absorb feed
Stress ulceration
Ileus, pseudo-obstruction
Diarrhoea
Acalculous cholecystitis
Liver dysfunction
Systemic inflammatory response syndrome

Stress ulceration

Stress ulceration may occur anywhere in the gastrointestinal tract but is most common in the duodenum and stomach. Bleeding from ulceration is common and may present as obvious haematemesis or as an unexplained fall in haemoglobin. Perforation needs to be considered in any patient with abdominal signs who deteriorates. The presence of free air on a plain abdominal X-ray confirms the diagnosis.

Stress ulceration is thought to be primarily due to inadequacy of mucosal blood flow. General resuscitation measures, including adequate fluid loading and maintenance of adequate perfusion pressures, together with early feeding are more important than prophylactic measures. (See Stress ulcer prophylaxis, p. 53, and GI bleeding, p. 144.)

Persistent ileus and pseudo-obstruction

Failure of gut motility is common in the critically ill. It is usually manifest as a simple ileus, with large nasogastric losses and failure to absorb feed. It will usually improve spontaneously as the patient's condition improves. Ensure that the patient's electrolyte balance is normal. Disturbances of potassium and magnesium in particular can contribute to gastrointestinal tract dysfunction. Prokinetic agents such as metoclopramide and erythromycin may promote the recovery of motility. (See Common problem: Feed not absorbed, p. 51.)

Occasionally ileus will progress to marked intra-abdominal distension, with obvious signs of gut obstruction in the absence of any apparent mechanical cause. This is called pseudo-obstruction. The diagnosis is supported by plain abdominal X-ray, which shows widely dilated loops of bowel. Cholinergic agents such as neostigmine have been used to provoke peristalsis. These agents can, however, produce severe gastrointestinal spasm (pain) and may have cardiovascular side effects (bradycardia). You should seek senior advice before using them.

If the colon is distended to greater than 10–12 cm in cross-section, there is a risk of colonic rupture. The use of prokinetic agents in this setting may be hazardous and mechanical decompression is usually necessary to prevent colonic rupture. This may be achieved by flexible sigmoidoscopy, or may require surgical intervention. Seek surgical opinion.

Ischaemic bowel

This should be considered as a possible cause of deterioration, particularly in the elderly patient with pre-existing vascular disease or vasculitis. Systemic inflammatory response, oliguria, persistent acidosis, raised amylase and bloody diarrhoea may all occur but none is specific. Thickened loops of bowel with gas present in the wall may be seen on plain abdominal X-ray. CT scan may be helpful but the diagnosis is usually made at laparotomy. Treatment requires resection of the ischaemic bowel. Difficulty, at laparotomy, in determining the demarcation between viable and non-viable bowel often necessitates a 'second look' laparotomy at 24–48 hours. Extensive infarction is often fatal.

Cholestasis and cholangitis

Cholestasis is common in the critically ill, particularly in the absence of enteral feed, and may result in jaundice. The alkaline phosphatase may be raised. This usually resolves as the patient's condition improves and enteral feeds are established. Abdominal ultrasound and endoscopic retrograde cholangiopancreatography (ERCP) may be necessary to exclude mechanical causes of biliary obstruction. Agents such as ursodeoxycholic acid may be used but there is little evidence for their benefit. Occasionally, cholestasis leads to ascending cholangitis, which may require antibiotic treatment.

Acalculous cholecystitis

Rarely, critically ill patients may develop an acute, necrotizing inflammation of the gallbladder, known as acalculous cholecystitis. The aetiology of this is multifactorial but includes bile stasis and splanchnic hypoperfusion. It should be considered in any patient with right upper quadrant pain, jaundice, raised alkaline phosphatase, abdominal signs and evidence of sepsis. There is no definitive test. Abdominal ultrasound or CT may demonstrate an enlarged, oedematous gallbladder with thickened wall. Management options include CT-guided drainage and acute cholecystectomy. Seek surgical opinion.

Liver dysfunction during critical illness

Liver dysfunction (as opposed to liver failure) is common during critical illness, particularly in association with severe shock states in which there is relative splanchnic and liver hypoperfusion. It is characterized by progressive rise in bilirubin, abnormalities of liver enzymes, coagulopathy with raised prothrombin time (PT) and delayed drug metabolism. Ultrasound or CT should be performed to exclude localized collections of infected fluid. The management is essentially supportive. Hepatotoxic drugs should be stopped. Liver function should improve as the patient's general condition improves.

Intra-abdominal collections of pus

Subphrenic, pelvic and other intra-abdominal collections are an ever-present threat in critically ill patients, particularly following any intra-abdominal surgery. The clinical signs and symptoms may be vague. Persistent ileus, with failure to absorb feeds, 'grumbling sepsis' and altered liver function tests, should raise suspicion. Assessment is by clinical examination followed by ultrasound or CT imaging. Management depends on the clinical condition of the patient. Options include radiologically guided drainage or open surgical drainage.

Abdominal compartment syndrome

The presence of blood, free fluid or gas in the abdominal cavity can lead to a progressive increase in the intra-abdominal pressure and decreased splanchnic perfusion. This may result in gut, renal and liver hypoperfusion with associated clinical features. If suspected, intra-abdominal pressure can be estimated via an indwelling urinary catheter. Between 50 and 100 ml of saline are instilled into the bladder and the catheter is clamped. The pressure in the bladder is measured by inserting a needle attached to a pressure transducer into the sampling port of the catheter (proximal to the clamp). Normally pressure should be less than 15–20 mmHg. If it is elevated, decompression of the abdomen may be required. Seek surgical advice. Once opened it may be impossible to close the abdomen at first laparotomy. The abdomen may be left 'open' under plastic coverings for later closure when the swelling has subsided.

IMAGING INTRA-ABDOMINAL PATHOLOGY

Plain abdominal X-rays

First-line investigation in most cases, e.g. failure to absorb feed, etc. Check position of nasogastric tube and any other intra-abdominal drains. Look for gastric air and normally distributed gas pattern throughout the large bowel. Check for distended loops of thickened bowel walls and for any air bubbles visible in the gut walls (implies ischaemic gut). Check outline of major viscera and psoas shadow. Look for free air, suggesting perforation of a viscus, and air in the biliary tree, suggestive of biliary tract sepsis.

Ultrasound

This is a valuable imaging technique, which can be performed at the bedside. It is particularly useful for imaging around the liver, biliary tract, kidneys, spleen and pelvic organs and can be used to identify intra-abdominal collections of fluid for drainage. It may be difficult to obtain good images because of obesity or the presence of excessive gas in the bowel.

CT scan

This is the definitive investigation for most acute intra-abdominal problems. CT generally requires oral and intravenous contrast. Its value may be limited in the very unstable patient by the need to transport the patient to the CT scanner.

GASTROINTESTINAL BLEEDING

Slow bleeding from the gastrointestinal tract may occur and is a common cause of reduced haemoglobin in the critically ill. Less commonly, but of greater immediate concern, acute massive GIT haemorrhage, which is life threatening, may occur. The source is usually the upper GIT. Common causes are listed in Table 6.2. Bleeding of this sort can result in haematemesis, melaena or even frank rectal blood loss. Lower GIT bleeding is less common but may still be life threatening.

Clinical features

History may be suggestive of the underlying diagnosis; predisposing factors include previous peptic ulceration, non-steroidal anti-inflammatory drugs (NSAIDs), corticosteroids, anticoagulants, liver disease, portal hypertension and critical illness. Brisk GI bleeding is complicated by hypovolaemic shock and oliguria. Myocardial ischaemia may occur. Patients with liver disease develop worsening encephalopathy. Patients with reduced conscious level are at risk of aspiration pneumonia.

Investigations

Full blood count and cross-match are followed by regular monitoring of haemodynamic status, urine output, haemoglobin, coagulation and electrolytes. The site of the bleeding may be identified by endoscopy or arteriography.

TABLE 6.2 Causes of upper GIT haemorrhage

Duodenal ulceration
Gastric erosion and ulceration
Oesophageal varices
Portal gastropathy/gastric varices
Aortoenteric fistulae
AV malformations
Other small bowel lesions

Management

- Large-bore vascular access is obtained and resuscitation of hypovolaemia commenced. In massive bleeds full haemodynamic monitoring, including arterial line, CVP or some other measure of volume status, are valuable.
- Coagulopathy should be corrected.
- Analgesics and anxiolytics are used judiciously in conscious patients. Massive bleeds, however, frequently necessitate intubation and ventilation.
- Endoscopy allows injection of bleeding ulcers and banding or sclerotherapy of varices. The co-administration of a proton-pump inhibitor (e.g. omeprazole 40 mg once or twice daily) is frequently all that is required to prevent recurrence.
- Persistent uncontrollable GI bleeding may necessitate surgery. Radiological embolization of actively bleeding vessels may occasionally be useful.

Variceal bleeding

Persistent variceal bleeding carries a high mortality (up to 50% from a first presentation). In addition to the above, management includes:

- Use of a Linton or Sengstaken–Blakemore tube to compress varices in the gastric fundus.
- The administration of vasopressin (up to 20 units by s.c. injection or slow i.v. infusion: beware vasopressor effects) and octreotide to reduce portal hypertension.
- Endoscopy and variceal banding once bleeding is controlled.

If these measures are ineffective, portosystemic shunting will be required. Transhepatic intravenous portosystemic shunt (TIPSS) is a radiological procedure that has a lower mortality than surgical shunt procedures, but is not considered definitive. Surgical options include splenorenal shunting, mesocaval shunting, oesophageal transection and liver transplantation. These interventions carry a high mortality. (See Practical procedures: Sengstaken–Blakemore tube, p. 358.)

HEPATIC FAILURE

Liver failure is defined as hyperacute where the onset of encephalopathy occurs within 7 days of the onset of jaundice, acute where the interval is 7–28 days, and subacute where it is between 28 days and 6 months. Longer intervals represent chronic liver failure. The term fulminant liver failure refers to an earlier classification where encephalopathy occurs within 8 weeks of the onset of jaundice. It thus encompasses acute and hyperacute liver failure.

Aetiology

The commonest cause worldwide remains hepatitis B. In the UK this is second to paracetamol poisoning. Other common causes include hepatitis A, drug idiosyncrasy and non-A non-B viral hepatitis. (Note: This does not equate to hepatitis C, which is not thought to be a cause of fulminant liver failure. Up to 20% of cases may, however, be hepatitis E.)

Pathophysiology

The final common pathway is hepatocellular failure with a reduction or loss of the synthetic, homeostatic and filter functions of the liver. This results in a failure of carbohydrate metabolism, depletion of glycogen stores and consequent hypoglycaemia. Deranged amino acid metabolism results in accumulation of ammonia and other intermediate compounds which account in part for the development of encephalopathy.

Protein synthesis is arrested, and this includes the synthesis of albumin and clotting factors. Coagulopathy is invariable. PT is the most sensitive index of hepatocellular failure and recovery. The coagulopathy may be exacerbated by activated fibrinolysis.

The filter (reticuloendothelial) functions of the hepatic Kupffer cells are central to the prevention of translocation of gut-derived endotoxin to the systemic circulation. In acute liver failure, there is systemic endotoxaemia. Further, the massive necrosis of hepatocytes releases high levels of tumour necrosis factor (TNF), platelet-activating factor (PAF) and other proinflammatory cytokines. The systemic inflammatory response syndrome (SIRS) and multisystem organ failure (MOF) thus ensue. The combination of these effects gives rise to failure of the blood–brain barrier, with cerebral oedema and altered consciousness.

Clinical features

Hypoglycaemia is common and develops any time in the first few days of the condition. It gradually resolves as the liver failure improves. Acid–base homeostasis is altered and either alkalosis or acidosis may complicate this. A metabolic acidosis is the more sinister.

Concurrently with the development of the metabolic derangement, conscious level may become impaired. Encephalopathy is graded as in Table 6.3.

The onset of encephalopathy is followed in some patients by cerebral oedema and raised intracranial pressure (ICP). The risk of raised ICP is greatest in hyperacute liver failure (in excess of 50% of cases), and much lower in acute failure. It is much less common in

TABLE 6.3 Grading of hepatic encephalopathy

0	Normal
1	Mild confusion (may not be immediately evident)
2	Drowsiness
3	Severe drowsiness, inappropriate words/phrases, grinding teeth
4	Unrousable

subacute failure (around 4%). A baseline elevation in ICP up to 20–25 mmHg may be followed by surges, which are transient but severe (up to 80–90 mmHg). This stage may be followed by inexorably rising ICP and brain death.

The haemodynamics of SIRS develop as conscious level reaches grade III–IV. The characteristic hypotension is associated with a high cardiac index and low systemic vascular resistance. Vasodilatation and increased capillary permeability contribute to reduced circulating volume and may predispose to renal failure. Acute tubular necrosis may also occur as a result of SIRS or directly as a result of the precipitating insult, e.g. paracetamol-induced renal damage.

The coagulopathy seldom gives rise to de novo bleeding, even though very high PT values are seen (> 100 s). Generalized oozing around cannulation sites is common but is seldom of great significance. Thrombocytopenia may also occur, either due to DIC or hypersplenism. It is occasionally necessary to perform invasive procedures under platelet cover.

True 'infective' sepsis may occur. A rising WCC, falling platelet count, a PT whose recovery becomes arrested or a worsening acidosis should all be regarded as suspicious.

Management

> ⚠ **Hepatic failure carries a high mortality. Treatment options include liver transplantation, so early discussion with and referral to a specialist centre are mandatory. PT is key prognostic indicator determining whether the optimal management is likely to be medical or surgical. Do not treat coagulopathy except in cases of life-threatening haemorrhage.**

- The development of grade III–IV encephalopathy or the onset of SIRS are indications for tracheal intubation and mechanical ventilation. This protects the airway, reduces the work of breathing and protects against the risk of secondary hypoxic damage.

- Fluid and haemodynamic management is guided by invasive monitoring. Maintain adequate filling to ensure optimal CO while avoiding the risk of interstitial oedema of the lung, brain and gut.
- Noradrenaline (norepinephrine) is used to keep the mean arterial pressure above 70–80 mmHg and the CPP > 50 mmHg (see below).
- Renal failure can make fluid balance difficult. Continuous renal replacement therapy is frequently necessary, but is often associated with transient haemodynamic instability and ICP surges.
- All patients should receive continuous N-acetylcysteine infusion (100 mg/kg/24 hours). This has been shown to improve outcome in fulminant liver failure irrespective of aetiology, even when instituted relatively late in the disease process.
- Stress ulcer prophylaxis with an H_2 antagonist or sucralfate should be prescribed.
- Prevention of sepsis is a major problem. Prophylactic antibiotics should be discussed with a microbiologist. Selective decontamination of the digestive tract is practised in some centres but is probably of marginal value.

Metabolic issues

- Hypoglycaemia is common. All infusions should be made up in dextrose solutions (5–20%), and dextrose (5–50%) infused to maintain a normal blood sugar.
- Nitrogenous feeds are avoided (no TPN or nasogastric feed should be administered until metabolic resolution of acute liver failure).
- Sodium and potassium are maintained within the normal range; this may involve judicious use of potassium infusions at 10–40 mmol/h.
- The liver will not metabolize citrate used as an anticoagulant in blood products. This chelates calcium, and may drastically reduce ionized calcium levels. Calcium chloride 10 mmol may be given by slow bolus to maintain the ionized calcium to above 0.8 mmol/l.
- Metabolic acidosis is a useful prognostic indicator and is in any case best left untreated on theoretical grounds. The exception to this is where a severe acidosis is associated with haemodynamic instability. It is acceptable to correct the pH slowly to 7.2 if this improves the haemodynamic status.

Control of ICP

- Nurse patient at a 20° head-up tilt.
- Keep physiotherapy, tracheal suctioning and turning to a minimum until the risk of ICP surges resolves (usually 5 days after the onset of grade IV encephalopathy).

- Ensure adequate sedation and paralysis.
- Primary surges in ICP (often followed by a reflex rise in arterial pressure) are treated acutely by hyperventilation. The response to hyperventilation is not maintained, so it should be discontinued as soon as a fall in ICP is seen. Mannitol 20% 100 ml is used to sustain the reduction in ICP and also where the baseline ICP remains above 25 mmHg.
- Even where the ICP remains very high, a good neurological outcome is possible provided CPP is maintained at or above 40–50 mmHg. Cooling the patient and liver support systems have been shown to help control ICP.

Prognosis

Without transplantation, the prognosis is poorest in the subacute group and best in the hyperacute group. Within this group, the prognosis is poorer in those at the extremes of age, those with non-A non-B hepatitis and drug dyscrasia. The overall mortality in patients with grade IV encephalopathy is 70%. With liver transplantation (i.e. in those patients at the highest risk of death with optimal medical management), the 1-year mortality is between 30 and 50%.

PANCREATITIS

Inflammation of the pancreas and autodigestion may be precipitated by a number of triggers, some of which are listed in Table 6.4. The commonest causes are alcohol and biliary obstruction. Frequently no cause can be identified.

Clinical features

A spectrum of severity exists from mild pain to severe shock. Epigastric pain radiating to the back and a history of risk factors (including previous episodes) suggest the diagnosis. Examination may reveal flank discoloration (Grey Turner sign) and peritonism. SIRS, ARDS, coagulopathy and renal failure may develop. The action of

---

TABLE 6.4 Causes of pancreatitis

Alcohol
Biliary obstruction (gallstones)/ERCP
Viral infection (CMV, EBV, etc.)
Surgical injury or trauma
Hypothermia
Cardiopulmonary bypass
Corticosteroids
Oral contraceptives

digestive enzymes on fat leads to 'soap formation' hypocalcaemia and hypomagnesaemia. Diabetes mellitus arising de novo may be permanent.

Investigations

A raised serum amylase (> 1000 IU/1) is diagnostic but is often absent. Values in the range 100–1000 suggest alternative intra-abdominal pathologies, including perforated viscus. Localized posterior perforations of duodenum or stomach may be difficult to distinguish. Chest and abdominal plain films should confirm the absence of free gas or pneumonia, and may show calcium deposition. In severe cases the typical radiographic features of ARDS may be present. Plain film and ultrasound may confirm the presence of gallstones or other underlying biliary lesion. Blood glucose and arterial gases should be closely monitored. As the condition progresses, serial CT scanning is valuable to monitor pancreatic viability and to diagnose pancreatic cysts and pseudocysts.

Management

Severe cases should be referred to specialist centres. In milder cases supportive treatment and analgesia are the main requirements. Pethidine theoretically causes less spasm of the sphincter of Oddi than does morphine. Hyperglycaemia is managed by sliding scale insulin infusion. Traditionally, the GI tract is rested by insertion of a nasogastric tube and regular drainage/aspiration. Total parenteral nutrition is frequently introduced early in the condition. These views are currently undergoing reappraisal; some studies suggest that very early enteral feeding reduces mortality.

In some centres, octreotide (25 µg hourly by infusion) is used to reduce exocrine activity. Patients who develop SIRS/ARDS require intubation, ventilation and haemodynamic optimization. These patients may benefit from antioxidant regimens. Acute renal failure may require renal replacement therapy. Particular attention should be paid to acid–base balance and electrolyte disorders. Repeated calcium, phosphate and magnesium supplementation is often required

Pancreatic cyst/pseudocyst formation requires expert surgical intervention. Treatment may be conservative, by radiologically guided drainage, or by surgical excision. The latter may require repeated laparotomy for intra-abdominal sepsis.

Prognosis

This depends on the severity and duration of the disease and the occurrence of SIRS, ARDS and ARF. In general, the prognosis is poorer in the elderly, in those with pre-existing diabetes mellitus and those with alcohol-related disease.

RENAL SYSTEM

RENAL DYSFUNCTION

Renal dysfunction is common in the ICU and frequently occurs as part of a syndrome of multiple organ failure. It is usually manifest as oliguria progressing to anuria, but high-output renal failure, in which there are large volumes of poorly concentrated urine, may also occur.

The mortality rate for patients in intensive care who develop ARF is increased to around 50%. This high mortality rate probably reflects the seriousness of the underlying condition, rather than mortality specifically attributable to renal failure. Patients usually die with renal failure rather than from renal failure.

Aetiology

In intensive care patients, the cause of renal dysfunction is often multifactorial. Pre-existing renal impairment may be worsened by the effects of critical illness, including release of cytokines, hypoperfusion, altered tissue oxygen delivery/extraction, and altered cellular function. In addition, many drugs used in intensive care are predictably nephrotoxic, while others have been implicated in idiosyncratic nephrotoxic reactions.

Classically, the causes of acute renal dysfunction are divided into prerenal (inadequate perfusion), renal (intrinsic renal disease) and postrenal (obstruction). These are summarized in Table 7.1.

Terminology

Prerenal failure. Decreased glomerular filtration rate (GFR) due to reduced renal perfusion. There is no tubular damage. May be reversed by adequate fluid resuscitation and reperfusion of the kidney.

Acute tubular necrosis (ATN). Decreased GFR due to reduced perfusion resulting in ischaemic renal tubular damage. No immediate reversal on restoration of perfusion. Usually improves over time. This

TABLE 7.1 Causes of renal failure

Prerenal	Renal	Postrenal
Dehydration	Renovascular disease	Kidney outflow
Hypovolaemia	Autoimmune disease	obstruction
Hypotension	SIRS and sepsis	Ureteric obstruction
	Hepatorenal syndrome	Bladder outlet obstruction
	Crush injury	(Blocked catheter)
	(myoglobinuria)	
	Nephrotoxic drugs	

Note: In many patients the cause of renal failure will be multifactorial.

is the commonest pattern of ARF (requiring renal replacement therapy) seen on ICU.

Acute cortical necrosis (ACN). Total and irreversible loss of renal function from severe prolonged ischaemia of kidneys. Rare.

INVESTIGATION OF ACUTE RENAL DYSFUNCTION

In many cases, the causes of acute renal dysfunction in the ICU can be determined from knowledge of the clinical background of the patient and by simple history and examination. Most cases of ARF will prove to be prerenal or ATN. Up to 10% of cases, however, will have other significant underlying pathologies.

History and examination
- Is there any indication of pre-existing renal disease? Vascular disease, diabetes, multisystem disease/vasculitis, chronic anaemia or previously abnormal U&Es are all suggestive. (Look for small shrunken kidneys on ultrasound or CT.)
- Is there any evidence for prerenal impairment, e.g. dehydration, hypovolaemia or hypotension?
- Is there any evidence for new intrinsic renal impairment, e.g. sepsis, nephrotoxic drugs?
- Is there any history or evidence of trauma or obstruction to the GU tract?

Investigations
Serial U&Es are used to monitor renal function and predict the need for renal replacement therapy. Avoid placing undue significance on single results. Take serial samples and look at trends. Some simple investigations can be performed to distinguish prerenal from intrinsic renal failure:

- Urinary U&Es.
- Urine and plasma osmolality.
- Urine microscopy: are there casts, red cells, crystals?

Normal urine osmolality depends on the hydration status of the patient and may vary from hypo-osmolar (less than normal plasma osmolality 280 mosmol/l) to highly concentrated hyperosmolar (> 1000 mosmol/l).

In prerenal failure, the kidney is functioning maximally to retain sodium and water in order to re-expand plasma volume. The urine sodium concentration is low and the urine is maximally concentrated, as indicated by high osmolality (600–900 mosmol/l), and a urine to plasma urea ratio greater than 10.

As ATN develops, the renal tubules are no longer able to function normally, and are unable to retain sodium or concentrate the urine. The urinary sodium rises, urinary osmolality falls and the urine to plasma urea ratio also falls. Eventually the urinary sodium and osmolality approach that of plasma. Renal tubular debris or casts may be seen in the urine. The distinguishing features of prerenal and renal failure are summarized in Table 7.2.

Other investigations may be indicated depending on circumstances:

- Serum creatinine kinase (CK) and urinary myoglobin may indicate rhabdomyolysis following trauma and crush injury (see p. 267).
- Vasculitic screen: renal disease may be associated with autoimmune conditions and vasculitidies. An autoimmune/vasculitic screen may be appropriate, particularly in the presence of coexisting pulmonary disease. Seek advice. Investigations are listed in Table 7.3.
- Plain abdominal films may show calcification or stones and give an impression of kidney size. Intravenous pyelogram (IVP) is not usually performed in ARF.

TABLE 7.2 Distinguishing features of prerenal and renal failure

	Prerenal	Renal (ATN)
Urinary sodium*	<10 mmol/l	>30 mmol/l
Urinary osmolality*	High	Low
Urine: plasma urea ratio	>10:1	<8:1
Urine microscopy	Normal	Tubular casts

*If patients have received diuretics, urinary sodium and osmolality are difficult to interpret.

TABLE 7.3 Investigations for autoimmune disease in renal failure

Vasculitis	Antineutrophil cytoplasmic antibodies (ANCA)
Goodpasture's syndrome	Antiglomerular basement membrane antibodies
Systemic lupus erythematosus (SLE)	Antinuclear antibodies (ANA) Anti-double-stranded DNA bodies
Rheumatoid disease	Rheumatoid factor

- Renal ultrasound may demonstrate small shrunken kidneys in cases with CRF. Ultrasound is useful to show obstruction (e.g. dilated ureters or renal pelvis).
- CT scan with contrast may be useful in trauma/obstruction.
- Renal biopsy and radioisotope perfusion scans may be useful in difficult cases.

OLIGURIA

Oliguria is defined as a urine output of less than 0.5 ml/kg/h for at least two consecutive hours. Most cases of oliguria do not progress to ARF if adequate steps are taken.

> **⚠ Check that the urinary catheter is not blocked, particularly if the oliguria is intermittent or there is total anuria. Flushing the catheter is not always sufficient. A few cases of 'renal failure' may be cured by recatheterization.**

- Review the biochemistry results. Is there evidence of deteriorating renal function over time (i.e. increasing serum urea and creatinine?)
- Review the clinical status of the patient. Is there evidence of dehydration/hypovolaemia suggested by: thirst, poor tissue turgor (pinch skin on back of hand), dry mouth, cool pale limbs, low CVP or wedge pressure, large respiratory swing on arterial line?
- Are CO and blood pressure adequate?
- Is there any obvious cause for renal failure, e.g. chronic renal insufficiency, nephrotoxic drugs, rhabdomyolysis?

Management
- Give volume according to the clinical signs. Even if the patient is apparently normovolaemic it is generally worth giving a fluid challenge (e.g. 500 ml colloid). Response may not be immediate. If there is no response consider the need for invasive monitoring to further assess volume status.
- Renal filtration is a pressure-dependent process. Elderly patients, and, in particular, those with hypertensive vascular disease, may require a higher than expected mean blood pressure. Consider the use of inotropes or vasopressors as appropriate to increase blood pressure towards the normal or admission blood pressure for the patient.

> ⚠ The practice of using dopaminergic agents
> specifically to improve renal perfusion has declined
> in recent years. There is no evidence that these agents
> improve GFR or prevent the onset of renal failure.

- If the cause of the oliguria is not clear from clinical evaluation and
  there is no response to simple measures, consider further
  investigations as above.
- Review the patient's prescription chart. Stop any potentially
  nephrotoxic drugs.
- Look for any sources of sepsis, necrotic muscle (rhabdomyolysis)
  and ischaemic gut.
- If the patient remains oliguric, give bumetanide 1–2 mg bolus i.v.,
  or furosemide (frusemide) 20–40 mg bolus i.v. (Bumetanide may
  be preferable to furosemide as it does not need to be filtered by the
  glomerulus to achieve its effect.) If there is a response, consider the
  use of an infusion to maintain urine output: bumetanide 1–2 mg/h
  or furosemide 20–40 mg/h.
- If there is no response, consider high-dose diuretics, e.g.
  bumetanide 5 mg or furosemide 250 mg over 1 hour, followed, if
  there is a response, by an infusion.

> ⚠ Urine output generated by diuretics may aid fluid
> balance but will often not be adequate for
> maintaining acceptable serum biochemistry. Renal
> replacement therapy may still be necessary.

- If there is still no response then ARF is established and renal
  replacement therapy is likely to be needed. Restrict fluid intake to
  the previous hour's urine output plus 30–50 ml to allow for
  insensible losses. Seek advice (See Renal replacement therapy,
  p. 158.)

ACUTE RENAL FAILURE

Oliguric renal failure

The management of a patient in renal failure may benefit from a
multidisciplinary approach. Seek senior advice and consider referral to
renal physicians or your local renal unit. The main problems
associated with acute renal failure (ARF) are inability to excrete fluid,

impaired acid–base regulation, hyperkalaemia and accumulation of
waste products.

- Inability to excrete fluid may result in progressive fluid overload.
  This may be manifest as hypertension, tissue and pulmonary
  oedema.
- Impaired acid–base balance results in progressive accumulation of
  hydrogen ions and metabolic acidosis.
- Impaired excretion of potassium leads to hyperkalaemia. This can
  develop rapidly, particularly in critically ill patients, and is a
  medical emergency. Other problems of electrolyte disturbance
  include abnormalities of sodium, phosphate and calcium balance.
- Accumulation of creatinine, urea and other molecules may produce
  clouding of conscious level, metabolic encephalopathy and
  myocardial depression. GIT side effects include gastric stasis and
  ileus. Coagulopathy may result from effects on platelet function.

Control of hyperkalaemia

The main concern in the acute phase is the development of ventricular
dysrhythmias associated with hyperkalaemia. Potassium levels can
rise quickly in the presence of severe sepsis and hypercatabolism.
Patients with chronic renal failure (CRF) may tolerate hyperkalaemia
much better than patients with ARF. A serum potassium greater than
6–6.5 mmol/l requires urgent treatment. Calcium, bicarbonate and
dextrose/insulin buy time prior to dialysis but do not alter the
underlying problem. (See Hyperkalaemia, p. 170.)

Indications for renal replacement therapy (RRT)

The indications for renal replacement therapy in acute renal failure are
shown in Table 7.4.

TABLE 7.4 Indications for renal replacement therapy (RRT)

Acute	Within 24 hours
K$^+$ >6.5 mmol/l	Urea >40–50 mmol/l and rising*
pH <7.2, deterioration of clinical state	Creatinine >400 μmol/l and rising*
Fluid overload/pulmonary oedema	Hypercatabolism, severe sepsis

*These are nominal values only, which are a guide to the probable
need for RRT in acute illness. Patients in chronic renal failure will
tolerate higher values. If values plateau and the patient is passing
adequate volumes of urine, RRT may be delayed in the hope that renal
function may recover.

High output (non-oliguric) renal failure

This is characterized by rising serum urea and creatinine despite adequate urine volumes. Urine biochemistry demonstrates a failure to concentrate urine. Indications for dialysis are as for oliguric renal failure but there are generally fewer problems with high potassium and fluid overload. Non-oliguric renal failure is said to have a better outcome than oliguric renal failure. Can accompany the recovery phase of ATN.

RENAL REPLACEMENT THERAPY

Which mode of renal replacement therapy?

Patients with chronic renal failure who require long-term renal replacement therapy usually undergo intermittent haemodialysis two or three times a week or alternatively receive long-term peritoneal dialysis. These modes are generally inappropriate for critically ill patients in intensive care.

Intermittent haemodialysis is associated with significant haemodynamic instability in critically ill patients. Continuous renal replacement systems that allow more gradual correction of biochemical abnormalities and removal of fluid are therefore preferred, at least during the acute phase of the illness. These systems also have the advantage that they can be safely used outside specialist renal dialysis centres. (See peritoneal dialysis below.)

Continuous venovenous haemofiltration (CVVHF)

The simplest form of continuous renal replacement is continuous venovenous haemofiltration (Fig. 7.1).

Blood from the patient is passed through a filter, which allows plasma water, electrolytes and small molecular weight molecules to pass through down a pressure gradient. This filtrate is discarded and replaced by a balanced electrolyte solution. Typically 200–500 ml/h of filtrate are removed and replaced. Overall negative fluid balance can be achieved by replacing less fluid than is removed. Older systems require hourly measurement and adjustment of outputs and fluid replacement. Newer systems are fully automated.

There has been a great deal of interest recently in the role of CVVHF in sepsis. Many of the proinflammatory molecules, toxins and cytokines, which are implicated in the pathogenesis of the systemic inflammatory response syndrome, are removed by haemofiltration. There is anecdotal evidence that some unstable patients have improved following the institution of CVVHF and many units now routinely haemofilter septic patients. (See Sepsis, p. 277.)

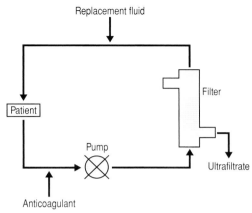

Fig. 7.1 Continuous venovenous haemofiltration.

Continuous venovenous haemodialysis (CVVHD)

One problem with CVVHF is that clearance of small molecules and solutes is inefficient and this can require large volumes of filtrate to be removed and replaced in order to achieve acceptable creatinine clearance.

In continuous haemodialysis (Fig. 7.2), dialysis fluid is passed over the filter membrane in a countercurrent manner. Fluids, electrolytes and small products can move in both directions across the filter, depending on hydrostatic pressure, ionic binding and osmotic gradients. Overall creatinine clearance is greatly improved compared with haemofiltration alone.

In CVVHD, provided the volume of dialysis fluid passing out from the system matches the volume of dialysis fluid passing in, there is no net gain or loss of fluid to the patient. By allowing more dialysate fluid to pass out of the filter than passes in, fluid can be effectively removed from the patient. In simple terms this can be achieved by using a side channel on the dialysis exit limb, controlled by a volumetric pump (Fig. 7.2). Rates of fluid removal up to 200 ml/h can be achieved. In reality, fluid removal is achieved in most CVVHD machines by increasing the rate of the dialysis pump controlling the exit side of the filter by the amount of fluid to be removed.

Continuous venovenous haemodiafiltration (CVVHDF)

This term is best used for systems that intentionally combine both haemodialysis and haemofiltration. Dialysis fluid is passed across the

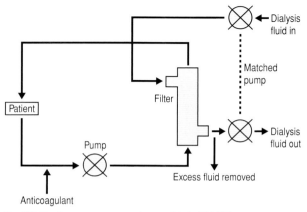

Fig. 7.2 Continuous venovenous haemodialysis (CVVHD).

filter to remove solutes by osmosis but at the same time ultrafiltrate is removed and replaced.

Venous access for renal replacement therapy

Venous access for venovenous renal replacement therapy is generally achieved using a large-bore double-lumen catheter (typically 11.5 Fr). These are sited using a Seldinger technique with the aid of a large, 'stiff' dilator. Care must be taken to avoid damage to the vessels and surrounding structures. Avoid siting in vessels with obvious tight corners, e.g. left internal jugular. Ideally, use right internal jugular or femoral veins. (See Central venous access, p. 326.)

These large-bore catheters are prone to 'clotting off' when not in use. When the catheters are inserted, or when extracorporeal circuits are discontinued, catheters should be flushed with heparin (1000 units/ml) to the priming volume of the catheter as printed on the hub.

Anticoagulant

In all systems where blood passes through an extracorporeal circuit, anticoagulation is needed to prevent clotting. All patients except those with a severe coagulopathy require anticoagulation. Typical regimens are heparin 1000 units loading dose then 100–500 units/hour or epoprostenol (prostacycline) 5 ng/kg/min. Infusions are run directly into the dialysis circuit. The effects of anticoagulation should be monitored regularly using activated clotting time (ACT) or activated partial thromboplastin time (APTT) and the anticoagulant regimen adjusted as necessary.

Excessive anticoagulation can result in bleeding problems. One approach to this has been the introduction of citrate as an anticoagulant for renal replacement therapy. As blood leaves the patient and enters the extracorporeal circuit, citrate is added. As the blood leaves the circuit the calcium is added to reverse the effects of the citrate, and prevent the patient becoming systemically anticoagulated. At the current time this technique is not in widespread use.

Problems associated with renal replacement therapy

The problems associated with renal replacement therapy are listed in Table 7.5.

TABLE 7.5 Complications of renal replacement therapy

Hypotension
Dysrhythmias
Haemorrhage
Platelet consumption
Errors of fluid balance
Infection
Rise in ICP
Air embolism

It is common to see a fall in blood pressure and CO and a deterioration in oxygenation when blood enters any extracorporeal circuit. Simplistically this is explained by fluid shifts, haemodilution and complement/cytokine activation from blood in the dialysis circuit. Hypotension generally responds to simple fluid loading but may require vasopressors/inotropes. Consider reducing the rate of fluid removal by the system.

The so-called dialysis disequilibration syndrome may occur when biochemical abnormalities are corrected too quickly. The rapid removal of plasma solute renders the plasma hypotonic with respect to the brain and acute cerebral oedema develops. It is usually associated with conventional intermittent haemodialysis and is rare with modern practice.

PERITONEAL DIALYSIS

Peritoneal dialysis is commonly used in children and adults for the management of CRF. In children it is frequently also used in the

TABLE 7.6 Potential advantages of peritoneal dialysis

No requirement for vascular access
No extracorporeal circuit
No need for anticoagulation
Little cardiovascular instability
Minimal direct effects on gas exchange in lung
Patients can remain ambulatory

management of ARF because of the difficulties of venous access. The potential advantages of peritoneal dialysis over other forms of renal replacement therapy are shown in Table 7.6.

In adult intensive care, peritoneal dialysis is rarely used for the management of ARF except in patients already established on this mode of dialysis. It is generally ineffective at controlling fluid and electrolyte balance in the septic, catabolic patient. Intra-abdominal pathology, particularly sepsis, is common, making peritoneal dialysis impractical. Fluid in the peritoneum can result in diaphragmatic splinting, which may impair ventilation.

OUTCOME FROM ACUTE RENAL FAILURE

Most cases of ARF in intensive care patients are due to ATN. The normal course of this condition is spontaneous recovery, although urine output does not usually improve until the underlying pathology has resolved. Oliguria (10–30 ml urine per hour, not anuria which is characteristic of obstruction) with a failure to concentrate urine persists for days or weeks followed by gradual recovery of urine output. A diuretic phase may follow. Eventually, there is usually complete recovery of renal function. The diuretic phase may produce large volumes of dilute urine, which may require replacement of fluid and electrolytes. Measure electrolyte losses in the urine to guide this.

MANAGEMENT OF CHRONIC RENAL FAILURE

Patients with chronic renal failure (CRF) may present to the ICU with intercurrent disease. The principles for managing these patients are very similar to those for managing patients with ARF. These patients, however, have a number of specific problems (Table 7.7).

Patients with CRF are invariably anaemic, but are generally well compensated (may be on erythropoietin, EPO). In the intensive care setting, the need for transfusion will depend on the overall clinical picture and the need for increased oxygen delivery. Hb less than 8 g/dl is a reasonable threshold for transfusion.

TABLE 7.7 Problems associated with chronic renal failure

Anaemia
Bone disease
Limited fluid tolerance
Hypertension
Accelerated CVS disease
Difficult vascular access

Patients with CRF who survive intensive care will need to return to long-term dialysis. This will require long-term AV access. Take great care to protect existing AV fistulae and avoid damage to potential future fistula sites. Minimize the number of arterial and venous punctures made. If central venous access is required, avoid the subclavian vein on the side of the fistula, due to risk of bleeding from the venepuncture site (arterialized high-pressure vessel) and because of the risk of late vein stenosis leading to blockage of the fistula. Radial artery lines may be best avoided.

PRESCRIBING IN RENAL FAILURE

Renal failure results in changes to both the pharmacodynamics (what the drug does to the body) and pharmacokinetics (what the body does to the drug) of many agents. Problems may include:

- Altered clearance of drugs and their metabolites can lead to toxicity.
- Altered sensitivity to some drugs even if clearance is unaltered.
- Reduced effectiveness of some drugs in the presence of renal failure.
- Many side effects may be tolerated poorly by patients in renal failure.

These changes are not necessarily corrected by renal replacement therapies. Prescribing drugs to patients in renal failure is therefore a complex issue. You should seek expert advice from pharmacists and renal physicians.

Nephrotoxic drugs

Caution should be used when prescribing drugs with nephrotoxic side effects (especially if their clearance is reduced in renal failure). A list of commonly prescribed nephrotoxic drugs is given in Table 7.8.

Where possible, nephrotoxic drugs should be avoided and alternative agents prescribed. Where either no alternative exists or none is suitable, close monitoring (e.g. of plasma levels) may be

TABLE 7.8 Commonly used drugs which impair renal function

ACE inhibitors
Aminoglycosides
NSAIDs
Cyclosporin
X-ray contrast media
Amphotericin
Cancer chemotherapy drugs

required and the risks and benefits of continuing treatment considered daily.

Drug clearance during dialysis

Drug clearance is dependent on molecular size, charge, volume of distribution and water solubility. In general, non-ionized drugs with high fat solubility and large volume of distribution will not be cleared efficiently by dialysis (e.g. CNS-acting sedative and analgesic drugs).

Opioids

The morphine metabolites (morphine-3-glucuronide and morphine-6-glucuronide) are both active and accumulate in renal failure. It is reasonable to give morphine derivatives as small intermittent intravenous injections but avoid infusing them over long periods of time. Pethidine is metabolized to norpethidine, which accumulates and may produce cerebral excitation and fits. Fentanyl/alfentanil/remifentanil accumulate less and may be used for continuous infusions.

Benzodiazepines

The two most commonly used benzodiazepines in intensive care are midazolam and diazepam. Both are metabolized by the liver but diazepam has an active metabolite that is excreted by the kidneys and may accumulate in renal failure.

Muscle relaxants

Some muscle relaxants may accumulate in renal failure. Atracurium and its isomer cis-atracurium undergo spontaneous (non-metabolic) degradation at body pH and temperature and are the best choice. (See Sedation and analgesia, p. 37.)

Antibiotics

The clearance of aminoglycosides is reduced in renal failure, and high levels are both nephrotoxic and cause deafness if maintained over time. Reduce the dosage/frequency and monitor levels. (See

Appendix, p. 381.) Penicillins may accumulate and produce seizures at high concentrations. High doses should be reduced after loading. Carbipenems, cephalosporins and other antibiotics may also need dose reduction. Seek advice.

Digoxin

Digoxin is unpredictable in renal failure. Levels may be substantially elevated compared with healthy patients. It is cleared to a variable extent by dialysis. Consider alternative agents, e.g. amiodarone.

PLASMA EXCHANGE

Simplistically, plasma exchange works by removing plasma, which contains immunologically active proteins. The plasma is typically replaced by 4.5% albumin solution or FFP. There are a number of established indications and it is occasionally used in ICU patients (Table 7.9). In general, for acute disease, benefit is only seen if performed in the first few days after presentation.

Typically in an adult a 40–50 ml/kg plasma exchange is performed daily (or alternate days) over 5–7 days using an extracorporeal circuit as in dialysis/haemofiltration. The problems associated with plasma exchange are similar to haemodialysis, i.e. need for large-bore venous access, hypotension, anticoagulation, fluid shifts and deterioration in oxygenation. Seek expert help and advice. Plasma exchange is generally performed by the blood transfusion service or renal medicine.

In some inflammatory conditions (e.g. Guillain–Barré syndrome) immunoglobulin solutions may be given as an alternative to plasma exchange. (See Guillain–Barré syndrome, p. 253.)

TABLE 7.9 Indications for plasma exchange	
Established indications include:	*Speculative uses include:*
Guillain–Barré syndrome	Severe sepsis
Myasthenia gravis	Pancreatitis
Systemic lupus erythematosus	
Other vasculitis (e.g. Goodpasture's syndrome)	
Thrombotic thrombocytopenic purpura (TTP – HUS)	

CHAPTER 8

METABOLIC AND ENDOCRINE PROBLEMS

INTRODUCTION

Metabolic and endocrine disturbances are common in the ICU. This may be the primary presenting condition of the patient or may be the result of the complexities of fluid management and/or the effects of prescribed or illicit drug use.

Some typical electrolyte disturbances seen on intensive care are discussed below. Long lists of possible causes have been deliberately omitted. In general, aim for slow correction of most abnormalities over a 24–48-hour period to avoid major fluid shifts.

SODIUM

(Normal range serum sodium 135–145 mmol/l)

Sodium is primarily an extracellular ion. Plasma or serum sodium concentrations are a result of the balance between the sodium and water content of the extracellular compartments. Most acute disturbances of sodium concentration represent changes in water balance rather than total body sodium.

Hyponatraemia

The causes of hyponatraemia are shown in Table 8.1.

Hyponatraemia is most commonly due to an excess of extracellular fluid (rather than sodium loss). This is often the result of excessive use of hypotonic intravenous fluids. Treatment is not usually necessary unless the serum sodium is below 130 mmol/l. Serum sodium below 120 mmol/1 may be associated with altered conscious level and fits.

TABLE 8.1 Causes of hyponatraemia

Excess water intake	Hypotonic fluids TURP syndrome Water intoxication
Reduced free water clearance	Stress response with raised ADH Syndrome of inappropriate ADH secretion Renal impairment Cardiac failure
Loss of body sodium	GI tract losses Renal losses including diuretic therapy Adrenal insufficiency Hyperpyrexia and sweating (inadequate salt replacement)

- Consider the underlying cause.
- Change maintenance fluids to 0.9% saline.
- Restrict fluid intake. Allow kidneys to clear excess fluid.
- If oliguria, consider the need for renal replacement therapy to remove excess fluid.

> ⚠️ **In severe cases rapid correction of hyponatraemia can cause central pontine demyelination (brainstem damage). It is recommended that sodium should not rise more than 2 mmol/l per hour and by not more than 12 mmol/l in 24 hours, to achieve a plasma sodium level of 120–130 mmol/l. The use of hypertonic saline solutions is controversial. Seek advice.**

Excessive antidiuretic hormone (ADH) secretion

This is a cause of dilutional hyponatraemia due to reduced free water clearance. It is most commonly seen as part of the syndrome of inappropriate ADH secretion (SIADH), which may accompany the neuroendocrine stress response to trauma, surgery and critical illness. Rarely, ectopic ADH secretion by tumours may produce a similar picture. Oliguria is accompanied by increased urine osmolality (> 500 mosmol/l) and reduced plasma osmolality (< 280 mosmol/l).

- Restrict fluids.
- Consider a trial of diuretic therapy.

Hyponatraemia due to sodium loss

Significant sodium depletion is associated with a reduction in extracellular fluid volume. This stimulates the release of aldosterone and causes the kidneys to retain salt and water and lose potassium. Urinary osmolality is raised and urinary sodium is low, less than 10 mmol/l (unless there is an intrinsic renal problem or use of diuretics).

- Replace sodium and ECF with isotonic (0.9%) saline.

Pseudohyponatraemia

Electrolytes are present and measured only in the aqueous phase of plasma but the concentration is expressed according to the total plasma volume. If there is a raised lipid or protein content in the plasma this can produce a spurious result.

Hypernatraemia

High serum sodium usually represents free water depletion. This is associated with a raised serum urea (without a significant corresponding rise in serum creatinine) and an increased serum osmolality (> 290 mosmol/l). In critically ill patients this situation can arise despite the apparent appearance of widespread oedema and 'fluid overload' as a result of fluid shifting between 'compartments'.

● Assess patient's clinical volume status (tissue turgor, sunken eyes, CVP, etc.).
● Review fluid balance regimen.
● Give additional free water as 5% dextrose (e.g. 1 litre over 6–12 hours) or water via NG tube. Consider diluting enteral feeds with sterile water.
● If additional fluid contraindicated or undesirable consider renal replacement therapy.

Hypernatraemia due to genuine sodium overload is uncommon. It is usually due to excess sodium chloride ingestion or administration and is therefore accompanied by a high serum chloride and a hyperchloraemic acidosis. Management is essentially the same. Increase free water to allow the kidneys to excrete the additional solute load.

> ⚠ **Rapid correction of hypernatraemia, particularly if serum sodium is >160 mmol/l, can result in cerebral oedema as water enters the brain. As with hyponatraemia, correct slowly.**

POTASSIUM

(Normal range serum potassium 3.5–5 mmol/l)

Potassium is primarily an intracellular ion. Small changes in serum concentration have significant effects on nerve conduction and muscle contraction.

Hypokalaemia

The causes of hypokalaemia are shown in Table 8.2.

Hypokalaemia is relatively common in the ICU. ECG changes include ST depression, flattening of the T wave and prominent U wave. If severe (< 2 mmol/l), cardiac arrhythmias, including supraventricular and ventricular extrasystoles, tachycardias, atrial

TABLE 8.2 Causes of hypokalaemia

Diarrhoea and vomiting
Nasogastric aspirates
Urinary losses (diuretics)
Dextrose and insulin
β Agonists
Hypomagnesaemia

fibrillation, and ventricular fibrillation, may occur. Ensure adequate potassium concentration in maintenance fluids. If additional potassium is required:

- Do not give rapid bolus injections of potassium, as there is a risk of sudden death.
- Give 20 mmol of K⁺ in 20–50 ml of saline over half an hour via a central line. Repeat as necessary. Monitor the ECG during infusion.

> ⚠️ **If adding potassium to bags of fluid, ensure that it is thoroughly mixed before administration. Strong potassium chloride solution is 'heavier' than standard i.v. solutions and tends to 'layer' at the bottom of the bag!**

Hyperkalaemia

The causes of hyperkalaemia are shown in Table 8.3.

ECG changes include peaked T waves, broad QRS complexes and conduction defects. Asystole may occur. Urgent treatment is required.

Treatment to reduce risk of immediate arrhythmia:

- 10 ml of 10% calcium chloride slow i.v. bolus will help to stabilize cardiac muscle.
- In the presence of metabolic acidosis, 8.4% bicarbonate as below.

TABLE 8.3 Causes of hyperkalaemia

Spurious (e.g. haemolysed blood sample, check result)
Iatrogenic (excess administration)
Renal failure
Acidosis
Muscle injury (including suxamethonium, crush injury, compartment syndrome)
Cell death (including haemolysis, chemotherapy)
Addison's disease

Treatment to lower serum potassium:

- Nebulized salbutamol 2.5 mg, repeated as necessary.
- 50 ml of 8.4% bicarbonate, particularly in the presence of metabolic acidosis.
- 20% dextrose infusion plus 10 units of short-acting insulin i.v. (e.g. Actrapid).
- Oral/rectal calcium resonium (chelating agent).
- Consider the need for urgent renal replacement therapy.

CALCIUM

(Normal range standard serum calcium 2.12–2.62 mmol/l)
(Normal range ionized serum calcium 0.84–1 mmol/l)

Most laboratories measure total calcium, which includes bound and unbound fractions. The unbound fraction (ionized Ca^{2+}), which is the physiologically active component, varies with the albumin concentration. Therefore, look at the corrected figure, which takes account of protein binding. Alternatively many blood gas analysers now measure ionized Ca^{2+} directly.

Hypocalcaemia

Hypocalcaemia is common on the ICU. The typical causes are shown in Table 8.4.

Hypocalcaemia causes depressed cardiac function, loss of vasomotor tone, muscle weakness, paraesthesia and tetany.

- Give 10 ml of 10% calcium chloride as slow IV bolus.
- Repeat as necessary or consider slow infusion.

In hypocalcaemia secondary to phosphate accumulation, there are risks of calcium phosphate deposition in tissues with overzealous calcium administration. Seek specialist advice.

> In cases of refractory shock, unresponsive to other drugs, I.V. calcium may be effective.

TABLE 8.4 Causes of hypocalcaemia

Large volume blood transfusion (accumulation of citrate)
Generalized failure of Ca^{2+} homeostasis in severe sepsis
Pancreatitis
Secondary to phosphate accumulation in renal failure
Parathyroid damage after head and neck surgery

TABLE 8.5 Causes of hypercalcaemia

Hyperparathyroidism
Excessive intake vitamin D or calcium
Malignancy
Sarcoidosis
Bone disease
Drug-induced (thiazide diuretics)

Hypercalcaemia

This occurs less commonly and is generally due to an underlying
disease process. Typical causes are listed in Table 8.5.

Symptoms include GI disturbance, confusion and polyuria.
Treatment is by rehydration and the use of calcium-binding agents:

- Give 0.9% saline to rehydrate the patient. Check plasma osmolality
  is within the normal range (280–290 mosmol/l).
- Forced diuresis may be used to aid excretion. Furosemide
  (frusemide) is administered and the urine output replaced with
  alternating 0.9% saline and 5% dextrose.
- Calcitonin 4 µg/kg s.c. 12-hourly. Calcitonin reduces the rate of
  calcium and phosphate release from the bones. It is useful in
  patients with hypercalcaemia associated with malignancy and
  generally reduces the calcium level within 2 hours.
- Bisphosphonates: e.g. disodium etidronate 7.5 mg/kg i.v. over
  4 hours daily for 3 days. These also reduce release of calcium from
  bones but generally take a few days to achieve maximum effect.
- Corticosteroids may be helpful in hypercalcaemia associated with
  sarcoidosis and malignancy.

PHOSPHATE

(Normal range serum phosphate 0.7–1.25 mmol /l)

Hypophosphataemia

This is common in the ICU. It is usually multifactorial, resulting from
reduced intake (particularly patients on TPN), redistribution and
increased losses (especially patients on renal replacement therapy).
Hypophosphataemia causes muscle weakness, which may lead to
difficulty in weaning from ventilators. It also causes failure of many
metabolic processes and, if severe, results in depressed conscious level
and seizures. It is debatable at what level replacement is required. In
most cases, as the patient's overall condition improves, phosphate
balance returns. Patients whose levels are below 0.8 mmol/l,

particularly if symptomatic, may benefit from additional phosphate either in feeds or intravenously.

- Use sodium phosphate or potassium phosphate depending upon requirements.
- Give 30–60 mmol phosphate diluted in 100–500 ml 5% dextrose. over 24 hours.

Hyperphosphataemia

Hyperphosphataemia is caused by excessive intake or decreased excretion (e.g. renal failure). Maintain adequate hydration with 5% dextrose. If severe, consider the need for renal replacement therapy. Phosphate is very effectively removed by continuous RRT techniques.

MAGNESIUM

(Normal range serum magnesium 0.7–1 mmol/l)

Hypomagnesaemia

Magnesium is the second most common intracellular cation and as such serum levels are a poor guide to the need for replacement. Serum magnesium is frequently depleted in critical illness. Causes of hypomagnesaemia are shown in Table 8.6.

Hypomagnesaemia is usually asymptomatic but can give rise to muscle weakness and cardiac arrhythmias. (Hypomagnesaemia exacerbates the effects of hypokalaemia.) The treatment is by magnesium supplementation:

- Give 10 mmol magnesium sulphate i.v. over half an hour.
- If severe can be followed by 50–100 mmol over 24 hours.

Magnesium can also be used for the control of seizure activity in eclampsia and for control of cardiac arrhythmias, particularly supraventricular tachycardia. (See Disturbance of cardiac rhythm, p. 73, and The obstetric patient, p. 305.)

TABLE 8.6 Causes of hypomagnesaemia

Diuretics
Insulin
Gastrointestinal tract losses
Parenteral nutrition

Hypermagnesaemia

This is less common and generally results from excessive administration, particularly in the presence of renal failure. Conscious level may be reduced. Cardiac conduction may be impaired with prolongation of the PR interval and broadening of the QRS complexes. At extreme levels this may result in cardiac arrest.

- 10 ml calcium chloride i.v. will temporarily improve cardiac conduction.
- Consider the need for urgent haemofiltration or haemodialysis.

ALBUMIN

Albumin is a plasma protein which is important in contributing to colloid oncotic pressure and as a binding protein for drugs and other substances.

Hypoalbuminaemia

Low serum albumin is common in critically ill patients. Causes of hypoalbuminaemia are shown in Table 8.7.

In the majority of cases low albumin should be considered as a marker of disease severity rather than a problem in its own right. Levels will generally recover as the patient's condition improves. Ensure adequate nutrition in order to encourage protein synthesis.

Use of albumin solutions

There are two albumin preparations that are readily available. They are relatively expensive compared to other synthetic colloids:

- 4.5% albumin (contains Na^+ 140 mmol/l)
- 20% albumin (contains Na^+ 60 mmol/l).

There has been considerable debate recently regarding the use of these solutions in critically ill patients. It has been suggested that the use of albumin-containing solutions may actually increase mortality. Although the meta-analysis that led to this suggestion has been heavily criticized, the use of 4.5% albumin solution purely for volume expansion purposes has declined. Albumin solutions may be used for volume expansion when serum albumin levels are < 20 g/l.

TABLE 8.7 Causes of hypoalbuminaemia

Malnutrition
Impaired protein synthesis (liver disease)
Increased losses; capillary leakage/renal disease

Twenty per cent albumin given as a bolus effectively raises the plasma oncotic pressure and expands the intravascular space by factor of 5 × the volume given, by drawing fluid in from extravascular spaces. It may be used, therefore, in association with diuretics in an attempt to correct oedema secondary to severe hypoalbuminaemia. Twenty per cent albumin is also frequently used in the nephrotic syndrome to replace protein losses.

METABOLIC ACIDOSIS

(See Interpretation of blood gases, p. 94, and Sepsis, p. 277)

Metabolic acidosis is common in intensive care. Common causes are shown in Table 8.8.

The effects of acidosis are increased respiratory drive (unless sedated/paralysed), and at low pH < 7.1 reduced CO, and reduced response to inotropes. Hydrogen ions move into cells and K^+ moves out in an attempt to buffer the acidosis, so hyperkalaemia may occur. Treatment depends on the severity, underlying cause and speed of response to interventions. In most cases the metabolic acidosis will correct as the underlying condition improves.

- Treat the underlying cause. (See Lactic acidosis below, Diabetic ketoacidosis, p. 179, and Poisoning p. 190.)
- If pH < 7.1 or the patient's clinical condition is deteriorating, give 50 ml 8.4% (50 mmol) sodium bicarbonate i.v. Check blood gases and repeat as necessary.

Alternatively, give a dose of bicarbonate as calculated below; then again check blood gases and repeat as necessary.

TABLE 8.8 Causes of metabolic acidosis

Accumulation of H+ (anion gap* >18 mmol/l)	Loss of bicarbonate (anion gap* <18 mmol/l)
Ketoacidosis	Vomiting or diarrhoea
Lactic acidosis (shock & tissue ischaemia)	Small bowel fistula
ARF	Renal tubular acidosis
Salicylate poisoning	

*Anion gap is calculated as follows: $[Na^+ + K^+] - [HCO_3^- + Cl^-]$. Normal anion gap is < 18 mmol/l. An increased anion gap implies the presence of an excess of a non-carbonic acid.

$$\text{Sodium bicarbonate} = \frac{1}{2} \times \frac{\text{base deficit (mmol/l)} \times \text{weight (kg)}}{3}.$$

> ⚠ **There are disadvantages to using sodium bicarbonate, including the large sodium load and the theoretical risk of worsening intracellular acidosis. Therefore, only use if the pH < 7.2 in an inotrope-resistant, hypotensive patient.**

There are a number of other alkalizing solutions commercially available, including tris buffered bicarbonate solution (THAM). Despite theoretical advantages they are not widely used. Ask for advice and seek local guidelines in your unit.

Measurement of lactate

Lactate measurements are increasingly available from blood gas analysers. There is considerable argument as to their value. Lactate levels > 2 mmol/l imply anaerobic metabolism. There are two situations in which lactic acidosis may occur.

Lactic acidosis

Type A

This is the commonest type of metabolic acidosis seen in the ICU and is due to inadequate delivery of oxygen to the tissue. This may occur, for example, as a result of cardiorespiratory arrest or from inadequate tissue perfusion, as seen in shock states. Inadequate oxygen delivery leads to anaerobic metabolism and the accumulation of lactate. (It is not uncommon, however, for patients with severe shock and acidosis to have a normal lactate.)

- Restore adequate oxygen delivery and tissue perfusion.
- Give bicarbonate as above if necessary.
- Consider the need for renal replacement therapy. (If already on RRT using lactate buffered replacement/dialysis fluid, consider changing to bicarbonate buffered solutions. Seek senior advice.)

Levels usually return to normal with adequate resuscitation. Failure to do so implies critically ischaemic or dead tissue.

Type B

This is uncommon and is due to the accumulation of lactate without evidence of tissue hypoxia. It may be precipitated by drugs, ingestion of ethanol or methanol, liver failure and some hereditary disorders.

- Treat underlying condition if possible.
- Give bicarbonate to correct the acidosis. Large amounts may be necessary.
- Consider the need for renal replacement therapy.

(See Methanol/ethylene glycol poisoning, p. 198.)

Hyperchloraemic acidosis

Elevated serum chloride levels, for example following resuscitation with large volumes of normal saline, produce a corresponding decrease in bicarbonate levels (in order to maintain anion balance) and hyperchloraemic acidosis. This usually resolves without the need for treatment as the chloride levels correct.

Renal tubular acidosis (RTA)

Metabolic acidosis arising from renal tubular dysfunction, in which there is excess loss of bicarbonate through the kidneys, with a corresponding increased serum chloride (normal anion gap). Type 1 (distal convoluted tubule) and type 2 (proximal convoluted tubule) are associated with hypokalaemia.

METABOLIC ALKALOSIS

This is relatively uncommon and is due either to the loss of acid (e.g. from vomiting of gastric acid), or from the excessive administration of alkali (e.g. sodium bicarbonate). The metabolism of citrate (an anticoagulant in transfused blood) may also produce metabolic alkalosis. (See Fulminant hepatic failure, p. 145.) Significant potassium loss alone (e.g. diuretic therapy) may also induce metabolic alkalosis.

Metabolic alkalosis typically occurs in young children following protracted vomiting (e.g. secondary to pyloric stenosis), but is also occasionally seen in adults. Massive losses of fluid, H^+, Cl^- and K^+ lead to a marked alkalosis and shock state. Profound hypoventilation occurs as the body retains CO_2 as a compensatory mechanism. The treatment is by volume resuscitation with 0.9% saline and added potassium. The use of acidifying agents like HCl or arginine hydrochloride is controversial and usually unnecessary. Seek advice.

If assisted ventilation is considered, beware of cardiovascular collapse when using sedative agents in profoundly dehydrated patients. Avoid hyperventilation, which will exacerbate alkalosis.

GLUCOSE INTOLERANCE

Both insulin and non-insulin dependent diabetes is common in hospitalized patients. In most cases, oral hypoglycaemic agents should be discontinued while patients are on the ICU. Blood sugar should be monitored closely and if necessary insulin infusion commenced.

Even in those patients who are not normally known to be diabetic, the effects of critical illness, the associated stress response and the effects of drugs such as exogenous catecholamines can lead to glucose intolerance. This may be further compounded by the use of high glucose loads in TPN. Consequently hyperglycaemia is common and frequently requires the use of insulin infusions to control the blood sugar.

- Start an insulin infusion sliding scale.
- Monitor potassium. β agonists and insulin all drive K^+ into cells.

It was previously considered that perfect control was not necessary, and indeed it may be impossible to achieve normal blood glucose levels in very sick patients. In this case avoid peaks and troughs in glucose levels caused by repeated changes in insulin dosage. Recent evidence, however, has demonstrated that the outcome of critically ill patients, particularly those with sepsis, may be improved by tightly controlling blood sugar within the normal range. (See Sepsis, p. 277.)

DIABETIC EMERGENCIES

Most diabetic emergencies are managed on general wards rather than ICU. Occasionally patients are moribund or have associated features, like sepsis, which require intensive care. The source of sepsis may be occult (e.g. renal abscess). Abdominal ultrasound and/or CT scan may be required.

Patients with hyperglycaemia or hyperosmolar coma have large deficits of water, sodium, potassium and other electrolytes. Manage these according to basic principles with rehydration, and the control of blood sugar and other metabolic derangements with insulin. Aim for gradual correction of deficits over 24–48 hours. There is a small but definite risk of cerebral oedema, which may in part be caused by over-rapid correction of electrolyte/fluid abnormalities.

DIABETIC KETOACIDOSIS

Diabetic ketoacidosis (DKA) is the most common diabetic emergency. It may be the presenting episode in a newly diagnosed diabetic, or

may be precipitated in existing diabetic patients by intercurrent illness
(increased insulin requirements) or by reduced insulin dosage.

Pathophysiology

Absolute or relative deficiency of insulin leads to an imbalance
between the hyperglycaemic effects of stress hormones and the
hypoglycaemic effects of insulin. Increased hepatic glycogen
breakdown and gluconeogenesis coupled with reduced cellular uptake
of glucose results in hyperglycaemia. This in turn leads to polyuria,
with loss of water, sodium and potassium. The hormonal changes also
result in lipolysis with release of triglycerides and fatty acids, which
are metabolized by the liver to ketones, which exacerbate the
metabolic acidosis.

Clinical features

- Polyuria.
- Polydipsia initially followed by anorexia, nausea and vomiting.
- Ketones on breath.
- Kussmaul respiration (hyperventilation in response to metabolic
  acidosis).
- Abdominal pain and tenderness.
- Severe dehydration and shock.

Management

> ⚠️ **Severe DKA is a life-threatening condition
> frequently occurring in young people. It requires
> careful management if a satisfactory outcome is to be
> achieved. Seek senior advice.**

- Give oxygen. Despite profound acidosis most patients manage to
  compensate well by hyperventilation and do not require artificial
  ventilation. If there is evidence of hypoxia, hypoventilation or
  compromised airway, intubate and establish ventilation, but beware
  of cardiovascular collapse!
- The need for invasive cardiovascular monitoring will depend on the
  severity of the condition but in general arterial access and CVP
  lines are appropriate.
- If severely shocked, colloid bolus and inotropic support may be
  required.
- Pass NG tube and urinary catheter.

- Take base line investigations. FBC, urea & electrolytes (sodium and potassium), glucose, and blood gases. Monitor glucose, potassium and arterial blood gases hourly.
- Look for precipitating cause. Send blood, urine and sputum for culture. Get ECG and CXR and send blood for cardiac enzymes if indicated. Abdominal pain is a common feature of DKA; consider abdominal ultrasound and send blood for amylase.
- Start i.v. infusion of 0.9% normal saline and aim to correct dehydration over 24 hours. The volume required can be estimated from the % dehydration (Table 8.9). Typically give 1 litre in the first 30 minutes and then 1 litre/hour over the next 2 hours, and assess response. Give the rest over the remaining 22 hours. If serum sodium is > 150 mmol/1 consider 0.45% saline as an alternative.
- In addition to resuscitation volume above, give maintenance fluids to provide the patient's normal daily requirements. Give this as a separate infusion. Initially give as 0.9% normal saline. This can be changed to dextrose solution when the blood sugar is under control (see below).
- Give 10 units of short-acting insulin i.v. Follow this with an insulin infusion 6–10 units/hour as necessary. The aim should be to reduce the blood sugar slowly over a number of hours.
- Acidosis will usually correct as the patient's overall condition improves. If severe metabolic acidosis pH < 7.1 and condition not improving, consider bicarbonate (see above).
- Monitor the potassium carefully. As the acidosis corrects, the potassium will fall. Start potassium infusion 20 mmol/h as required.

TABLE 8.9 Estimation of % dehydration

	Mild (<5%)	Moderate (5–10%)	Severe (>10%)
Dry mucous membranes	+	++	+++
Reduced tissue turgor	+	++	+++
Reduced urine output	+	++	+++
Pulse	Normal	Tachycardia	Tachycardia
Blood pressure	Normal	Normal/mild hypotension	Significant hypotension
Conscious level	Normal	Normal	Reduced

Fluid requirement (ml) is calculated as: % dehydration x weight in kg x 10.
Example: 70 kg patient 10% dehydrated deficit = 7000 ml

- When plasma glucose falls to 12–14 mmol/l change maintenance fluids to dextrose 4%/saline 0.18% to prevent hypoglycaemia. Continue insulin as a sliding scale infusion and potassium replacement as necessary.

HYPEROSMOLAR NON-KETOTIC STATES

Some diabetic patients may have sufficient residual insulin activity to prevent ketogenesis but not to prevent hyperglycaemia. Polyuria develops, which leads to dehydration and hyperosmolar states. Hyperglycaemia, hyperosmolality and hypernatraemia are typical and these eventually lead to reduced conscious level and seizure activity. Severe dehydration may lead to raised haematocrit and increased risk of thromboembolic disease. Hyperosmolar non-ketotic states are more common in the elderly. They may be precipitated by the stress response to surgery or infection, and the effects of some drugs, including diuretics, phenytoin and glucocorticoids.

Management
- Similar to DKA above.
- Give oxygen. Secure airway and institute ventilation if necessary.
- Invasive cardiovascular monitoring. NG tube. Urinary catheter.
- If severely shocked, colloid bolus and inotropic support may be required.
- Use 0.9% saline as rehydration fluid (0.45% saline in severe cases). Correct dehydration more slowly than in DKA, typically over 24–48 hours. Rapid correction may be associated with cerebral oedema.
- Insulin as in DKA but typically give lower doses, e.g. 3 units/hour.
- Monitor potassium and replace as necessary. Potassium requirements are usually less than for DKA because of the absence of significant acidosis.

HYPOGLYCAEMIA

Hypoglycaemia can be defined as a blood glucose less than 3 mmol/l. It occurs most commonly as a consequence of insulin or oral hypoglycaemic therapy in diabetic patients but may also be associated with some disease states. Causes are shown in Table 8.10.

Management
- Consider the cause. Reduce or discontinue hypoglycaemia agents as appropriate.

TABLE 8.10 Causes of hypoglycaemia

Insulin administration
Oral hypoglycaemics
Hepatic failure
Adrenal cortical failure
Hypopituitarism
Excessive insulin secretion (insulinoma)
Hypothermia

- Give 50 ml of 20% dextrose and repeat as necessary. (Boluses of 50% dextrose may be associated with significant disturbances of osmolality and are best avoided.)
- Commence infusion of 10–20% dextrose as necessary to maintain blood sugar. (See Hepatic failure, p. 145.)

ADRENAL DISORDERS

ADRENAL INSUFFICIENCY

Addison's disease

Addison's disease (primary adrenal cortical failure) is rare, but should be considered in 'shocked' patients who do not respond to treatment. The typical clinical features are increased pigmentation, weakness, abdominal pain, vomiting, diarrhoea and hypotension. Biochemical findings include hyponatraemia, hyperkalaemia, hypoglycaemia and hypercalcaemia. Aside from general support measures:

- If possible perform a short Synacthen test. (Synacthen is an ACTH analogue.) Give Synacthen 0.25 mg i.m. Measure plasma cortisol before and 30 minutes after. Cortisol level should rise by 2–3 times the basal level.
- Give steroid replacement therapy. Basal replacement doses hydrocortisone 20 mg a.m., 10 mg p.m. In stress states give larger doses, e.g. 100 mg three times daily.
- Consider mineralocorticoid replacement, e.g. fludrocortisone 50–300 µg daily.

Patients on long-term steroid therapy

Many patients will already be on long-term oral corticosteroids for management of various disease processes. The significance of pituitary adrenal suppression by longer term steroid therapy is still debatable but most authorities recommend increasing doses of steroids during critical illness. Equivalent anti-inflammatory doses are:

hydrocortisone 20 mg = prednisolone 5 mg

TABLE 8.11 Conditions in which steroids may be indicated

Asthma, COAD
Pneumocystis pneumonia
Fibroproliferative ARDS
Spinal cord injury
Airway swelling
Cerebral tumours
Meningitis
Autoimmune conditions

Functional adrenal insufficiency

While primary adrenal failure is rare, it is increasingly recognized that critically ill patients may have inadequate levels of cortisol production for their needs. This can contribute to refractory shock. Low-dose steroid replacement may improve outcomes in these patients and there are currently large clinical trials underway to evaluate this.

- Measure random cortisol or perform short Synacthen test (above).
- Give low (physiological) replacement doses of hydrocortisone, e.g. 50 mg b.d.

High-dose steroid therapy

High-dose steroid therapy has been trialled in shock states but studies tend to show it worsens outcomes. Likewise there is no benefit in traumatic acute brain injury. Steroids have been reported to improve outcomes in some conditions (Table 8.11).

PHAEOCHROMOCYTOMA

This adrenal secretory tumour is a rare cause of hypertension/heart failure in young adults. Patients are most likely to been seen in ICU situation in the postoperative period. Patients are typically volume depleted due to the long-term effects of endogenous catecholamine secretion.

Management

- Patients are commenced on α-blocking agents preoperatively. These prevent the hypertensive effects of catecholamines. Relative hypovolaemia is unmasked and fluid loading is required until postural changes in blood pressure are abolished.
- If tachycardia develops, β blockers may be added only after full α blockade.
- Perioperative dysrhythmias are common and may require magnesium, β blockers or lidocaine (lignocaine).

- Once the tumour is removed, patients may require replacement of catecholamines (e.g. adrenaline (epinephrine) or noradrenaline (norepinephrine) infusion) to maintain blood pressure. These can then be gradually reduced over 2–3 days.

THYROID DYSFUNCTION

The accurate clinical and laboratory assessment of thyroid function is difficult in a normal outpatient/inpatient setting. Laboratory results are tempered by clinical impressions. In the ICU, symptoms of thyroid under/overactivity are mimicked by many other conditions, making diagnosis difficult.

Most patients will have reasonably controlled thyroid disease and present with other conditions. For patients on oral thyroid replacement therapy, the effects of oral thyroxine last 7–10 days so that it is reasonable to wait for gut function to return rather than moving to parenteral preparations, which are usually only available as T3. If the oral route cannot be used, change to T3. (20 µg T3 is approximately equivalent to 100 µg T4.)

Sick euthyroid syndrome
Thyroid function tests are often abnormal in the critically ill patient. Most sick patients will have results consistent with the so-called sick euthyroid syndrome. The pattern is low T3, low T4, and inappropriately low/normal TSH. This pattern persists until recovery occurs. The current consensus is that it does not reflect clinical hypothyroidism so thyroid replacement therapy is not usually warranted.

Hypothyroidism
Hypothyroidism should be considered in the elderly patient presenting with hypothermia, coma or other non-specific illness. Treat with replacement therapy in the form of oral/parenteral T3, or thyroxine.

Hyperthyroidism
Uncontrolled hyperthyroidism is rarely seen. Management includes antithyroid drugs, e.g. carbimazole, β blockers and general supportive measures. (See Management of the postoperative patient, p. 292.)

TEMPERATURE CONTROL

Disturbances in temperature regulation are common in ICU. Often the cause will be multifactorial, combining abnormalities of central temperature control and environmental causes.

Measurement of temperature

Core temperature measurements may be obtained from the tympanic membrane, nasopharynx, oesophagus, bladder and rectum or from an indwelling pulmonary artery catheter. These reflect the patient's true temperature more reliably than axillary, oral or peripheral temperature measurements. The core–peripheral temperature gradient gives an indication of the cardiovascular condition of the patient and the degree of peripheral vasoconstriction.

Hyperthermia

Hyperthermia is important as a marker for infection or other disease processes. Causes of hyperthermia are shown in Table 8.12.

The exact mechanisms that produce hyperthermia are not known but in many cases it can be viewed as a physiological response to critical illness rather than a significant part of the disease process. There is debate, therefore, about the need to treat a mildly raised temperature < 39°C except in brain-injured patients, where increased temperature is associated with a worse outcome. Measures such as regular paracetamol and tepid sponging for low-grade pyrexia may, however, improve patient comfort.

Urgent treatment is required if core temperature exceeds 39°C. Prolonged core temperatures of > 42°C are associated with cardiovascular collapse, rigors, seizures, coagulopathy, multiple organ failure and death.

- Ensure adequate hydration (increased insensible losses).
- Give regular rectal paracetamol. (Ibuprofen is also effective if there are no contraindications to NSAIDs.)
- Institute passive cooling: wet drapes, ice packs, fans, and gastric, peritoneal or bladder lavage with cold fluids.
- Consider sedation, intubation, ventilation and muscle relaxation to reduce metabolic rate.

TABLE 8.12 Causes of hyperthermia

Infection
Systemic inflammatory response syndrome
Adverse reactions to drugs or blood products
Sympathomimetics
Brain injury
Seizures
Malignant hyperthermia*
Heatstroke*
Neuroleptic malignant syndrome*

*Rare.

- If severe hyperpyrexia, consider an extracorporeal circuit to actively cool the patient. Seek senior advice.

Dantrolene is a muscle relaxant that works distal to the neuromuscular junction. It has an established role in malignant hyperpyrexia, and appears to work after ecstasy ingestion but not other conditions; however, it has limited side effects in ventilated patients so should be tried when other measures fail:

- dantrolene 1 mg/kg bolus repeated every 10 minutes up to 10 mg/kg.

(See Malignant hyperpyrexia, p. 187.)

Hypothermia

Hypothermia is defined as a core temperature below 35°C. To avoid missing hypothermia you should always have a high index of suspicion and use a low-reading rectal thermometer in at-risk patients. Common causes are given in Table 8.13.

Hypothermia is associated with a number of adverse effects. These include: arrhythmias, myocardial depression, vasoconstriction, coagulopathy, increased risk of wound infections and wound dehiscence, prolonged drug clearance, altered acid–base balance and prolonged ICU stay.

In the surgical context prevention is better than cure. The use of fluid warming devices, warming blankets and heated humidifiers perioperatively all help to reduce the risk. In severely hypothermic patients:

- Exclude other injuries, drug ingestions, myxoedema, pressure necrosis of limbs, rhabdomyolysis and renal failure (measure CK). Treat appropriately. (See Trauma, p. 258.)
- Most patients respond to passive slow rewarming with a slow rise in core temperature of about 1°C per hour. Utilize a warm environment, hot-air warming blankets, and warm i.v. fluids for volume replacement.

TABLE 8.13 Common causes of hypothermia

Environmental (particularly elderly)
Exposure (e.g. trauma victims)
Cold water immersion
Drug overdosage
Prolonged surgery with massive fluid/blood losses
Deliberate cooling during cardiac bypass
Brain protection (neurosurgery)

- For severely hypothermic patients, core temperature below 32°C, consider more active warming measures such as peritoneal lavage with warm fluids, instillation of warm fluids into the bladder, or partial (femoral–femoral) bypass with a heat exchanger.
- Patients may develop dysrhythmias on rewarming, usually at around 31°C, and may need repeated cardioversion. It may, however, be difficult to restore sinus rhythm while the patient remains hypothermic. Occasionally under these circumstances profoundly hypothermic patients will be warmed utilizing cardiopulmonary bypass.

In profoundly hypothermic patients it may be difficult to determine whether the patient has actually died. This follows cases of patients making a full recovery from prolonged circulatory arrest and deep hypothermia after cold water immersion. Therefore, resuscitation efforts should be continued until the patient approaches normothermia. Remember the maxim, 'you can't be dead until you're warm and dead'. Seek senior advice.

CHAPTER 9

OVERDOSE, POISONING AND DRUG ABUSE

OVERDOSE AND POISONING

The problems associated with overdose and poisoning (deliberate or accidental) are responsible for a significant portion of the acute medical workload in hospitals. While most overdoses and poisonings are not serious and can be managed on medical wards, some patients will require admission to intensive care. This may be the result of the specific nature and effects of the substance involved, respiratory or cardiovascular complications or occasionally due to the onset of multiorgan failure. Common complications associated with overdose and poisonings are shown in Table 9.1.

This chapter provides general advice only. There are a number of poisons information centres in the UK which are manned 24 hours a day to provide advice on the management of specific types of overdose, poisonings and difficult cases. You should call these for additional advice. Telephone numbers are given in Table 9.2 or are available in the *British National Formulary* (*BNF*).

INVESTIGATIONS

In the unconscious patient it is still essential to exclude other treatable causes of loss of consciousness (e.g. head injury, subarachnoid haemorrhage, hypoglycaemia, meningitis), even if patients have left

TABLE 9.1 Potential complications of overdose	
General	Hypothermia/hyperthermia Pressure sores Crush syndrome/rhabdomyolysis Dehydration
Respiratory	Respiratory depression Aspiration Hypostatic pneumonia
Cardiovascular	Dehydration Hypotension/hypertension Dysrhythmias
CNS	Coma Hypoxic brain damage Seizures Confusional states/aggression
Kidney	ATN secondary to hypotension/dehydration Effects of rhabdomyolysis Direct toxic effects
Liver	Acute liver failure

TABLE 9.2 Poisons information centres (24-hour service)	
Centre	Telephone
Belfast	0123 224 0503
Birmingham	0121 507 5588
	0121 507 5589
Cardiff	0422 270 9901
Dublin	Dublin 837 9964
	Dublin 837 9966
Edinburgh	0131 536 2300
London	02071 635 9191
	02071 995 5095
Newcastle	0191 232 0300

suicide notes or are known to have taken overdoses previously. If in doubt, organize a CT scan of the brain and consider lumbar puncture and other investigations as appropriate.

The response to a challenge of naloxone or flumazenil may occasionally be helpful in identifying opioid and benzodiazepine overdose, respectively (see below).

Aspirin (salicylates) and paracetamol assays are performed in all cases. Alcohol levels can be measured in most centres and may be useful to distinguish intoxication from brain injury. The majority of other assays are unavailable at short notice and are sent to regional centres. Aside from paracetamol it is rare for assays to alter clinical management. Ask the laboratory to save serum in uncertain cases for later analysis and send urine for toxicology screen.

MEASURES TO REDUCE ABSORPTION AND INCREASE ELIMINATION

Gastric lavage

Gastric lavage may be performed in an attempt to remove tablet debris from the stomach. This is now performed much less frequently than before. Unless life-threatening quantities of drug have been ingested, gastric lavage is usually only performed when the patient presents within 1 hour of ingestion. Those drugs for which delayed gastric lavage (beyond 1 hour) may be of benefit are shown in Table 9.3. Contraindications to gastric lavage include ingestion of corrosive and refusal of consent. Gastric lavage is not usually performed in children.

Gastric lavage is dangerous in the patient who cannot protect the airway or cough adequately, because of the risk of pulmonary

TABLE 9.3 Possible indications for delayed gastric lavage

Aspirin
Dextropropoxyphene
Digoxin
Ethylene glycol
Methanol
Paracetamol
Phenobarbitone
Theophylline
Tricyclic antidepressants

aspiration. Assess the patient's general status, ability to cough, gag and maintain the airway. If there is any doubt about the patient's safety, seek help from an experienced anaesthetist prior to gastric lavage.

- If the patient is very obtunded it may be possible to intubate the trachea without any anaesthetic drugs.
- If not, perform a rapid sequence induction with preoxygenation, cricoid pressure, an intravenous induction agent and suxamethonium.
- Pass the gastric tube under direct vision and then perform lavage. Consider extubation in head-down, left lateral position.
- If the patient is not fit to extubate and/or send to the ward, keep the patient intubated and send to ICU. If respiratory effort is feeble it is better to support ventilation for a few hours than leave the patient to breathe spontaneously with poor tidal volumes. This helps to maintain lung expansion, minimizes the tendency to atelectasis and provides ongoing airway protection.

Activated charcoal

Activated charcoal (oral or via a nasogastric tube) has two effects. It binds free drug within the lumen of the bowel and also actively absorbs drug from the circulation. It is absorption of ingested drug from the bloodstream that is the rationale for repeated use of activated charcoal in some cases. Indications for multiple dose activated charcoal are shown in Table 9.4.

A typical dose regimen is as shown:

- 50 g 4-hourly oral/NG.
- If nausea/vomiting are a problem, can be given as 12.5 g hourly.

Forced alkaline diuresis

Traditionally this has been used to increase the renal clearance of soluble, acidic drugs, particularly salicylates and barbiturates. It is

---

TABLE 9.4 Overdoses for which multiple dose activated charcoal may be useful

Barbiturates
Carbamazepine
Clormethiazole
Digoxin
Phenobarbital
Phenytoin
Quinine
Salicylates
Theophylline

---

now controversial due to problems with fluid overload and acid–base disturbance. Seek senior advice. A typical regimen is as follows:

- Use CVP to guide volume loading with normal saline/colloid.
- Give 0.25–0.5 g/kg mannitol 20% to promote diuresis > 200 ml/h.
- Give sodium bicarbonate (8.4%) 1 mmol/kg/h to achieve urinary pH > 7.5.

The role of loop diuretics to increase urine flow in this setting is controversial. Some authors recommend them if the response to mannitol is inadequate. They can, however, produce acidification in the renal tubule and promote precipitation of acid-soluble drugs and compounds such as myoglobin. (See Rhabdomyolysis, p. 267.)

Haemodialysis and haemoperfusion

Haemodialysis and haemoperfusion over activated charcoal are useful for some life-threatening overdoses. These are listed in Table 9.5. Seek specialist advice.

SPECIFIC ANTIDOTES

Some overdoses/poisonings have specific antagonists or antidotes which reduce the toxic effects and mortality. These should generally only be used for potentially life-threatening situations when the nature

---

TABLE 9.5 Role of haemodialysis and haemoperfusion in overdose

Haemodialysis	Haemoperfusion
Ethylene glycol	Barbiturates
Lithium	Theophylline
Methanol	
Salicylates	

TABLE 9.6 Antagonists and antidotes to common overdoses and poisonings

Benzodiazepines	Flumazenil
Copper	Penicillamine
Digoxin	Digoxin-specific antibodies
Ethylene glycol	Ethanol, fomepizole
Iron	Desferrioxamine
Lead	Sodium calcium edetate
Methanol	Ethanol, fomepizole
Opioids	Naloxone
Organophosphates	Atropine, pralidoxime
Paracetamol	N-acetylcysteine
Warfarin	Vitamin K, fresh frozen plasma, prothrombin complex

of the overdose or poison is known. Available antagonists/antidotes are shown in Table 9.6.

INTENSIVE CARE MANAGEMENT

In the majority of overdoses/poisonings there is no specific antidote and care is supportive with the aim of preventing or reversing the onset of complications. Indications for admission to intensive care are shown in Table 9.7.

● Secure the airway and support respiration with IPPV if necessary. Sedative drugs can usually be avoided and the patient extubated once the conscious level improves.
● Monitor ECG and blood pressure. A number of common overdoses are associated with cardiac rhythm disturbances. Avoid central

TABLE 9.7 Indications for admission to intensive care following overdose/poisoning

Need for tracheal intubation/assisted ventilation
Reduced conscious level (GCS <8) or seizures
Need for invasive monitoring/cardiovascular support
Dysrhythmias
2nd or 3rd degree heart block
QRS >0.12 s or QTc >420 ms
Need for renal replacement therapy or other organ support

venous access and cardioactive drugs, which may trigger a dysrhythmia. Use fluid in the first instance to manage hypotension.

- Some patients may be severely dehydrated and require significant fluid therapy.
- Monitor body temperature. Hypothermia is common following prolonged unconsciousness and after overdose with some centrally acting drugs. Hyperthermia may follow some overdoses.
- Single short convulsions do not require treatment. Prolonged seizure activity should be treated with diazepam initially followed by phenytoin. (See Brain injury: Seizures, p. 245.)
- Beware of pressure-related injuries from prolonged immobilization. Pressure sores, tissue necrosis and compartment syndromes are common following prolonged unconsciousness. Rhabdomyolysis and myoglobinuria can precipitate renal failure.
- (See Compartment syndrome, and Rhabdomyolysis, p. 267.)

The typical course is for a patient to require 12–24 hours of supportive care before discharge to the ward. All patients who are admitted following deliberate overdose should be seen by a liaison psychiatrist. This is not usually appropriate while the patient is on the ICU but should be considered on return to the general ward when the patient is in a fit state to be seen. Many patients will, however, self-discharge against medical advice.

PARACETAMOL

Paracetamol poisoning is important, as it is the leading cause of hyperacute liver failure in the UK. Relatively low doses of drug may produce fatal liver failure in susceptible patients, such as those with pre-existing liver disease. In addition, the ingestion of other drugs (e.g. anticonvulsants) may increase the toxicity of paracetamol.

The need for treatment is determined by plasma paracetamol concentrations. For those who fall above treatment thresholds, intravenous N-acetylcysteine is an effective antidote if started within 0–12 hours of ingestion. For treatment thresholds and dosage schedules, see BNF or contact poisons advice centre.

For those patients who present more than 12 hours after significant ingestion of paracetamol, N-acetylcysteine may still be of some benefit. Advice should be obtained from the poisons centre and/or the local liver unit.

Patients who develop liver failure will often have few visible signs of problems for about 48 hours, and then will rapidly deteriorate. Established liver failure follows, with hepatic encephalopathy, increasing prothrombin time or INR, falling platelet count, jaundice

TABLE 9.8 Indications for liver transplant following paracetamol overdose

Either:	Or (all of the following):
pH <7.3 after fluid resuscitation	Creatinine >300 μmol/l PT >100 s Grade III or IV encephalopathy

and renal dysfunction. These patients must be urgently transferred to a regional liver unit for further management, including possible acute transplantation. Do not wait until patients are moribund with multisystem failure. Indications for immediate transplantation (within 24 hours) are shown in Table 9.8. (See Fulminant hepatic failure, p. 145.)

SALICYLATES (ASPIRIN)

The features of salicylate poisoning are hyperventilation, tinnitus, deafness, vasodilatation and sweating. Hyperventilation and sweating result in dehydration. Coma is uncommon but indicates severe overdose. Gastric emptying is delayed and gastric lavage is useful to retrieve tablet debris up to 4 hours after ingestion. For the same reason, plasma levels may be misleading if taken within 6 hours.

Blood gases and electrolytes should be monitored. Treatment is by rehydration. If plasma levels are above 500 mg/l (3.6 mmol/l) in adults or 350 mg/l (2.5 mmol/l) in children then forced alkaline diuresis with 1.26% sodium bicarbonate should be used to improve urinary excretion.

In very severe cases, levels above 700 mg/l (5.1 mmol/l) in adults, haemodialysis is the treatment of choice.

SEDATIVE AND ANALGESIC DRUGS

Overdoses with benzodiazepines or opioids usually require no specific therapy other than assisted ventilation and supportive care until conscious level and respiratory drive improve. Flumazenil and naloxone may be used to confirm the diagnosis in benzodiazepine and opioid overdose but may precipitate seizures, arrhythmias and hypertension. Do not use these antidotes in an attempt to avoid the need for tracheal intubation, assisted ventilation and ICU admission. They are short acting. If the infusion stops or the cannula is pulled out then the patient's conscious level will rapidly deteriorate, with potentially fatal consequences. Worse still, the patient may awaken

---

TABLE 9.9 Effects of tricyclic overdose

Confusion
Seizures
Coma
Dehydration
Tachycardia/dysrhythmias
Widely dilated pupils
Hyperthermia

---

and self-discharge to collapse once again outside the hospital.
(See Intravenous drug abusers, p. 202.)

TRICYCLIC ANTIDEPRESSANTS

The tricyclic antidepressant drugs have sympathomimetic effects,
which cause the main problems following overdose. Potential effects
are shown in Table 9.9.

Treatment is supportive, with resuscitation, control of seizures and
rehydration. Tachydysrhythmias are common and may require
repeated cardioversion. Antidysrhythmic drugs are best avoided. Once
hypoxia, acidosis and dehydration are corrected, cardiac rhythm will
usually settle to sinus tachycardia. Correction of acidosis with
bicarbonate is thought to help by reducing unbound free drug (pK_a
effect). Typically, even after severe problems (e.g. dysrhythmia
requiring repeated cardioversion), patients are stable enough to be
extubated after 12–24 hours. Often the patient will require no sedation
for the first few hours. Short-acting sedatives/anticonvulsants (e.g.
propofol infusion) may be required for a few hours until the patient is
stable.

CARBON MONOXIDE AND CYANIDE POISONING

Carbon monoxide

Carbon monoxide is a product of incomplete combustion. Carbon
monoxide poisoning may be seen in combination with burns, from
smoke inhalation, from inadequately ventilated heating appliances
(unexplained collapse) and following suicide attempts. Apparently
unburned victims from house fires may present with carbon monoxide
poisoning.

Carbon monoxide bonds avidly to haemoglobin, resulting in
carboxyhaemoglobin, which does not carry oxygen. Severe cases may
suffer anoxic brain damage. The clinical features are shown in
Table 9.10.

TABLE 9.10 Clinical features of carbon monoxide poisoning

Cherry red colour (unreliable)
Headaches
Nausea and vomiting
Arrhythmias
Seizures
Coma, confusional states

Diagnosis is made by measurement of carboxyhaemoglobin levels. Many blood gas analysers now include a co-oximeter that can measure carboxyhaemoglobin (normal levels < 5%).

Treatment is supportive. If the inspired oxygen concentration is increased to 100% the half-life of carboxyhaemoglobin is 1 hour; therefore, blood levels will quickly return to normal. Tissue levels and levels bound to other globulins may remain elevated for longer, however. There is some evidence that, in patients who have had recorded carboxyhaemoglobin levels > 20% and/or neurological symptoms at any time, the incidence of late neurological sequelae may be reduced by hyperbaric oxygen therapy. The benefits of hyperbaric oxygen need to be weighed against the risks of transfer to a specialist centre. Seek senior advice.

> ⚠️ **Not all hyperbaric facilities are based on hospital sites: check before agreeing to go, as you may find yourself in the middle of nowhere!**

Cyanide poisoning

Cyanide is a product of combustion of some foam materials. Cyanide poisoning may therefore occur in patients with smoke inhalation/carbon monoxide poisoning. The clinical features, which may be rapid in onset, include anxiety, vomiting, headache and reduced consciousness. Metabolic acidosis is common.

In mild cases, treatment is supportive only. Give 100% oxygen. In severe cases with loss of consciousness, sodium thiosulphate is used to convert cyanide to thiocyanate:

● sodium thiosulphate 150 mg/kg i.v. followed by 30–60 mg/kg/h infusion.

METHANOL AND ETHYLENE GLYCOL

These agents may be ingested accidentally or deliberately.

Methanol

Methanol is available as a solvent, in methylated spirits and is present in de-icers and antifreeze solutions. Clinical features are progressive confusion, ataxia and visual disturbance. Metabolism to formaldehyde and then formic acid leads to severe metabolic acidosis 12–18 hours after ingestion. The direct toxic effects of formate on the optic nerve can result in blindness. Plasma osmolality and anion gap are increased.

Ethylene glycol

Ethylene glycol is a sweet-tasting liquid used alone or in combination with other alcohols in antifreeze. Clinical features are similar to alcohol intoxication, followed by nausea, vomiting and haematemesis. Focal neurological signs, seizures and a gradual deterioration in conscious level then occur. While most of the ethylene glycol is excreted unchanged in the urine, metabolites include oxalic acid. This accumulates, resulting in severe metabolic acidosis, increased anion gap and hypocalcaemia. Oxalate excretion in the urine leads to the formation of oxalate crystals and renal failure.

Treatment of both methanol and ethylene glycol poisoning is based on supportive care, correction of the underlying acidosis and inhibition of the metabolism with ethanol or fomepizole. Ethanol competes with methanol/ethylene glycol as a substrate in the metabolic pathway, while fomepizole is an expensive, newly introduced, alcohol dehydrogenase inhibitor. In both cases, the metabolism of methanol/ethylene glycol and the production of toxic metabolites is reduced. Haemodialysis to remove methanol/ethylene glycol should be considered in severe cases. Seek specialist advice.

ALCOHOL

Alcohol (ethanol) is the most commonly used and abused non-prescription drug. Acute alcohol intoxication is a factor in many patients admitted to intensive care, particularly following trauma.

Acute alcohol intoxication

Acute alcohol intoxication produces coma, hypothermia, hypoglycaemia and in severe cases metabolic acidosis. Other causes of coma (e.g. extradural haemorrhage) must be excluded. Other injuries should also be excluded. Treatment is supportive. Consider:

intubation to protect the airway and ventilation as necessary
gastric lavage to reduce alcohol absorption (alcohol delays gastric emptying)
dextrose infusion to correct hypoglycaemia.

TABLE 9.11 Problems associated with chronic alcohol abuse

Decreased resistance to infection
Severe chest infections are common (TB should be excluded)
Self-neglect/poor nutrition (give B group vitamins)
Alcoholic cardiomyopathy (atrial fibrillation common)
Cirrhosis/liver failure
Gastrointestinal bleeding
Pancreatitis
Acute confusional states
Autonomic neuropathy
Acute withdrawal states/delirium tremens/seizures

Chronic alcohol abuse

Chronic alcohol abuse is associated with a number of medical problems (Table 9.11).

Management of alcohol withdrawal on ICU

Acute withdrawal from alcohol may result in insomnia, tremor, agitation and seizures. Delirium tremens, in which patients develop visual hallucinations, is the most serious withdrawal phenomenon. This may occur 1–5 days after withdrawal and may be life threatening. Treatment comprises adequate sedation together with supportive care:

● Standard ICU sedative regimens (particularly benzodiazepine based) are usually adequate. Chlormethiazole given by infusion is difficult to titrate, provides a substantial fluid load, and is probably best avoided. (See Sedation and analgesia, p. 30.)
● All chronic alcoholics should receive vitamin B supplements parenterally.

RECREATIONAL DRUG ABUSE

The abuse of drugs by all routes is widespread. Some of the commonly abused 'recreational' drugs and their effects are shown in Table 9.12.

ECSTASY

This and other amphetamine derivatives are increasingly seen as a cause of severe toxic reactions. Patients present with signs of sympathetic overactivity similar to tricyclic overdose. These reactions appear more idiosyncratic rather than dose related. It is not clear what triggers the response in a particular individual who may have been exposed to the

TABLE 9.12 Common drugs of abuse and their effects

Substance	Effects
Cannabinoids	Euphoria, slowed reaction time, impaired balance/co-ordination/anxiety and panic attacks
Gammahydroxybutyrate (GHB)	Reduced pain and anxiety, feeling of well-being, drowsiness, nausea/vomiting, loss of consciousness, depressed reflexes, seizures, coma and death
Ketamine	Tachycardia, hypertension, impaired motor function; high doses, respiratory depression
Phencyclidine (PCP)	Panic, aggression, violence, bradycardia, hypotension
Lysergic acid diethylamide (LSD)	Altered states of perception, hyperthermia, tachycardia, hypertension
Opioids	Pain relief, euphoria, drowsiness, unconsciousness, respiratory depression/arrest
Amphetamines	Stimulant effects, increased metabolic rate, weight loss, tachycardia, hypertension, dysrhythmias, hallucinations, paranoia, aggression
Methylenedioxymetamphetamine (MDMA) (group includes ecstasy)	Similar to amphetamines. Mild hallucinogenic effects, impaired memory and learning, hyperthermia, idiosyncratic hyperacute liver failure
Cocaine	Stimulant effects similar to amphetamines Tachycardia, hypertension, seizures, CVA, coma
Anabolic steroids	No intoxication effects. Occasional acute psychosis; long-term risks associated with steroids
Solvents	Stimulants. Headaches, loss of coordination, nausea/vomiting, dysrhythmias, sudden death

drug before without problems. Hyperpyrexia, rhabdomyolysis, acute renal failure and multiple organ failure are seen in severe cases. Treatment is supportive with cooling measures and dantrolene may be helpful. Seek advice from poisons centre. (See Hyperthermia, p. 185.)

INTRAVENOUS DRUG ABUSERS

Intravenous opioid drug abusers frequently require admission to intensive care. This may be due to the effects of the drugs, trauma occurring while under the influence of drugs, or as a result of medical problems from the side effects of drug abuse. Common medical problems in this group are shown in Table 9.13.

It may not be evident on admission that patients are drug abusers, and neither the patient nor the friends or relatives may disclose this. There is a significant risk of such patients being carriers of hepatitis, HIV and other infectious diseases. This highlights the need to use universal precautions at all times when carrying out procedures. (See Universal precautions, p. 310.)

Managing opioid withdrawal

Patients may develop symptoms and signs of drug withdrawal.

- Avoid precipitating withdrawal phenomena by unnecessary discontinuation of drugs.
- Where acute withdrawal is likely, symptoms can generally be controlled by the use of standard ICU sedative regimens.

Occasionally a reformed intravenous opioid drug abuser may want to avoid opioid-based sedative or analgesic regimens to prevent relapse in habit. Consider the use of peripheral, regional or central axial blockade and other analgesic drugs for pain relief.

TABLE 9.13 Problems associated with intravenous drug abuse

Self-neglect/malnutrition
HIV/hepatitis
Thrombosed veins (difficult venous access)
Abscess formation
Endocarditis
Pneumonia
Sepsis
Pancreatitis

HAEMATOLOGICAL PROBLEMS

INTRODUCTION

Haematological problems are common in the ICU. Most are related to blood loss, the need for large volume blood transfusions and the development of coagulation disorders. Bone marrow failure and immune suppression are also problems.

BLOOD PRODUCTS

In the UK, blood is donated by unpaid volunteers, who undergo general health screening. Whole blood is collected into a citrate-based anticoagulant solution (chelating calcium to prevent clotting) and then further separated to yield platelets, fresh frozen plasma (FFP), cryoprecipitate, etc.

All donations are serologically tested for HIV-1 and HIV-2, hepatitis B and C, syphilis and cytomegalovirus (CMV). CMV-free blood components are used for immunosuppressed patients and those under 1 year of age.

Recently there has been concern about the risk of transmission of new variant Creutzfeldt–Jakob disease (vCJD). It is likely that in the near future screening of donors for vCJD will become available. Currently in the UK all blood products have white cells removed (leucodepletion) as a precaution against vCJD transmission. (White cell count $< 5 \times 10^6$.) Continuing concerns regarding the potential for carriage and transmission of vCJD by the UK blood donor pool has resulted in some plasma products being sourced from outside the UK, principally from the USA.

Red cell replacement

Whole blood was traditionally used for the replacement of blood loss. There are no functional platelets, and factors V and VIII are at 20% of normal levels. Other clotting factors and albumin are present at near-normal levels. Whole blood is rarely available now but may be useful where simultaneous replacement of clotting factors is also required.

More usually, red cell concentrates are used. The plasma component of whole blood is removed (removes clotting factors and albumin) and the red cells are suspended in an additive solution to maintain their integrity during storage. The two commonly used additive solutions are:

● citrate, phosphate, dextrose and adenosine (CPDA)
● sodium chloride, adenosine, glucose and mannitol (SAGM).

The blood products available for red cell replacement are shown in Table 10.1.

TABLE 10.1 Red cell products

	Whole blood	Packed red cells	Red cells Additive solution
Volume (ml)	470 ± 50	270 ± 50	550 ± 70
Source	Single donor	Single donor	Single donor
Haematocrit (%)	35–45	55–75	50–70
Leucocytes	Depleted	Depleted	Depleted
Additives	CPDA	CPDA	SAGM

Plasma replacement

Fresh frozen plasma (FFP) may be from a single donor or recovered from pooled donors. The volume of units provided therefore varies from 150 to 500 ml. FFP contains both labile and stable factors, including albumin, gamma globulin, fibrinogen, factor VIII. Usually 2–4 units are given when required for coagulopathy (prolonged PT). Should be ABO compatible.

Recent concerns regarding virus transmission have resulted in treated plasma products becoming available. There are currently two: methylene blue treated and solvent detergent treated. These are compared in Table 10.2.

Recent reports of procoagulant complications with solvent detergent-treated FFP are thought to be due to relative protein S deficiency. This, together with the problems associated with pooled donors (1000 donors per batch), is likely to limit its widespread use.

Cryoprecipitate

Cryoprecipitate is provided as 1–6 single donations per pack, suspended in 10–20 ml plasma. It contains fibrinogen and factor VIII. It is used to correct coagulopathy where fibrinogen levels are depleted. six units generally raise fibrinogen levels by approximately 1 g/l.

TABLE 10.2 Fresh frozen plasma products

	Standard FFP	Methylene blue-treated FFP	Solvent detergent-treated FFP
Source	Single donor	Single donor	Pooled donor
Volume (ml)	180–300	235–305	200
Coagulation factor content	Variable	Variable	Constant

Platelets

Platelets may be single donor (apheretic), or pooled (5–6 donors). six units raise platelet count by approximately $10–20 \times 10^9/l$. Platelets should ideally, but not necessarily, be ABO compatible.

ADMINISTRATION OF BLOOD PRODUCTS

The complications of blood transfusion are discussed below. The biggest cause of major ABO incompatibility reactions is human error. Most commonly these result from failure to follow approved procedures. The following notes are applicable to all blood products. When ordering and administering blood products you should:

- Ensure that you follow local procedures and guidelines.
- Ensure blood samples are carefully labelled and that the accompanying request forms are accurately completed.
- Ensure that blood products are appropriately prescribed.

Before administering any blood product it is essential that the product is matched to the intended recipient. The product label always states the nature of the contents (e.g. whole blood, FFP), its storage temperature, expiry date and time, ABO and RhD grouping, donation or batch number and details of the patient against whom it has been cross-matched.

Check recipient identity

- If possible, ask the patient to confirm his or her identity and that the details on the identification band are correct.
- Ensure that the patient's name and identification number on the wristband match those on the intended blood product and also those on the form sent with the product.
- Ensure that the ABO blood group, rhesus blood group and unit identification number are all correct.

Administration

Blood should ideally be given through a large cannula (minimum 18 gauge) to avoid haemolysis. Standard giving sets with 170 µm filters are adequate. Microaggregate filters are not necessary and must never be used when giving platelets. If blood is given through the same set as other fluids, calcium-containing solutions should be avoided. Consider the use of a blood warmer.

Blood products are stored under carefully controlled conditions in the blood bank. Once removed from controlled storage they must be used within set time frames, as indicated on the pack, generally as shown in Table 10.3.

TABLE 10.3 Storage and use of blood products				
	Red cells	*FFP*	*Cryo-ppt.*	*Platelets*
Stored	2–6°C	–30°C	–30°C	22°C on agitators
Shelf life	35 days	1 year	1 year	5 days
Once removed from storage complete transfusion within:	5 hours	4 hours	4 hours	2 hours

INDICATIONS FOR BLOOD TRANSFUSION

Critically ill patients may require transfusion for a host of reasons, including the anaemia of chronic disease, the effects of repeated blood sampling, haemorrhage and bone marrow suppression. There is much debate over the haemoglobin at which transfusion should be instituted. When considering tissue perfusion, haematocrit (%) is an important consideration. This is approximately given by Hb × 3. Prime considerations are:

- Oxygen carriage and delivery. The oxygen content of blood is given by Hb × SaO_2, × 1.34. Raising haemoglobin is an effective way of improving oxygen content and delivery. (See Oxygen delivery and oxygen consumption, p. 57.)
- Myocardial function. Myocardial ischaemia and diastolic dysfunction occur in the stressed heart where haematocrit falls below 0.18. In the presence of coronary artery disease the threshold is 0.24 or higher.
- Rheology. In vitro and probably in vivo, blood viscosity is reduced as Hb falls below 8 g/dl, and rises above 10 g/dl. This may have implications for perfusion of the microcirculation, particularly in critical illness and following vascular surgery. Recent evidence suggests that both very low and very high haematocrits are associated with impaired tissue perfusion.
- Immunology. There is some evidence that transfusion induces a degree of immune suppression, particularly massive transfusion. This is important following any major surgery, and especially so where surgery has been performed for malignant disease.

Recent work suggests that restrictive transfusion strategies produce the best outcome in critically ill patients and that the optimal level in most cases is Hb of 8–10 g/dl. (See Oxygen delivery and oxygen consumption, p. 57.)

MANAGEMENT OF MAJOR HAEMORRHAGE

Key considerations are:

- Where possible control the source of the bleeding, for example by direct pressure.
- Ensure adequate vascular access: at least 2×14-gauge peripheral lines or single large-bore cannulae such as 8.5-Fr pulmonary artery catheter introducer sheath. This need not necessarily be inserted into a central vein; a peripheral vein may well be easier to cannulate in an emergency, and just as adequate.
- Continue background or maintenance fluids to provide free water, glucose and electrolyte requirements.
- Commence initial volume replacement with a crystalloid or simple colloid such as modified gelatin (e.g. Gelofusine or Haemaccel).
- Continue with packed cells to maintain a haematocrit of 0.26–0.32.
- After 5 units of blood, consider changing to whole blood if available and/or giving FFP to minimize the effects of dilutional coagulopathy.
- Recheck FBC, U&Es, clotting and thromboelastogram (TEG) if available.
- Ensure adequate treatment of coagulopathy. In particular, keep the ionized calcium above 0.85 mmol/l. Maintain normothermia with active warming of the patient if necessary.
- After 10 units, recheck clotting. Consider cryoprecipitate, platelets and further FFP. (See Coagulopathy below.)

RISKS AND COMPLICATIONS OF BLOOD TRANSFUSION

The greatest risk in major haemorrhage is the non-availability of appropriate blood when needed. Other complications include fluid overload, hypothermia, hypocalcaemia, acidosis and dilutional coagulopathy; ARDS and multiple organ failure are also considered to be complications of massive transfusion. Bacterial contamination of blood occurs rarely and is usually fatal. (Platelet transfusion carries the greatest risk of bacterial contamination because of the need to store at room temperature.)

Recent figures suggest the risk of HIV transmission is around 1 per million donor exposures. Risk of hepatitis C, E and seronegative hepatitides is probably higher.

Acute transfusion reactions are relatively uncommon. They include:

- haemolytic (75% due to ABO incompatibility)
- anaphylactic (antibodies to IgA in IgA-deficient patients)

- febrile white cell reactions (antibodies to leucocyte antigens)
- transfusion-related acute lung injury (antibodies to leucocyte antigens)
- urticaria (1–2% of transfusions).

Severe haemolytic reactions due to ABO incompatibility are rare and usually result from the wrong blood being given. Febrile reactions are less common with leucocyte-depleted blood but may still occur.

Transfusion-related acute lung injury (TRALI)

This is a relatively rare cause of acute lung injury following transfusion of blood (or any plasma-containing blood product). Antibodies in the transfused blood product cause activation of the recipient's white cells. leading to an inflammatory response. The onset is typically within a few hours of transfusion and the clinical features are that of non-cardiogenic pulmonary oedema which may lead on to the development of ARDS. If TRALI is suspected, the blood transfusion service should be advised so that donors can be screened for white cell antibodies. Treatment is supportive, as for any acute lung injury/ARDS.

Management of acute transfusion reactions

Minor febrile/urticarial transfusion reactions may settle following hydrocortisone 100 mg and chlorphenamine 10 mg and it may be possible to cautiously continue the transfusion. Major transfusion reactions require transfusions to be discontinued. Blood bags should be returned to the transfusion laboratory, together with a sample of the patient's blood, for further evaluation. Seek the advice of the haematology department.

THE JEHOVAH'S WITNESS

Jehovah's Witnesses have strong religious views regarding the acceptability of blood and blood products. While it is appropriate to clarify the individual's wishes in each case, their religious views and wishes should be respected. Failure to do so may constitute an assault. The Jehovah's Witness patient in intensive care may of course be unable to express their wishes and to give or withhold informed consent. In the case of adults, advice may be sought from the Jehovah's Witness hospital liaison committee. (See Ethical and legal issues, p. 28, and Death and different cultural views, p. 372.)

The following notes are broad guidelines only, and may not be completely acceptable to all individuals:

- Blood (red cells, whole blood), FFP, platelets may not be given to Jehovah's Witnesses under any circumstances.
- Predonated blood is generally not acceptable.
- Albumin and cryoprecipitate is accepted by some (but not all) Jehovah's Witnesses.
- Factor concentrates: concentrates of specific factors (for example, factor XI, IX and VII) are generally accepted. Seek the advice of your hospital liaison committee.
- Extracorporeal circuits. The majority of Jehovah's Witnesses accept blood that has been passed through an extracorporeal circuit. This allows for cardiac surgery (cardiopulmonary bypass) and for renal dialysis. Intraoperative cell salvage is generally acceptable provided the blood is reinfused immediately, at the time of surgery, and not several hours later on the ICU.
- An individual contract/management plan may be prepared before treatment to clarify treatment options, where the patient is well enough to do this.

Management

- Patients with an anticipated major haemorrhage should receive supplementation of iron and other haematinics preoperatively.
- Erythropoietin (EPO) may be prescribed to stimulate red cell production. Side effects are uncommon but include hypertension, headache and stroke. Not all patients respond.
- Minimize any potential blood loss during surgery.
- Consider aggressive hypervolaemic haemodilution to reduce the haematocrit of any blood lost during surgery. Haemoglobin concentrations as low as 4 g/dl may be tolerated.
- Consider techniques such as elective hypotension to further reduce blood loss.
- Avoid unnecessary blood sampling.

Jehovah's Witnesses who develop a coagulation disorder pose a special problem. The use of antifibrinolytic drugs (such as aprotinin) is generally acceptable and should be considered early on. If there is evidence of endogenous heparins (as evidenced by a prolonged APTT), consider giving protamine (see below). Management of the coagulopathy will depend on which clotting factors (if any) the individual is prepared to accept.

NORMAL HAEMOSTATIC MECHANISMS

In order to understand coagulation disorders you need to understand the mechanisms by which haemostasis is normally achieved. Following injury to a blood vessel, a series of events is initiated:

- Vasoconstriction reduces blood flow in the damaged vessel.
- Platelets adhere to exposed collagen in the vessel wall and release a number of mediators, including ADP. More platelets are attracted, which rapidly form a temporary haemostatic platelet plug.
- The coagulation cascade is triggered, which results in the conversion of fibrinogen to fibrin. Cross-linking of fibrin molecules results in conversion of the primary platelet plug to an organized clot.

The normal coagulation cascade is shown in Figure 10.1.

There are also mechanisms within the body to prevent clot formation in healthy vessels and to dissolve established clots. These fibrinolytic pathways are shown in Figure 10.2.

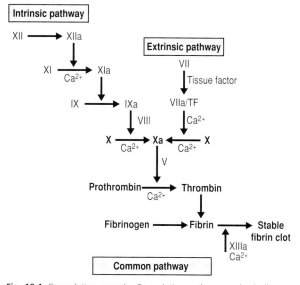

Fig. 10.1 Coagulation cascade. Coagulation pathway as classically described, showing intrinsic, extrinsic and common (shown in bold type) pathways. In vivo binding of factor VII to exposed tissue factor may be the primary initiating mechanism.

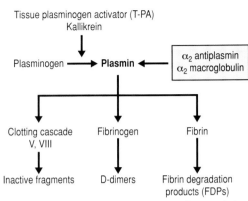

Fig. 10.2 Fibrinolytic pathways. Plasmin is a non-specific proteolytic enzyme which degrades factors V and VIII, fibrinogen and fibrin and also inhibits both the coagulation cascade and the conversion of fibrinogen to fibrin. α_2-Antiplasmin and α_2-macroglobulin inhibit plasmin.

Under normal circumstances, therefore, there is a constant balance maintained between procoagulant mechanisms and anticoagulant mechanisms. If this balance becomes disturbed, bleeding or thrombosis may result.

COAGULOPATHY

The term coagulopathy is generally used in respect of those disorders of haemostasis that produce a bleeding tendency. (Prothrombotic disorders are considered below.)

Causes
Coagulopathy may result from failure of clot formation, failure of clot stabilization or excessive activation of fibrinolysis. Often more than one process is involved and the early involvement of a haematologist is advisable. Typical causes of coagulopathy are shown in Table 10.4.

TABLE 10.4 Typical causes of coagulopathy

Congenital	Acquired
Haemophilia A (factor VIII)	Acquired/functional factor deficiency
Haemophilia B (factor IX)	Dilutional coagulopathy
von Willebrand's disease	Thrombocytopenia
Other factor deficiencies	Sepsis
	Hypothermia
	Hepatic dysfunction
	Vitamin K deficiency/malabsorption
	Renal failure
	Drugs

In intensive care, acquired causes of coagulopathy are much more common than congenital causes:

- Sepsis may produce bone marrow suppression (thrombocytopenia) and triggers inflammatory cascades, which activate both coagulation and fibrinolysis.
- Reduced gastrointestinal absorption of fat-soluble vitamins (A, D, E, K) leads to reduced manufacture of vitamin K-dependent factors (II, VII, IX, X, protein C).
- Reduced hepatic reticuloendothelial function permits increased circulating levels of endogenous heparinoids (potentiating antithrombin III and inhibiting factors V, X).
- In renal failure uraemia impairs platelet function.
- Massive transfusion and vigorous fluid loading can result in 'dilutional coagulopathy'.
- Citrate anticoagulants may persist in the circulation for some time, chelating calcium and potentially reducing cardiac contractility. Additionally, some synthetic colloids may impair platelet function (dextrans, hetastarch in particular).
- Activated fibrinolysis leads to consumptive coagulopathy.

Investigations

Basic investigations include platelet count, prothrombin time (PT), activated partial thromboplastin time (APTT), thrombin time (TT), fibrinogen, and fibrinogen breakdown products (FDPs/D dimers). If a specific factor deficiency is considered likely then individual factor assay may be appropriate. Seek haematological advice. Normal ranges are shown in Table 10.5.

Thromboelastography (TEG)

While the in vitro tests listed above can be useful diagnostically to determine the likely cause of a coagulopathy, they test individual

TABLE 10.5 Coagulation tests

	Normal range	Significance
Platelets	150–450 × 10⁹/l	See thrombocytopenia below
PT	12–14 s (INR = PT/control; normal INR = 1)	Extrinsic and common pathway Marker of hepatic dysfunction/vitamin K deficiency Used to monitor warfarin therapy
APTT	30–40 s	Intrinsic and common pathway Used to monitor heparin therapy
TT	10–12 s	Tests conversion of fibrinogen to fibrin Prolonged by heparin/FDPs/D dimers
Fibrinogen	>2 g/l	Reduced in dilutional coagulopathy, liver failure, fibrinolysis (DIC)
D dimers	<0.2 g/l	Increased in presence of fibrinolysis (DIC)

aspects of the coagulation process rather than reflect the overall process of clot formation. The thromboelastograph can be used to provide a dynamic test of coagulation and fibrinolysis. This can be used to help identify the need for FFP, cryoprecipitate, platelets or antifibrinolytic therapy. Typical TEG traces are shown in Figure 10.3.

Management

In general, coagulation abnormalities should only be treated if there is active bleeding or when the potential consequences of bleeding may be disastrous.

- Ensure that the patient is adequately resuscitated. Oxygen, i.v. access and adequate volume or blood replacement. Correct hypothermia.
- The commonest cause of bleeding in the postoperative patient is failure of surgical haemostasis. Surgical causes of bleeding must be excluded. Seek surgical advice.
- Other underlying causes of bleeding and coagulopathy should be addressed. Do not forget inherited causes, e.g. the haemophilias, although these are rare.
- Perform basic investigations of haemostasis, as above. The diagnosis should be clear from a combination of history, examination and the results of these tests.

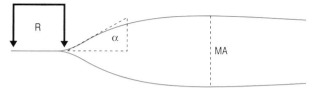

R = Lead time reflects time for activation of clotting cascade
α = Angle reflects rate of clot formation
MA = Maximum amplitude reflects clot strength

Fig. 10.3 Thromboelastogram (TEG) from a normal healthy (non-pregnant) adult.

- If the APTT is prolonged, suspect heparinoids or other inhibitors. The laboratory may be able to repeat the APTT in the presence of a heparinase to help distinguish this.
- If heparin is present, but you do not know how much has been given, give protamine 50 mg then repeat the APTT. If you know the dose of heparin given, then protamine 1 mg per 100 units of heparin given should provide adequate reversal.
- If the PT and APTT are prolonged in the absence of exogenous anticoagulants give FFP, which should be administered in 2–4 unit aliquots until PT falls below 20 seconds. Additionally, if fibrinogen depletion is marked, consider cryoprecipitate 6 units initially.
- If the platelet count is $< 80 \times 10^9/l$, give 4 units platelets, although more may be required if the count is lower or where the response to transfusion is limited, for example in DIC. In renal failure, platelet function may be abnormal even if platelet numbers are adequate. Desmopressin (DDAVP) 20 µg as a one-off bolus releases peripheral stores of factor VIII:RAg. This increases platelet 'stickiness' and thereby improves function.
- Check the ionized calcium: if below 0.85 mmol/l this may contribute to coagulopathy. Give 2.5–10 mmol calcium chloride slowly. (See Hypocalcaemia, p. 172.)
- In malabsorption states and liver disease, vitamin K 10 mg can partially correct clotting disorders.

Recombinant factor VIIa

There has been a great deal of interest recently in the role of activated factor VII in the management of coagulopathy and uncontrolled bleeding. Activated factor VII binds to exposed tissue thromboplastin on damaged endothelial surfaces and activates the common pathway leading to localized fibrin production and clot formation. There is increasing evidence that VIIa is effective in reducing bleeding when other measures have failed.

THROMBOCYTOPENIA

Thrombocytopenia is a common finding in critically ill patients. Causes of thrombocytopenia are shown in Table 10.6.

The normal range is $150–400 \times 10^9/l$. A normal platelet count does not, however, necessarily imply normal platelet function. Furthermore, patients with hypersplenism may exhibit reduced platelet count, but with relatively well-preserved platelet function. Consider a functional test (for example, TEG).

In general terms, significant bleeding secondary to thrombocytopenia is uncommon unless the count is very low. Therefore do not give platelets unless the platelet count is less than $20 \times 10^9/l$. Below this level there is a risk of spontaneous intracranial haemorrhage.

> ⚠ In some situations thrombocytopenia is associated with increased microvascular thrombotic processes. Under these circumstances, giving platelets may increase the risk of clinically significant thrombosis. Do not give platelets unless there is active bleeding, or the platelet count is less than $20 \times 10^9/l$ and the risk of thrombosis has been excluded (see below).

TABLE 10.6 Causes of thrombocytopenia

Reduced production	Increased destruction/sequestration
Bone marrow failure	Infection
Drugs, toxins	Disseminated intravascular coagulation (DIC)
Viral infections	Mechanical destruction (balloon pump/CVVHD)
	Heparin-induced thrombocytopenia (HIT)
	Immune thrombocytopenia purpura (ITP)
	Thrombotic thrombocytopenia purpura (TTP)
	Sequestration (e.g. splenomegaly)

In the presence of active bleeding it is reasonable to give platelets in order to keep the platelet count above $80-100 \times 10^9$/l. In all cases attention should be paid to addressing the underlying cause of the thrombocytopenia.

Heparin-induced thrombocytopenia (HIT)

Heparin-induced thrombocytopenia is an immune-mediated phenomenon which occurs in up to 5% of patients receiving unfractionated heparin and up to 1% patients receiving low molecular weight heparin. Antibodies to the heparin–platelet complex lead to platelet activation and release of procoagulant mediators, resulting in both thrombocytopenia and thrombosis.

Consider the diagnosis if the platelet count falls by more than 50% after exposure to heparin (usually occurs within 4 days), or if thrombosis occurs despite heparinization and/or thrombocytopenia. (Includes deep vein thrombosis, pulmonary embolism, arterial thrombosis, thrombotic stroke, myocardial infarction.)

- Send blood for HIT screen. (Discuss with haematology service.)
- Discontinue all heparin, including unfractionated and low molecular weight heparin.
- Avoid platelet transfusion; bleeding is uncommon.
- Consider anticoagulation with an alternative agent (e.g. lepirudin) (see BNF).

TTP-HUS

In thrombotic thrombocytopenic purpura (TTP), thrombocytopenia is associated with thrombosis (typically cerebral vascular). In the haemolytic uraemia syndrome (HUS), thrombocytopenia is associated with renal dysfunction. In adults, TTP and HUS are considered to be different presentations of the same underlying pathological processes.

Congenital or acquired deficiencies of plasma protease result in an abnormally large von Willebrand molecule, which activates platelets and causes (microvascular) thrombosis. Depending on the site of this, the clinical picture may be predominantly of renal failure (HUS) or neurological deficit (TTP).

Management is supportive. Do not give platelets. This is associated with increased intravascular thrombosis and a worse outcome. Fresh frozen plasma and/or plasma exchange is of benefit.

DISSEMINATED INTRAVASCULAR COAGULATION

Disseminated intravascular coagulation (DIC) is a complex process arising as a result of generalized activation of the inflammatory cascade. It involves activation of clotting within the microvasculature, with consequent tissue damage. There is a consumptive coagulopathy, where normal clotting fails to take place because of depletion of circulating factors. The process is generally accompanied by activated fibrinolysis, with clot instability. The breakdown products of fibrinogen (D-dimer) and fibrin (FDPs) are in themselves anticoagulant, thus adding an extra level of complexity.

The management of DIC presents a challenge. Early involvement of a haematologist is essential. The principles of management revolve around treating the underlying cause and adequate replacement therapy with FFP, cryoprecipitate and platelets. Some units employ antithrombin III in the treatment of DIC; seek advice. There is no role for heparinization.

THROMBOTIC DISORDERS

A number of factors predispose to thrombosis in ICU patients (Table 10.7).

Despite these predisposing factors, clinically significant venous thrombosis is relatively unusual in ICU patients. The incidence of venous thrombosis detected by ultrasound or venography is, however, higher, and therefore all patients should receive prophylactic anticoagulation. (See DVT prophylaxis, p. 54.)

Some patients are particularly at risk of thrombosis. These include the pregnant, the obese and those with carcinomatosis, myeloproliferative disease, systemic lupus erythematosus (lupus anticoagulant) and conditions such as TTP-HUS.

(See TTP-HUS, p. 217.)

There are also some familial disorders that lead to increased risk of thrombosis, including protein C deficiency, protein S deficiency, and antithrombin III deficiency. If these are suspected, advice on investigation and management should be sought from a haematologist.

TABLE 10.7 Factors which predispose to venous thrombosis	
Vascular endothelial damage	Trauma/surgery Central venous catheters
Altered blood flow	Immobilization Central venous catheters Shock states Effects of vasoactive drugs
Altered platelet activity and coagulation state	Underlying disease processes

Management

Arterial thrombosis may require embolectomy and/or surgical exploration. Seek advice.

All patients with venous thrombosis will require anticoagulation initially with heparin:

- Start an infusion of (unfractionated) heparin 20–40 000 units/ 24 hours.
- Monitor APTT and aim to keep 2–3 × normal.
- Alternatively start therapeutic dose low molecular weight heparin.

Underlying pathology may require specific treatment, e.g. plasma exchange for TTP. (See Pulmonary embolism, p. 89.)

THE IMMUNOCOMPROMISED PATIENT

Immunocompromised patients are increasingly common in the ICU. Immune deficiency may be inherited (e.g. severe combined immune deficiency, SCID) or acquired. Most commonly, it is seen in patients with depressed bone marrow function, either as a result of an underlying disease process or as a result of treatment. Typical causes of immune suppression in ICU patients are shown in Table 10.8.

Most immunocompromised patients referred to ICU will have had their underlying diagnosis established. Referral is usually precipitated either by respiratory failure, febrile neutropenia or sepsis syndrome. Often the time course is short, and the precipitating events may be unclear.

Management

The principles of management are largely the same as for the immune competent patient. Resuscitation and stabilization are the initial priorities.

Cross-infection with potentially resistant organisms is a major problem in intensive care, and can be disastrous in the immunocompromised patient. Patients should be barrier nursed in side

---

TABLE 10.8 Causes of immune compromise

Cancer chemotherapy
Haematological malignancy
Bone marrow infiltration from any malignant process
Immune suppressant drugs
HIV infection/AIDS
Chronic illness
Aplastic anaemia (idiosyncratic drug reactions)

rooms, ideally with positive pressure airflow, to protect them from further risk of infection. (See Infection control, p. 17.)

Some patients (e.g. those with haematological malignancy or on long-term chemotherapy) will have dedicated long-term venous access (Hickman, Portacath, etc.). These can be used for resuscitation purposes; however, avoid accessing them for general purpose use, to reduce the risk of infection in the catheter. If possible, site a separate central venous catheter for general use.

Base line blood count including WBC count may give some clue as to the nature and severity of the immune compromise. Temperature and C-reactive protein are useful markers of infection in neutropenic patients. Once the patient is adequately resuscitated, sources of sepsis must be sought. Clinical history and examination may give a strong clue to this. (See Pneumonia in immunocompromised patients, p. 119.)

- Obvious sites of sepsis should be cultured and any abscesses drained.
- Send blood cultures. Remember previous multiple broad-spectrum antibiotic therapy may mask growth, predispose to resistant organisms, and further increase the risk of fungal infection.
- Suitable culture media should be used (e.g. bottles with antibiotic-binding resins). Alert the microbiology laboratory to this, so they can culture for unusual organisms.
- Protozoal infection: discuss media with laboratory.
- Urine culture.
- Stool culture.
- Serology for viral infection, CMV, herpes, EBV, etc., should be sent.
- *Candida* and *Aspergillus* antigen tests.

Antibiotic therapy is guided by culture results. In the first instance broad-spectrum antibiotics are usually required. Typical regimens are:

- Piperacillin/tazobactam and tobramycin as first-line agents.
- Imipenem and vancomycin as second-line agents.
- Fluconazole may be added as prophylaxis against fungi.
- Co-trimoxazole may be added as prophylaxis against PCP.

Haematological malignancy

Patients with haematological malignancy are a tremendous diagnostic and therapeutic challenge in the ICU. A frequent problem is neutropenia following marrow ablation and transplantation. Recovery of WBC count may occasionally be hastened by administration of granulocyte-colony stimulating factor (GCSF).

The combination of haematological malignancy and requirement for IPPV carries a high mortality, especially where the pneumonia remains undiagnosed. (Patients with proven PCP often survive.) When renal failure is added to this constellation, the mortality is even higher. As a result of this, some people are reluctant to admit patients with haematological malignancy to intensive care. Blanket policies of this sort are not appropriate and each patient should be considered on their merits. Those who are referred early and those who can be managed on non-invasive forms of respiratory support can do well.

AIDS

Patients with AIDS who develop PCP pneumonia can have a reasonably good prognosis provided multiple organ failure does not supervene. CD4 count is a valuable guide to the likelihood of response to therapy.

Organ transplant recipients

Solid organ transplant recipients no longer require special protection in the ICU during their perioperative course. The same is probably true should they develop opportunistic infections, surgical sepsis or pneumonia, as their immunosuppression is less severe than those with true immunocompromised states. If necessary, immune suppression can be withdrawn and patients managed on steroids during an acute illness. Maintenance immunosuppressive therapy can then be reintroduced following recovery or in the event of rejection. (Seek advice from the transplant team.)

BRAIN INJURY, NEUROLOGICAL AND NEUROMUSCULAR PROBLEMS

PATTERNS OF BRAIN INJURY

The brain is extremely susceptible to injury from many causes. Typical causes and patterns of injury are shown in Table 11.1.

Primary versus secondary insult

The brain, unlike many other organs of the body, is highly sensitive to the effects of trauma, hypoxia and hypoperfusion and has very limited powers of regeneration. Following the initial insult, there is often little that can be done to reverse the effects of the primary injury and management is largely centred on preventing secondary damage.

KEY CONCEPTS IN BRAIN INJURY

The principles of management of brain injury are to:

- limit where possible the effect of the primary injury
- identify and treat conditions amenable to surgical intervention
- identify and treat conditions amenable to medical treatment
- prevent secondary injury.

The prevention of secondary injury is mainly dependent on the maintenance of adequate brain perfusion and oxygenation. There are a number of key concepts relating to brain perfusion that underpin the management of the brain-injured patient.

TABLE 11.1 Causes and patterns of brain injury

Traumatic brain injury	Diffuse swelling
	Diffuse axonal injury
	Acute intracerebral haematoma
	Acute subdural haematoma
	Acute extradural haematoma
	Contusions (bruising)
Spontaneous haemorrhage	Subarachnoid haemorrhage
	Intracerebral haemorrhage
Cerebrovascular disease (embolic)	Stroke
Infection	Meningitis, encephalitis, abscess
Hypoxic/ischaemic injury	Watershed infarction
	Global infarction
	Hypoxic encephalopathy
Metabolic	Encephalopathy

Cerebral perfusion pressure

Cerebral perfusion pressure is effectively the driving pressure across the cerebral circulation. It is calculated as shown:

cerebral perfusion pressure = mean arterial BP − intracranial pressure
    (CPP)   (MABP)   (1CP)

Cerebral blood flow and autoregulation

Cerebral blood flow is normally maintained at a constant level over a wide range of cerebral perfusion pressures, a phenomenon known as autoregulation (Fig. 11.1). In normotensive patients autoregulation occurs at cerebral perfusion pressures between 50 and 150 mmHg. In previously hypertensive patients the curve is shifted to the right and autoregulation occurs at a higher blood pressure.

Following significant brain injury, autoregulation is often deranged and cerebral blood flow becomes directly related to cerebral perfusion pressure (CPP). Inadequate CPP results in inadequate cerebral blood flow. The maintenance of adequate CPP is therefore crucial. Typical target values for CPP are shown in Table 11.2.

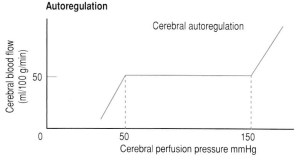

Fig. 11.1 Cerebral autoregulation.

TABLE 11.2 Typical target values for cerebral perfusion pressure (mmHg)

Adults	>60
3–12 years	>50
<3 years	>40

Intracranial compliance

The skull can be conceptually considered as a rigid box containing the brain, CSF and blood. If the volume of one of these components is increased, e.g. by cerebral oedema, then the volume of the others must be reduced. Initially, CSF is displaced into the spinal canal, followed by a reduction in blood volume. Eventually, when no further compensation is possible, the ICP will rise rapidly, impairing cerebral perfusion. If the pressure is not relieved, the brain itself may become displaced, leading to so-called herniation or coning. (See Raised ICP, p. 234.)

In the presence of reduced intracranial compliance, the cerebral blood volume is an important determinant of ICP. If the cerebral circulation becomes vasodilated, cerebral blood volume increases and ICP may increase. Hypercarbia and hypoxia both cause cerebral vasodilatation and should be avoided. Brain-injured patients are normally ventilated to a $PaCO_2$ of 4–4.5 kPa. Hyperventilation to lower levels of $PaCO_2$ may cause significant cerebral vasoconstriction and ischaemia and should be avoided.

IMMEDIATE MANAGEMENT OF TRAUMATIC BRAIN INJURY

The following notes relate to the management of traumatic brain injury. The principles apply equally well to the management of other forms of brain injury.

Depending on local policy, you may be required to assist with the management of head-injured patients in the resuscitation room. You should be familiar with Advanced Trauma Life Support (ATLS) protocols as well as the acute management of the brain-injured patient. (See Trauma, p. 258.)

Primary survey

The initial assessment includes:

- **A** Airway (with cervical spine control)
- **B** Breathing
- **C** Circulation
- **D** Disability (neurological assessment).

Airway (with cervical spine control)

The maintenance of a clear airway and the prevention of hypoxia and hypercarbia are paramount. Indications for intubation and ventilation are shown in Table 11.3.

TABLE 11.3 Indications for intubation and ventilation of brain-injured patient

GCS less than 8 or falling rapidly
Hypoxia
Hypercarbia (PaCO$_2$ >6.5 kPa), or hypocarbia (PaCO$_2$ <3.0 kPa)
Inability to protect the airway
Significant facial injuries and bleeding (swelling may make intubation very difficult if delayed)
Seizures
Major injuries elsewhere, especially chest injuries
Evidence of shock state (tachycardia, low BP, acidosis, etc.)
A restless patient who requires transfer to CT
Any patient requiring interhospital transfer

Intubation/ventilation of brain-injured patients

(See Practical procedures: Intubation of the trachea, p. 337.)

Laryngoscopy and intubation is a major stimulus and may produce a significant rise in blood pressure and ICP. Adequate anaesthesia and muscle relaxation must be provided to blunt this response in order to avoid potential worsening of the brain injury.

- Establish intravenous access. Give volume loading, particularly if haemorrhage and other injuries. Blood, colloid or crystalloid as appropriate. If possible, establish direct arterial pressure monitoring.
- Check all intubation equipment, breathing circuits, ventilators and suction, etc. Monitor should be available for BP, ECG, SaO$_2$ and ETCO$_2$.
- Note the baseline GCS score and pupil size for reference. The pupils are the principal clinical monitor of the brain following anaesthesia and paralysis.
- Assume there is cervical spine injury until proved otherwise. A second person should provide inline immobilization of the neck. (It is useful to use a gum elastic bougie to facilitate intubation without extending the neck.)
- Assume a full stomach and perform rapid sequence induction. Preoxygenate with 100% oxygen. Get an assistant to apply cricoid pressure. Use etomidate if the BP is low, otherwise thiopentone or propofol are suitable induction agents. Suxamethonium is used to provide muscle relaxation. Fentanyl 100 µg increments help to block the hypertensive response to intubation.
- Intubate the patient and pass an orogastric tube to drain stomach contents. Change to nasogastric only after excluding a base of skull fracture. (There is a risk of a nasogastric tube entering the cranium in the presence of a base of skull fracture.)

> ⚠ **Suxamethonium causes a transient rise in intracranial pressure. However, in the context of the multiply-injured patient with brain injury, securing the airway rapidly and safely is essential. Suxamethonium is usually the drug of choice.**

- Ventilate to normocapnia or moderate hypocapnia ($PaCO_2$ 4–4.5 kPa). Monitor the SaO_2 and $ETCO_2$. Measure direct arterial blood pressure and blood gases as soon as possible. Maintain adequate cerebral perfusion pressure with fluids and vasoactive drugs (see below).
- Maintain sedation with benzodiazepines, propofol and opioids. During the early resuscitation and stabilization phase continue paralysis with an atracurium or vecuronium infusion.

Circulation

It is vital to maintain adequate cerebral perfusion pressure in brain-injured patients:

- Give colloid or normal saline to restore circulating volume.
- Give blood if Hb low and correct any coagulopathy.
- Consider inotropes/vasopressors early to maintain blood pressure.

(See intensive care management below.)

Neurological assessment

Neurological assessment requires serial documentation of conscious level, pupillary signs, lateralizing limb signs (suggesting space-occupying lesion), tone and posture. Fundal haemorrhages, papilloedema, CSF rhinorrhoea/ottorrhoea and bleeding from the ear should be documented.

Conscious level

The simplest assessment of conscious level utilizes a four-point scale:

- **A** <u>A</u>lert
- **V** Responds to <u>V</u>ocal stimuli
- **P** Responds to <u>P</u>ainful stimuli
- **U** <u>U</u>nresponsive.

This score is insufficiently sensitive for neurological assessment of the brain-injured patient and is only used during A&E resuscitation to give a broad indication of conscious level. Response to pain only represents a significant decrease in conscious level equivalent to a GCS score of 8 or less.

The Glasgow Coma Scale

The Glasgow Coma Scale (GCS), shown in Table 11.4, is a more comprehensive neurological assessment, which is universally used to describe conscious level and has prognostic value. It should be performed as soon as the patient is stabilized. It is repeated throughout the resuscitation process to identify any deterioration in the patient's condition, which may suggest expanding intracerebral haematoma or brain swelling.

Pupils

Pupillary size and response to light (direct and consensual) should be documented regularly. Any asymmetry greater than 1 mm or a change in response to light must be assumed to be due to the effects of an intracranial space-occupying lesion causing compression of the ipsilateral third nerve. Urgent CT scan of the brain is required. Bilateral, dilated and unresponsive pupils in the context of a brain injury and in the absence of mydriatic agents is a grave sign.

Reassessment and secondary survey

Having completed a primary survey and stabilized the patient, the patient should be reassessed before moving on to secondary survey.

TABLE 11.4 Glasgow Coma Scale (GCS)		
Eye opening	Spontaneously	4
	To speech	3
	To pain	2
	None	1
Best verbal response	Orientated	5
	Confused	4
	Inappropriate words	3
	Incomprehensible sounds	2
	None	1
Best motor response (arms)	Obeys commands	6
	Localization to pain	5
	Normal flexion to pain	4
	Spastic flexion to pain	3
	Extension to pain	2
	None	1

Maximum score 15. Minimum score 3. (A modified GCS is used for children under 5 years.)

PRIORITIZING MANAGEMENT IN TRAUMATIC BRAIN INJURY

Traumatic brain injury may be an isolated injury but this should never be assumed. The care of the brain injury must proceed alongside the continuing re-evaluation and resuscitation of the other injuries according to ATLS protocols. In particular, remember:

● cervical spine injury (immobilize, X-ray lateral cervical spine)
● cardiothoracic trauma (CXR, ± drains)
● abdominal injuries (diagnostic peritoneal lavage, US, CT, laparotomy)
● pelvic fractures (X-ray, early external fixation)
● splint limb injuries (assess neurovascular integrity).

Which injury should take priority?
In the multiply-injured patient with a brain injury priorities must be decided. The following are important considerations:

● Many brain injuries do not require neurosurgical intervention.
● Any brain injury will be worsened by significant hypoxia or hypotension.

Any injury that compromises the airway, breathing or circulation takes priority. In particular, life-threatening bleeding from the chest or abdomen requires immediate surgical intervention and should not be delayed by CT head scan or neurosurgery. In exceptional cases blind burr holes or craniotomy can be performed simultaneously with other surgery, and a CT scan performed before transfer to ICU.

> ⚠ **Priorities will depend upon the nature of the injuries and the local expertise and facilities. The death of a patient from bleeding during a CT scan is a disaster. Only transfer patients when you are sure they are stable. Seek senior help.**

INDICATIONS FOR CT SCAN

Plain skull X-rays may be useful in the initial evaluation of patients with mild head injuries, as the presence of a skull fracture greatly increases the risk of subsequent intracerebral haematoma. In the severely head-injured patient, however, CT scans are required to:

● Confirm diagnosis, e.g. head injury, subarachnoid bleed, tumour.

TABLE 11.5 Indications for CT scan
All patients with moderate/severe injury
GCS <13
Neurological signs
Inability to assess conscious level, e.g. due to anaesthetic drugs
Any patient with mild injury plus any of the following
High-risk mechanism of injury
GCS <15 for more than 2 hours
Skull fracture
Vomiting
Age >60 years

- Identify space-occupying lesions.
- Direct surgery to the site of injury.

CT scans should not be delayed by taking plain X-rays. Indications for CT scan are shown in Table 11.5.

Following CT scan and depending upon other injuries, options for the further management of the patient can be decided. These may include:

- CT findings, normal or minimal changes only: stop sedative drugs; allow the patient to wake up and reassess neurological state.
- CT findings diffuse, or non-operable injury (e.g. diffusely swollen brain): admit patient to ICU for further management, including monitoring of ICP.
- CT findings, space-occupying lesion with a mass effect: requires urgent neurosurgical referral and craniotomy.

> ⚠ **CT scans require skilled interpretation. Do not make clinical decisions until senior experienced staff have reviewed them. Minor subarachnoid bleeding, mild cerebral oedema, early cerebral infarction, pituitary lesions and brainstem lesions are all easily missed.**

INDICATIONS FOR REFERRAL TO NEUROSURGICAL CENTRE

The facilities available for dealing with the head-injured patient vary. Hospitals may have no CT scanner, a CT scanner but no neurosurgery, or all facilities. The decision to transfer a patient will, therefore, be influenced not only by the patient's condition but also by the local

---

TABLE 11.6 Indications for referral to neurosurgical centre

CT scan indicated but not available locally
CT scan findings intracranial haemorrhage/midline shift
CT scan findings suggest diffuse axonal injury
CT scan findings suggest raised intracranial pressure/hydrocephalus
GCS <15 for more than 24 hours
GCS deteriorates 2 points or more
GCS <9
Basal skull fracture or compound skull fracture

---

availability of resources. Indications for referral are summarized in Table 11.6.

Identification of a vacant ICU bed space should not delay transfer of patients who require urgent CT scan or craniotomy for evacuation of a haematoma. Most neurosurgical units try to adopt an open admission policy, taking all seriously injured patients who have not had a CT scan and those who require operative intervention, regardless of the availability of ICU beds. Once appropriate interventions have been performed, any delay in finding an intensive care bed will not place the patient at further significant risk. Patients can if necessary be transferred back to the referring hospital once the need for further intervention has been excluded.

Indications for less urgent transfer include:

- isolated depressed skull fractures with no neurological deficit
- isolated CSF leaks
- patients with lesser injuries who fail to improve neurologically over time.

ICU MANAGEMENT OF TRAUMATIC BRAIN INJURY

The ICU management of brain injury is based upon maintenance of adequate cerebral perfusion and oxygenation in order to prevent secondary brain damage. Limitation of cerebral oedema and surges in ICP may help to prevent brain herniation. Other general principles of management are the same as for any patient:

- Maintain adequate sedation and analgesia. Paralysis is usually required in the early phases of treatment but should only be continued in unstable patients, those with raised intracranial pressure or when required to enable satisfactory ventilation.
- Ventilate to maintain adequate oxygenation and normocapnia, or mild hypocapnia ($PaCO_2$ 4–4.5 kPa).

- Nurse the patient 15–20° head-up to ensure adequate venous drainage. Avoid tight tapes to secure endotracheal tube, which may occlude jugular veins.
- Establish monitoring. Arterial blood pressure and CVP, urinary catheter, NG tube. Avoid internal jugular routes of cannulation except for jugular bulb cannula. Insertion difficulties may impair cerebral venous drainage and also risk carotid injury. The femoral route has some advantages, avoiding the need for head-down tilt during insertion.
- Give maintenance fluids as 0.9% saline (plus K^+) initially. In the past maintenance fluids were restricted, but maintenance of cerebral perfusion is now considered paramount. Hyponatraemia and hyperglycaemia worsen outcome and should be avoided.
- Prevent rises in temperature. Give regular paracetamol and use surface cooling (tepid sponges, fans, cool air blankets). There may be some benefit from mild hypothermia 35.5–36.5°C.
- Stress ulcer prophylaxis. Commence enteral feeding as soon as practicable. Otherwise NG sucralfate should be prescribed.
- There is no indication for routine use of prophylactic anticonvulsants.

There is little evidence that specific regimens designed to produce cerebral protection, e.g. the use of barbiturates, or steroids, alter the outcome of brain-injured patients. Hypothermia is known to produce cerebral protection in some settings, e.g. near drowning, but studies of induced hypothermia in brain injury have failed to show any benefit beyond that afforded by maintaining normothermia (i.e. preventing pyrexia).

Maintenance of cerebral perfusion pressure (CPP)

Maintain the CPP above 60 mmHg in adult patients. It may need to be even higher in elderly hypertensive patients (normal autoregulation curve shifted to the right). Similarly CPP may need to be higher if there is evidence of cerebral vasospasm (e.g. in subarachnoid haemorrhage) or inadequate perfusion (e.g. low SjO_2). (See Jugular venous bulb oxygen saturation, p. 239.)

- Titrate fluid therapy according to CVP. If there is no improvement or if the patient is haemodynamically unstable, consider the use of a pulmonary artery catheter.
- After adequate fluid resuscitation if CPP remains low, use vasopressors, e.g. noradrenaline (norepinephrine) or phenylephrine to increase mean arterial pressure and improve CPP.
- Adrenaline (epinephrine) may be used if invasive monitoring indicates that the primary reason for a low MAP is low CO.

- The use of progressively higher doses of vasopressors in order to maintain a target CPP may produce subendocardial myocardial ischaemia and other end-organ damage. If increasingly higher doses are required, seek advice.

Control of intracranial pressure (ICP)

The measurement of ICP is now routine practice in the management of head injury. It is also being increasingly applied to other conditions where there is likely to be raised ICP, for example in the management of metabolic conditions such as liver failure. It is used to give an indication of increasing cerebral oedema, the re-accumulation of haematoma, and to calculate CPP.

Normal ICP is less than 10 mmHg and a sustained pressure higher than 20 mmHg is associated with worse outcomes. If ICP is greater than 20–30 mmHg then intervention may be necessary, particularly in the first 24–48 hours following injury. Table 11.7 provides a checklist of causes of a raised ICP. Exclude measurement errors and avoidable rises before starting treatment.

If all factors are optimized, exclude development or re-accumulation of haematoma. Consider repeat CT scan and seek neurosurgical opinion. Correct any coagulation defects. Other measures to control ICP include the following.

1st line

- Mannitol 0.5 g/kg over 20 minutes, and/or furosemide (frusemide) 0.5 mg/kg. Any benefit tends to be temporary.

TABLE 11.7 Management of raised ICP

Problem	Action
Accuracy of measurement	Reposition, flush and recalibrate device
Inadequate sedation or paralysis	Give bolus of sedation, analgesia and/or relaxants Increase infusion rates
Hypoxia or hypercarbia	Check blood gases Alter FiO_2 and ventilation appropriately
Inadequate CPP	Give additional i.v. fluids Increase vasopressors/inotropes
Impaired venous drainage from head and neck	Check head twisted, endotracheal tube tapes too tight Nurse 15–20° head up
Seizures	Often masked by muscle relaxants Check CFM trace or EEG. Treat appropriately
Pyrexia	Give antipyretics

- Moderate hyperventilation to lower $PaCO_2$ > 4 kPa. Lower levels may result in excessive cerebral vasoconstriction and may produce areas of ischaemia. Any benefits will tend to disappear over a few hours.
- CSF drainage via external ventricular drain.
- Ensure that adequate CPP is maintained at all times. If there is no response to simple measures, consider further increasing CPP. The benefit of this may not be immediate and may take a few hours.

2nd line

- Thiopentone infusion. 15 mg/kg 1st hour, 8 mg/kg 2nd hour, 5 mg/kg/h thereafter. Monitor levels over time.
- Decompressive craniotomy. Removal of bone flap and lobectomy.
- Induced hypothermia.
- Aggressive hyperventilation to $PaCO_2$ < 3 kPa. See note above.

COMMON PROBLEMS IN TRAUMATIC BRAIN INJURY

Cardiovascular instability

Haemodynamic instability is common and may be seen in association with neurogenic pulmonary oedema (see below). The importance of an adequate cerebral perfusion pressure has already been stressed. Hypotension may be due to a combination of factors. You should exclude causes such as hypovolaemia, pneumothorax and sepsis.

All patients should have direct arterial pressure and CVP monitoring. In complex cases insert a PA catheter to guide fluids, inotropes and vasopressor therapy, as for any shock state.

Dilated pupil

Sudden increases in pupil size, particularly if unilateral and non-reactive to light, may be due to stretching of the IIIrd cranial nerve and may herald brainstem herniation. This is an indication for urgent repeat CT scan. Dilated pupils may reflect underlying seizure activity. Bilateral fixed dilated pupils are an ominous sign, suggesting impending brain death, but should not be considered in isolation.

Seizures

Generalized or focal seizures are common with brain injury from any cause. In the complicated ICU patient the distinction between focal and generalized seizures is indistinct and usually of little relevance. Such patients with repeated seizures will almost always be ventilated. The peripheral manifestations of seizures will be masked by the use of

Normal   Seizure activity

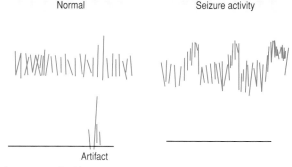

Artifact

Fig. 11.2 Cerebral function monitoring.

muscle relaxants but their damaging effects on the brain will continue
if left untreated.

A cerebral function monitor (CFM) may be used to detect
abnormal seizure activity. The simplest of these displays two
channels, base line activity (to detect artefacts) and global cerebral
electrical activity. Typical traces are shown in Figure 11.2. The 'saw
tooth' pattern is typical of seizures.

Newer forms of cerebral function monitors have multiple channels
and display the electrical activity of each cerebral hemisphere separately.
You should seek advice on the interpretation of these. If in doubt in the
paralysed patient request a formal EEG. Alternatively there is usually
little harm in temporarily reducing/stopping muscle relaxants to assess
seizure activity; ensure adequate doses of sedative/analgesic drugs first!

Continued seizure activity increases the oxygen requirement of the
brain and worsens brain injury, therefore seizures should be treated
promptly.

● Exclude any treatable precipitating cause such as hypoxia,
  hypercarbia, hyperthermia or electrolyte disturbance.

1st line
● Intravenous benzodiazepines, e.g. diazepam 5–10 mg or
  clonazepam as necessary. Large cumulative doses may be needed.
  Midazolam is also effective.
● Intravenous phenytoin. Loading dose 15 mg/kg. Give 300 mg
  loading dose over 1 hour and then 1200 mg over next 24 hours.
  Daily dose 300 mg thereafter. Measure levels over time. Phenytoin
  may cause disturbances of cardiac rhythm in some patients.

- Intravenous propofol, bolus followed by infusion 200–400 mg/h may also be effective.

2nd line

- If seizure activity is not controlled, then additional anticonvulsant agents such as sodium valproate, phenobarbital, clormethiazole, paraldehyde or magnesium, may be required. Seek advice and check dose regimens in BNF.
- Consider thiopental bolus 500 mg over 5 minutes, followed by infusion 2.5–5 g daily. Check levels over time.

Prophylactic anticonvulsants are commonly given to at-risk patients; for example, patients with significant contusions on CT or documented seizures after injury. Phenytoin is the usual drug as it does not produce significant sedation (see doses above).

Diabetes insipidus (DI)

Neurogenic DI results from failure of the posterior pituitary to produce antidiuretic hormone (ADH). It may result from either localized damage to the pituitary/hypothalamic area or from diffuse brain injury, as in brain death. It is usually seen in the first 24–48 hours post injury and is manifest as an excessive urine output due to inability to concentrate the urine. Untreated, this results in progressive dehydration and hypernatraemia.

DI should be considered if urine outputs persist at greater than 300–400 ml/h in the absence of diuretics. Other causes of excessive urine output include excretion of resuscitation fluids, use of dopamine/dopexamine, mannitol and diuretics.

- To confirm the diagnosis check urine/plasma osmolalities. Normal plasma osmolality is 286 mosmol/l. If increased > 310 mosmol/l then urine should be highly concentrated. In this context urine osmolality < 500 mosmol/l implies DI.
- Give DDAVP 1–2 µg i.v. as required.
- Replace urinary losses with 5% dextrose with added K^+.

> ⚠ **If DI is severe, patients may have significant dehydration and hypernatraemia. Avoid rapid correction which may lead to acute cerebral oedema. (See Sodium, p. 168.)**

Poor gas exchange

Respiratory problems are very common in the presence of brain injury and are often a reason for initial ICU admission or delayed discharge. The precise mechanisms are multifactorial but may include inadequate cough and gag reflexes, pulmonary aspiration, chest infection (particularly staphylococcal), pulmonary capillary leak and depressed immune function. (See Nosocomial pneumonia, p. 118.)

Most patients with severe brain injury will require a tracheostomy to facilitate airway management for short- to medium-term care. Neurological function is typically assessed 48–72 hours post injury. Consider early tracheostomy in the seriously brain-injured patient. Try to avoid the scenario of repeated extubation and reintubation and then subsequent tracheostomy. Tracheostomy protects the airway, is more comfortable for the patient, allows early reduction in sedative and analgesic drugs, aids nutrition and mobilization, and allows easier weaning of ventilatory support.

Neurogenic pulmonary oedema

Pulmonary oedema is an unusual but well-recognized complication of brain injury. In its severest form it is characterized by extreme cardiovascular instability with profuse pink frothy pulmonary oedema. Simplistically, it is thought to result from a rapid rise in ICP, which produces a catecholamine surge, with subsequent pulmonary hypertension and leakage of pulmonary capillaries. A similar clinical scenario may follow strangulation or acute airway obstruction.

The management is supportive with IPPV, high FiO_2 and PEEP. Diuretics are not usually effective and the volume of fluid leaking into the alveoli and out of the lung may lead to marked hypovolaemia. Cardiac instability will often require invasive monitoring with a PA catheter, inotropes and vasopressor therapy. The pulmonary oedema usually settles over time but may develop into severe ARDS. (See ARDS, p. 128.)

Cerebrospinal fluid (CSF) leaks

Clear or blood-stained fluid from nose or ear may represent a CSF leak, which is a feature of injuries to the frontal sinus and base of skull. CSF tests positive for glucose on test strips. In the past, antibiotic prophylaxis was thought to be necessary but most centres have stopped this practice. It is usual to wait about 10 days to see if the leak will cease spontaneously, then consider craniotomy and placement of a dural patch.

The irritable brain-injured patient

Irritability and restlessness are common in patients with minor brain injury or in the recovery phase of more severe injuries. In the latter there will often be severe movement disorders in the form of extensor spasms. Despite the theoretical risks of masking neurological signs it is often necessary to give sedatives (benzodiazepines) and major tranquillizers (chlorpromazine/haloperidol) to such patients to allow nursing care and prevent further injury. The patient with extensor spasms will need a tracheostomy to stop him or her biting on the endotracheal tube and causing obstruction, and may require very large doses of drugs to settle. Consider nursing such patients on a mattress on the floor to avoid them falling out of bed (cot sides do not always prevent this and increase the height of the fall!).

NEW MONITORING MODALITIES IN BRAIN INJURY

You may encounter a number of newer monitoring modalities that are currently under evaluation in brain injury. Most are intended to provide additional information regarding perfusion, oxygen delivery and oxygen consumption in the brain. The majority of these techniques are limited either by technical difficulties or by inability to detect small, critically ischaemic areas within the brain.

Jugular bulb oxygen saturation (SjO_2)

Measuring the saturation in venous blood from the brain gives an indication of the adequacy of oxygen delivery and utilization by the brain. The normal range is 55–75%. Changes are more valuable than isolated values and reflect global/regional perfusion and oxygenation.

A low SjO_2 implies inadequate oxygen delivery. Consider measures to improve cerebral blood flow, in particular raising CPP. If the saturation is high then the brain is either hyperaemic or failing to extract oxygen. Barbiturates may be helpful to control ICP in the presence of hyperaemia. In brain death the saturation may approach 100% as the brain ceases to extract oxygen.

Near infrared spectroscopy

This technique uses light absorption to measure brain tissue oxygenation. Light of a particular wavelength is passed through the skull and the absorption by brain cell cytochromes is detected. The technique is limited by the depth to which the incident light is able to penetrate effectively. Changes probably reflect perfusion/oxygen delivery in superficial areas of the brain only.

Brain tissue PO$_2$

Brain tissue PO$_2$ can be measured directly using a miniaturized electrode placed within or on the surface of the brain through a cranial burr hole.

Brain tissue microdialysis

A microdialysis catheter is placed into brain parenchyma through a small cranial burr hole. Fluid is passed through the catheter and allowed to equilibrate with brain tissue interstitial fluid. This is then aspirated and analysis of the chemical content of the fluid retrieved provides an indication of local tissue perfusion and oxygenation.

TYPICAL COURSE AND OUTCOME FOLLOWING BRAIN INJURY

Following severe brain injury, patients typically require tracheal intubation, assisted ventilation and sedation/paralysis. Cerebral perfusion pressure and other parameters are optimized for a period of 48–72 hours in the hope of minimizing secondary brain injury. If after this period they remain unstable, have high ICP or other ongoing system failure, further time will be required to allow for the patient's condition to improve. Otherwise, a decision is usually made to stop sedatives and to allow patients to waken, so that their neurological status can be assessed.

If such patients respond purposefully to commands, move both sides normally and are haemodynamically stable, a trial of weaning and extubation can be commenced. If, however, they fail to waken, to obey commands, have a hemiparesis, abnormal flexion or extensor posturing, then rapid weaning and extubation is unlikely to be successful. Consideration should be given to tracheostomy as an aid to weaning.

Once weaned from mechanical ventilation the neurologically damaged patient can usually be managed on a high dependency unit. Tube feeding will usually be required initially via a fine-bore nasogastric tube or gastrostomy (PEG). Neurological improvement may occur over time and long-term rehabilitation is important.

Outcome

Outcome following brain injury depends on a number of factors, including the mechanism and severity of the initial injury, subsequent episodes of hypotension, hypoxia or hypercarbia, adequacy of resuscitation, and the presence of other injuries. Age is important, young patients have a substantially better outcome than elderly

TABLE 11.8 Glasgow Outcome Scale for brain-injured patients

Description	Classification
Return to preinjury levels of function	Good recovery
Neurological deficit but self-caring	Moderately disabled
Unable to care for self	Severely disabled
No higher mental function	Vegetative
	Dead

patients for a given injury. In particular, young children may make a good recovery from an apparently devastating injury. There is a wide spectrum from mild to devastating injury. The Glasgow Outcome Scale (Table 11.8) can be used to classify outcomes.

It is relatively easy to predict outcomes at either end of the spectrum but not in between. The passage of time (weeks/months) is essential to assess potential for recovery. Clinicians learn from experience that it is often impossible to predict longer-term outcome in any individual patient. Furthermore, even apparently good physical recovery may mask subtle underlying cognitive deficits or psychological impairment and these problems may be manifest even after apparently trivial injuries.

SPONTANEOUS INTRACRANIAL HAEMORRHAGE

Patients may require intensive care following spontaneous intracranial haemorrhage, to protect the airway or support ventilation. Often the requirement may be precipitated by the need to transfer the patient to a neurosurgical centre.

The outcome will depend upon the site and nature of the bleed, the neurological state and conscious level of the patient, age and coexisting medical problems. Subarachnoid haemorrhage is distinct in that there is an established benefit in early surgical or radiological intervention (see below). The role of surgery for intracerebral bleeds (haemorrhagic stroke) is less clear and is associated with a high morbidity and mortality, especially in elderly patients.

SUBARACHNOID HAEMORRHAGE

Patients with spontaneous subarachnoid haemorrhage (SAH) frequently require intensive care, either early at presentation, after surgery or some time later due to respiratory or other complications.

Patients present with sudden onset of headache, neurological deficit and collapse. Subarachnoid haemorrhage is confirmed by CT scan and/or lumbar puncture. The site and appearance of bleeding may suggest an aneurysm or arteriovenous malformation. There are associations with other diseases, e.g. atheromatous vascular disease, polycystic kidney disease, collagen/connective tissue disease and other congenital malformations.

Management and outcome is determined by grading. Two common grading systems are shown in Tables 11.9a and 11.9b. Grading is difficult once the patient is sedated/ventilated. Rebleeding or vasospasm may rapidly worsen neurological state.

Surgical management

Large intracerebral haematomas may require emergency surgical evacuation. Intraventricular drainage may be used to decompress the brain and treat hydrocephalus.

All patients with potential for recovery will require cerebral angiography to delineate the site and nature of the lesion. The timing and indications for angiography and subsequent definitive intervention depend upon the patient's age (increasing risk of cerebrovascular

TABLE 11.9a Hunt and Hess grading system for subarachnoid haemorrhage

Description	Grade
Unruptured aneurysm	0
Asymptomatic, minimal headache or nuchal rigidity	1
Moderate headache or nuchal rigidity No neurological deficit except cranial nerves	2
Drowsiness, confusion or mild focal deficit	3
Stupor, hemiparesis	4
Deep coma, decerebrate rigidity, moribund appearance	5

TABLE 11.9b World Federation of Neurological Surgeons scale

Glasgow Coma Scale	Motor deficit	Grade
15	No	1
13–14	No	2
13–14	Yes	3
7–12	Yes or no	4
3–6	Yes or no	5

disease and cerebral infarction) and preoperative status. Aneurysms may be embolized under radiological control or clipped surgically, depending on the site of lesion, and local facilities and expertise.

In operable cases, early surgery reduces the risk of rebleeding, and the development of intercurrent medical problems, but is technically more difficult and increases the risk of vasospasm. Delayed surgery (10–14 days post bleed) is technically easier, carries less risk of vasospasm but increases the risk of bleeding in the intervening period. In general, early angiography and clipping of aneurysms is indicated in the younger patient with milder grade 1–2 signs and aneurysms in the anterior cerebral circulation.

ICU management

The management of SAH is essentially no different from other causes of brain injury. Cerebral vasospasm may occur. The exact mechanism by which this occurs is unclear but it can result in areas of ischaemic infarction. It is diagnosed by angiography or transcranial Doppler. Management is centred on prevention.

- Maintenance of cerebral perfusion pressure using fluids and vasopressors is crucial. Aim for mean systemic pressure of 90–100 mmHg. It is not usual to monitor ICP. Vasopressor therapy is usually used and may be required for up to 3 weeks.
- The Ca^{2+} channel blocker nimodipine has been shown to improve neurological outcome. Its effect is thought to be independent of any antivasospasm action. Its systemic vasodilator effects may worsen CPP and require vasopressor therapy. It is available in oral and i.v. preparations.
- Cardiac dysrhythmias are common in SAH. These do not usually require treatment.

Typically many patients are managed in an HDU/ward area. More severe cases may need a period of ventilation in ICU, followed by a period of weaning and tracheostomy.

HYPOXIC BRAIN INJURY

Hypoxic brain injury is most commonly seen following resuscitation from prolonged cardiac arrest. Other causes include:

- profound hypotension/hypoxaemia from any cause prolonged seizures
- carbon monoxide poisoning
- attempted strangulation or hanging near drowning.

Patients who are resuscitated following cardiac arrest are usually referred for intensive care because of haemodynamic instability or inadequate respiratory effort. There is no evidence to suggest that periods of elective ventilation, or the use of so-called cerebral protection agents (e.g. barbiturates/steroids), affect neurological outcome. The emphasis should be on prevention of secondary insults.

● Ventilate for 12–24 hours, without sedation if possible, then reassess neurological state. If the patient begins to get agitated then short-acting agents, e.g. propofol, allow subsequent periodic reassessment of neurology.
● Purposeful or semipurposeful movements are a good sign and usually herald recovery. Absence of respiratory effort, myoclonic jerking and fixed dilated pupils usually indicate severe hypoxic damage and a poor long-term outlook.

A similar scenario is also seen following prolonged hypoglycaemia. This usually follows deliberate overdosage with insulin.
(See Management of patients following cardiac arrest, p. 90 and Hypoglycaemia, p. 179.)

Outcome
The prediction of long-term outcome after hypoxic brain injury is difficult. In the patient who does not awaken, longer-term management will depend upon the patient's background health, age, previous wishes (advance directives, etc.). The patient's relatives and family need to be kept aware of the situation and their wishes must also be considered. Unless a consensus is reached regarding withdrawal of active management, the patient should be stabilized, weaned off IPPV, usually via a tracheostomy, established on enteral feeding and transferred for ward-based care awaiting neurological change over time. If the patient does not improve over time and all parties agree that further treatment is futile, then it is reasonable to wean from assisted ventilation, extubate the trachea, and await events. (See Do not resuscitate orders, p. 364.)

INFECTION

Meningitis
It is rare for adults to require intensive care when meningitis is the primary presenting diagnosis. In the case serious enough to warrant intensive care it is advisable to perform CT scan prior to lumbar puncture to exclude cerebral oedema and the potential risk of coning after lumbar puncture. If lumbar puncture is contraindicated, empirica

antibiotic therapy can be started. Steroids have been shown to reduce longer-term neurological sequelae in both adults and children presenting with *Haemophilus*, pneumococcal and recently meningococcal meningitis and should be given on presentation.

Occasionally more severe cases develop secondary hydrocephalus and benefit from intraventricular CSF drainage; therefore, perform a CT scan in patients who deteriorate or who fail to improve over time.

Encephalitis

As for meningitis, it is rare for adults to require intensive care. Occasionally encephalitis needs to be considered as a diagnosis of exclusion in cases of coma. There are characteristic EEG changes with herpes encephalitis. A brain biopsy may be indicated to confirm the diagnosis. Start empirical aciclovir (in addition to broad-spectrum antibiotics) until diagnosis is proved/disproved. (See Empirical antibiotic therapy, p. 282.)

Brain abscess

Occasional cause of ICU admission. Look for embolic sources of infection, e.g. endocarditis, and local sources, e.g. middle ear infection. Check tuberculosis status. Immunosuppressed patients (e.g. HIV) may present with unusual CNS abscesses/meningitis e.g. toxoplasmosis and cryptosporidiosis. Large abscesses will require surgical drainage. Seek neurosurgical advice.

STATUS EPILEPTICUS

Seizures are common in the critically ill, either as a presenting diagnosis of epilepsy or as a secondary complication of other disorders. Some of the more common causes are listed in Table.11.10.

Status epilepticus can be defined as seizures lasting longer than 30 minutes, or so frequently that no recovery occurs between attacks. Patients are at risk of brain injury, cerebral oedema, hypoxia and aspiration. Typically, intensive care referral occurs when first-line drug

---

TABLE 11.10 Conditions precipitating seizure activity

Worsening of existing seizure disorder
Alcohol or other drug withdrawal
Drug overdose, e.g. tricyclic antidepressants
Brain injury
Brain abscess or tumour
Metabolic, e.g. hypoglycaemia/hypomagnesaemia
Hypoxia

treatment has failed and the patient becomes increasingly obtunded due to the effects of ongoing seizures and sedative drug accumulation. If untreated, patients may suffer complications of immobility, hypothermia, hyperthermia and rhabdomyolysis.

Occasionally patients will present with convincing pseudoseizures as part of a Munchausen-type syndrome. If there is doubt as to whether jerky movements or loss of consciousness represent a true seizure, request an EEG.

Management

Most cases severe enough to require admission to ICU will require a period of tracheal intubation and assisted ventilation. Consider CT scanning and/or lumbar puncture to exclude treatable disorders. Correct any metabolic abnormality or derangement of body temperature. Anticonvulsant therapy should be optimized. Seek advice from a neurologist.

BRAINSTEM DEATH

Brainstem death is caused by irreversible damage to the brainstem, which is the control centre for the autonomic functions of the brain. Its description in 1959 followed the introduction of assisted ventilation in brain-injured patients. The intention was to reliably identify hopeless cases that had nothing to gain from further treatment. There have been no verified cases of recovery or long-term survival in patients fulfilling criteria for brainstem death, as stated in the UK. Brainstem death is a clinical diagnosis and does not require confirmatory tests such as EEG/angiography in the UK. Doctors in training should not be expected to formally diagnose brainstem death (i.e. perform brainstem death tests) but should understand the process.

It will usually be clear from clinical bedside observations that brainstem death has occurred. The typical features of brainstem herniation are tachycardia and hypertension, followed by bradycardia, hypotension and pupil dilatation. A lack of response to endotracheal suctioning, turning and mouth care, with fixed dilated pupils, suggests the diagnosis of actual or impending brainstem death. All are performed routinely during nursing care. Formal brainstem death tests are then used to confirm that brainstem death has already occurred. It looks unprofessional to do formal tests and then find that the patient is not brain dead after all!

Preconditions

Before brainstem tests are performed there are a number of preconditions that must be satisfied in order to exclude potentially

---

TABLE 11.11 Preconditions to performing brainstem death tests

Known cause of brain damage, e.g. trauma, intracerebral
haemorrhage, hypoxia
Absence of neuromuscular blocking drugs
Absence of any residual CNS depressant drugs
Normothermia (core temp. >35.5°C)
Normal metabolic and endocrine state
No significant electrolyte or blood glucose disturbance

---

reversible causes of brainstem dysfunction. These are shown in
Table 11.11.

Active measures to maintain blood pressure, temperature and
normal electrolytes may be required if the patient is to fulfil
preconditions, and to be potentially suitable for organ donation. This
may require fluids, inotropes, vasopressors and DDAVP in the hours
prior to tests (often overnight). Replacement of the large urine
volumes seen with diabetes insipidus with isotonic saline or synthetic
colloid solutions will lead to progressive hypernatraemia. Use DDAVP
and fluid replacement with dextrose solutions (with added K$^+$) to
avoid this. (See Diabetes insipidus, p. 237.)

Before performing tests ensure that all preconditions are satisfied.
Always confirm the integrity of the neuromuscular junction and
exclude the effects of muscle relaxants by use of a nerve stimulator
(see p. 37). Scrutinize the drug chart and intensive care chart to ensure
that sufficient time has elapsed for any centrally acting drugs to have
been metabolized and eliminated. Beware of active metabolites, which
may have long half-lives. Check the patient's core temperature and
recent biochemistry results.

> ⚠ **The preconditions for the diagnosis of brainstem
> death are absolutely fundamental to the process and
> must be satisfied before consideration of the diagnosis.**

Conduct of brainstem death tests

In the UK, the tests are carried out by two doctors who are 5 years
post registration. This is usually two consultants or one consultant and
one senior trainee. At least one of the doctors should have been
responsible for the patient during the admission and neither should be
associated with the transplant services. The tests may be performed
together or separately, providing each doctor satisfies himself or
herself of the results. The tests are usually repeated at a suitable

TABLE 11.12 Brainstem death tests

Test	Brainstem function (cranial nerves)
Pupil light reflex	II , III
Corneal reflex	V, VII
Caloric tests	VIII, IV, VI, III
Gag reflex	IX, X
Tracheal suction	X
Response to pain (see text below)	Sensory afferents Motor efferents
Apnoea tests	Respiratory centre

interval to confirm the findings. Following the completion of the second set of tests, brainstem death is confirmed.

Occasionally families will ask to observe the tests being done. This is acceptable providing that staff have taken the time to explain the process and they understand the nature of the tests. The whole process of testing, counselling the family and explaining the concept of brain death and organ donation is, of necessity, extremely time consuming.

Most hospitals have preprinted documentation for brainstem death tests and organ donation. The tests required are listed in Table 11.12.

Response to pain
Deep pain is produced peripherally by pressure on sensitive points such as the nail beds and centrally by pressure over the supraorbital nerves, while observing for a response within the cranial nerve distribution. Peripheral non-purposeful movements in response to peripheral pain represent spinal reflexes and are not indicative of brainstem function. Simplistically these reflect the loss of descending control over the spinal cord from higher centres and may become exaggerated over time. Relatives and attending staff should be warned of these and their significance explained.

Apnoea test
The patient is preoxygenated with 100% O_2, and then disconnected from the ventilator and connected to a breathing circuit with high flow 100% O_2. If the lungs are healthy, oxygenation is maintained and the $PaCO_2$ rises gradually. The $PaCO_2$ must be allowed to rise to a level at which the patient could be expected to breathe ($PaCO_2$ of 6.6 kPa for a previously healthy patient, higher in patients with chronic lung

disease and CO_2 retention). The rise in CO_2 usually takes about 10 minutes. If pulmonary function is poor, there is a risk of profound hypoxia and cardiac arrest during apnoea testing. In such cases ventilate slowly with 100% oxygen and added CO_2, or add a deadspace into the circuit, then briefly disconnect the ventilator to look for respiratory movement.

Completion of tests

Following the confirmation of brainstem death, the patient is legally dead. The death should be reported to the coroner if this is required (see p. 371). Arrangements may be made to retrieve organs for transplantation if consent has been obtained, or alternatively ventilation may be withdrawn. The family should be offered the opportunity to sit with the patient and allowed time for distant relatives to visit. At the time of ventilator disconnection they may choose to stay with the patient. Alternatively, some prefer to say their farewells before the event and leave or visit later.

If during brainstem testing residual brainstem function is demonstrated (usually residual cough or respiratory effort), ventilatory support should be continued and the situation reassessed. Assuming catastrophic brain injury has occurred, residual brainstem activity will usually disappear over 24–48 hours and then repeat brainstem tests can be performed to confirm brainstem death.

> ⚠ **Do not use the terms pass or fail in relation to brainstem death tests. This creates too much confusion. Brainstem death is either confirmed or not confirmed.**

Management of catastrophic brain injury

Some patients, despite suffering an apparently catastrophic and presumed fatal brain injury, retain some residual brainstem function. They cannot be declared brainstem dead, yet appear to have no prospect of meaningful survival. Honest discussions with the family regarding the benefits of continuation or withdrawal of treatment should take place so that decisions can be reached over a period of time that are in the best interests of the patient. If a consensus is reached that further active management is inappropriate, then treatment should be withdrawn. Such patients may be suitable for consideration as asystolic or non-beating heart organ donors (see p. 372).

ORGAN DONATION

Once brainstem death has been established, the possibility of
(cadaveric) heart beating organ donation arises.

Consent to donation

Theoretically, an organ donor card signed by the patient, or an entry in
the national donor register, is all that is required to enable organ
donation to take place after the establishment of brainstem death. The
donation of organs, however, is crucially dependent on positive public
perceptions of the scheme. As a result, in the UK, relatives are almost
always asked to give consent, and organs are not taken in the absence
of relatives' consent. Regrettably, in the UK, up to half of all relatives
will refuse donation.

> ⚠ **You must also seek the coroner's permission for
> organ donation from those patients whose death
> would normally require referral to the coroner. (See
> Reporting deaths to the coroner, p. 371.)**

The most appropriate time to approach the subject of organ
donation will depend upon the individual circumstances of the case.
Relatives will often discuss the subject informally with staff and it is
reasonable to explain about the possibility of donation at any time
once the possibility of brainstem death and tests are raised. However,
the diagnosis of brainstem death and the request for organ donation
are separate issues. You certainly should not make any formal
approach until brainstem death has been confirmed. Most transplant
coordinators are willing to come and speak to relatives about donation
if required.

Practicalities of donor management

Transplant surgeons are accepting organs (particularly kidneys) from
more unstable and elderly patients than in the past, and in addition
there is increasing utilization of tissues such as bone, skin and heart
valves. If in doubt about what can be used, ask the transplant
coordinator. Each region has one or more transplant coordinators who
will liaise between the organ retrieval teams and the referring hospital.
They will also provide advice on the management of the donor.

The management of a potential organ donor is no different from
that of other ICU patients, in particular those with brain injury. The
optimization of physiological parameters, particularly oxygen

delivery, and the avoidance of secondary physiological insults to organ systems is similar in both situations.

Problems after brainstem death include:

- Haemodynamic disturbances, with low CO and/or SVR. Oxygen uptake and CO_2 production may be abnormally low. Large volumes of fluid may be required to maintain adequate filling pressures, and inotropes/vasopressors are frequently necessary to maintain adequate perfusion pressures. Optimization of the cardiovascular system may require invasive monitoring.
- Poor gas exchange is common (e.g. neurogenic pulmonary oedema), and frequently lungs are unsuitable for transplantation. Ventilation should be optimized.
- Pituitary function is impaired. There is no evidence, however, that donor organ function is improved by the administration of steroids or thyroid hormones. Diabetes insipidus is common, use DDAVP (0.5–1 µg i.v.) as necessary to reduce urine output to sensible volumes (see p. 237).
- Temperature regulation is lost. Use warmed i.v. fluids, inspired gases and warm air blankets to maintain normothermia.

Special investigations

A number of tests need to be carried out before organ donation. These are shown in Table 11.13. There are increasing concerns about the risks of donor-transmitted infection and malignancy. The transplant coordinator will give advice, as this is a changing area, particularly in relation to hepatitis serology. Usually all tests are sent to a single regional laboratory.

TABLE 11.13 Tests prior to donation
Tissue typing
HIV
Hepatitis screening
U&Es
Glucose
LFTs and amylase
ECG
CXR
Height, weight and girth measurements

SPINAL CORD INJURY

Spinal cord injury may occur as a result of trauma, vertebral collapse, infection, tumours, infarcts and other pathologies. In all cases of trauma assume that the spine (cervical, thoracic or lumbar) is injured until proven otherwise and immobilize it as part of initial resuscitation.

> ⚠️ **X-rays of the spine do not exclude instability resulting from ligament injury. Spinal cord damage can only be fully excluded by clinical examination in an awake, co-operative patient. Therefore, even if X-rays are normal you should maintain immobilization until the spine can be assessed clinically.**

Early management

- Immobilize the spine to prevent secondary damage. Use a cervical collar, sandbags and tape for cervical spine, plus spinal board. (Log roll with inline stabilization to control head and neck movement.)
- Establish i.v. access to support blood pressure. Sympathetic blockade from cord injury will produce hypotension and bradycardia, depending upon the level of cord injury. Patients rarely require inotropes to maintain the circulation following isolated spinal injury. Look for haemorrhage from other injuries (e.g. the 'silent' denervated abdomen).
- Tracheal intubation and assisted ventilation may be required for respiratory insufficiency or surgery. Consider awake intubation using local anaesthesia (fibreoptic or conventional). Alternatively, intubate the anaesthetized patient with inline immobilization of the neck. Use of a bougie and McCoy laryngoscope limits the need to extend the neck. Use of suxamethonium is allowed in the first few hours after injury. Avoid after 24 hours because of the potential for massive K^+ release. (See Suxamethonium, p. 37.)
- Urinary retention is a significant cause of spinal hyperreflexia. Perform early urinary catheterization.
- Gastric stasis is common: pass a nasogastric/orogastric tube.

High-dose steroids (methylprednisolone), if given early, may have beneficial effects in spinal injury. Discuss the management with the local spinal injuries unit or spinal surgeon. The indications for early spinal decompression and surgical stabilization are controversial. Transfer to a spinal injury unit only after exclusion and stabilization of other injuries in a general/neurosurgical unit.

Patients with high spinal injuries will have impaired ventilation and cough reflexes and will have predictable difficulties weaning from artificial ventilation. Early tracheostomy may be of benefit. Those

with injuries affecting the phrenic nerve (C3,4,5) may remain
ventilator-dependent in the long term.

NEUROMUSCULAR CONDITIONS

Both acute and chronic neuromuscular conditions are important in
intensive care practice. The characteristics of the various conditions
vary in detail and many patients will never have a definitive diagnosis
made. However, you should consider all such patients to be at risk
from the following:

- Incipient respiratory failure. Commonly follows chest infections or
  major surgery.
- Bulbar palsy leading to recurrent pulmonary aspiration.
- Autonomic neuropathy leading to cardiovascular instability.
  Bradycardias, tachycardias, hypertension or hypotension may all
  occur.
- Cardiomyopathy. There is a risk of arrhythmias and sudden death.
- Profound sensitivity to muscle relaxants. There may be longlasting
  weakness after non-depolarizing drugs. Massive K^+ release after
  suxamethonium is well recognized even before clinical
  manifestations are seen (avoid using it!).

In the presence of most neuromuscular conditions patients will retain
a normal conscious level. If they are paralysed and ventilator-
dependent they may be unable to move or show any sign of distress.
(The only means of communication may be by blinking the eyelids.)
It should be assumed that they are conscious until proved otherwise.

Patients with neuromuscular conditions require supportive care
(assisted ventilation, tracheostomy, non-invasive ventilation, nutrition,
physiotherapy, etc.). Increasing numbers of such patients are managed
on non-invasive home ventilation. Severe kyphoscoliosis is a
significant feature in many patients. Occasionally patients who have
difficulty in weaning from assisted ventilation are found to have
previously undiagnosed neuromuscular disease. The commoner
conditions encountered are discussed below.

Myasthenia gravis

This autoimmune disease results from antibodies to the cholinergic
receptors in the neuromuscular junction. The mainstay of treatment is
with anticholinesterase drugs, which increase the level of
acetylcholine available at the cholinergic receptors.

Deterioration, increasing muscle weakness and subsequent
respiratory failure may result from intercurrent disease, surgery or

overdosage of anticholinesterase drugs (cholinergic crisis). The short-acting anticholinesterase edrophonium may be given to test whether muscle function can be improved ('tensilon test'). In practice, by the time myasthenic patients require intensive care it is often difficult to distinguish a cholinergic crisis from other causes of muscle fatigue.

Acute exacerbations are treated by increases in anticholinergic drugs, steroids and plasma exchange. Azathioprine, cyclophosphamide and thymectomy are useful treatments in the longer term.

Guillain–Barré syndrome

This condition of ascending muscle paralysis usually follows an intercurrent illness. The early use of intravenous immunoglobulin and plasmapheresis may reduce the need for assisted ventilation. Patients who require assisted ventilation may take weeks or months to recover, and recovery is not always complete. Autonomic disturbances and neuropathic pain are common. A variant of this condition, known as Miller Fisher syndrome, predominantly affects the cranial nerves.

Tetanus

This is very rare in the UK, due to successful immunization programmes. It is, however, a major problem abroad. The toxins produced by the bacteria disrupt normal neuromuscular control and produce severe spasms and autonomic disturbances. The management is supportive, with wound debridement, antibiotics, immunoglobulins and control of spasms and autonomic problems. Severe cases may require protracted sedation and assisted ventilation.

CRITICAL ILLNESS NEUROMYOPATHY

As more and more critically ill patients survive, increasing numbers of patients are developing residual neuromuscular problems: the so-called 'critical illness neuromyopathy'. The exact aetiology is unclear but severe sepsis, prolonged immobility, poor nutritional status, neuromuscular blocking drugs and elderly medically unfit patients are all considered risk factors. Typically it is first noticed when a critically ill patient is in the recovery phase of illness and is unable to move limbs. It is important to recognize the diagnosis and appreciate that the patient may be completely awake but unable to move. Craniofacial movements are often relatively spared and the patient's only means of communication or response may be to blink.

It is important to rule out other causes of weakness like cervical cord problems. Neurological examination usually reveals a flaccid paralysis. EMG indicates a mixed picture of neuropathy and myopathy. Biopsy, although not routine, shows axonal degeneration with preservation of myelin sheaths. The condition usually improves over weeks or months but recovery may be incomplete and neuropathic pain is common.

TRAUMA

INTRODUCTION

The successful management of major trauma requires the early identification and treatment of life-threatening injuries followed by systematic evaluation and treatment of all other injuries. Best outcomes are achieved by a co-ordinated team approach and protocol-based management.

Depending upon local policy, you may be called to assist in the initial resuscitation of major trauma victims. Although an A&E doctor or trauma surgeon will generally lead trauma resuscitation, you should be familiar with advanced trauma life support protocols.

PRIMARY SURVEY

The purpose of the primary survey is to identify and begin the treatment of any immediately life-threatening injuries. These include:

- airway obstruction
- tension pneumothorax
- cardiac tamponade
- massive haemorrhage.

The principal elements of the primary survey are A, B, C and D, as follows.

(A) Airway (with cervical spine control)
- Assess the adequacy of the airway. Clear upper airway with suction and simple airway manoeuvres and provide 100% oxygen using a mask with reservoir bag.
- If necessary, secure the airway by intubation or cricothyroidotomy, depending on clinical situation and degree of urgency.

> ⚠ **The cervical spine should be assumed to be unstable and must be protected at all times. Use inline immobilization; sandbag and tape the head to prevent unnecessary movement.**

(See Spinal cord injury, p. 251.)

(B) Breathing
- Support ventilation if necessary.
- Expose the chest and examine for adequacy of respiration. Identify and treat life-threatening conditions such as flail chest, tension pneumothorax and massive haemothorax.

(C) Circulation

- Stop major haemorrhage by direct pressure.
- Assess the adequacy of circulation; in particular, pulse rate, BP, and capillary refill.
- Insert two 14-gauge peripheral intravenous cannulae. If this is not possible then cannulate the femoral vein or consider peripheral venous cut down (e.g. saphenous vein). In ATLS doctrine CVP lines are used for monitoring and not for resuscitation purposes.
- Send blood for cross-matching.
- Give 2–3 litres of crystalloid. If there is no response, continue with colloids and blood products. Fully cross-matched blood is preferable but group-specific, or non-cross-matched O negative can be used, depending upon circumstances.
- If volume loading does not restore perfusion, consider adrenaline (epinephrine) bolus followed by an infusion.

(D) Disability (neurological assessment)

- Assess conscious level, pupil size and note any obvious neurological deficit. A deteriorating Glasgow Coma Score, or GCS of 8 or below, is an indication for intubation and ventilation. (See Immediate management of brain injury, p. 226.)

Reassessment

- Reassess A, B, C and D to ensure continued stability and appropriate response to treatment before moving on to the secondary survey.

EXPOSURE AND SECONDARY SURVEY

Once the initial survey is complete and the patient is stabilized ensure that appropriate monitoring is established and that necessary investigations have been organized (Table 12.1).

TABLE 12.1 Investigations and monitoring

Routine investigations	Monitoring
FBC	ECG
U&Es, glucose	Blood pressure (non-invasive or invasive)
Arterial blood gas	Pulse oximeter
(Pregnancy test)	CVP
ECG	Urine output
Lateral cervical spine X-ray	
CXR	
Pelvic X-ray	
Urine (stick test)	

Ensure that an adequate medical history has been obtained. At minimum, this should include the patient's past medical history, medications, allergies, time of last meal and the mechanism of injury. The mechanism of injury is particularly important in providing important clues as to the likely injuries that may have been sustained.

● Completely expose the patient, while at the same time taking steps to avoid hypothermia.
● Systematically examine the patient from head to toe, looking for other injuries. Log roll the patient to examine the back and spine, and perform rectal and vaginal examinations.
● Urinary catheters and nasogastric tubes may be inserted if there are no contraindications.

Following resuscitation, stabilization and re-evaluation of the patient, further management can be planned. This may include immediate surgery for life-threatening injuries, or further investigations such as diagnostic peritoneal lavage, ultrasound or CT scan.

Ultrasound is increasingly used by A&E staff to identify free fluid (blood) in the peritoneal pleural and pericardial spaces. In this context, its value is in identifying a problem (e.g. peritoneal fluid) rather than the definitive diagnosis (e.g. ruptured spleen).

Blunt versus penetrating trauma

Blunt and penetrating trauma produce different patterns of injury. Blunt trauma is associated with significant soft-tissue injury and haemorrhage into tissues and body cavities. In penetrating trauma, tissue injury may be quite localized and haemorrhage may be tamponaded by the presence of a foreign object. There is ongoing debate about resuscitation strategies in the two groups.

Aggressive intravenous fluid resuscitation with blood, colloid or crystalloid may raise blood pressure, disturb blood clots and restart bleeding. There is some evidence, particularly in penetrating trauma, that restrictive fluid strategies, which limit the volume of resuscitation fluid given until surgical control of bleeding can be achieved, are associated with better outcomes. Similar considerations may apply in other surgical situations, such as that of leaking aortic aneurysm.

INTENSIVE CARE MANAGEMENT

Patients with multiple injuries will frequently require transfer to an intensive care unit after initial resuscitation, stabilization and surgery. Care of the multiply-injured patient is essentially no different to care of any other ICU patient. Multiple trauma is by its nature a multisystem disorder, rather than a collection of isolated injuries. Treatment is generally supportive, with appropriate intervention for problems as they are identified.

Multiple organ failure

Multiple organ failure is common after massive trauma. Typically patients develop SIRS 24–48 hours after apparently adequate resuscitation, which then leads on to multiple organ failure. Tissue damage, massive blood transfusion and activation of the cytokine cascade are all implicated but exact mechanisms are unclear. Treatment is largely supportive. Possible sources of any ongoing inflammatory response, including necrotic tissue and foci of infection, must be excluded. (See Multiple organ failure, p. 277, and SIRS, p. 277.)

The management of specific groups of injuries is discussed below.

HEAD AND NECK INJURIES

Head injury
(See Traumatic brain injury, p. 246.)

Facial injury

In the unconscious or obtunded patient the airway should be secured early by intubation. With time, swelling may make subsequent reintubation or airway manipulation impossible. Therefore, in severe injuries consideration should be given to early tracheostomy. In the presence of facial or base of skull fractures avoid nasal intubation or nasogastric tubes as these may pass into the cranium. Use the oral route.

Heavy bleeding from facial injuries should not be underestimated. Bleeding from the nose may require nasal packing and use of Foley catheters to tamponade bleeding. Seek ENT/maxillofacial surgical advice. Injuries to the jaw often require internal fixation and jaw wiring. Do not be afraid to cut the wires in the event of airway problems. When extubating these patients ensure they are awake and have full return of protective reflexes.

Broken or dislodged teeth may have been aspirated. These may be visible on X-ray, particularly if there are amalgam fillings. A lateral film may help to confirm position (note position of NG tube to delineate the oesophagus). Bronchoscopy may be required for the location and removal of radiolucent teeth/fragments. Removal usually requires rigid bronchoscopy. (See Airway obstruction, p. 113.)

Cervical spine injury
(See Spinal cord injury, p. 251.)

Cervical soft-tissue injury
Direct injury to soft tissues of the neck can result in airway compromise, due either to haematoma/tissue swelling causing compression of the airway or to direct injury to the larynx or trachea. Secure the airway by early intubation and seek expert surgical help. Vascular injuries in the neck may compromise the cerebral circulation. Dissection of the carotid arteries by blunt injury from seatbelts or other trauma is easily missed. Bleeding may track down into the chest, resulting in haemothorax or haemomediastinum and rarely cardiac tamponade.

THORACIC INJURIES

Pneumothorax
All traumatic pneumothoraces should be drained. (See Practical procedures, p. 353.)

Massive air leaks may require bronchoscopy to exclude bronchial rupture. Bronchial rupture should be suspected in the presence of deceleration injury, mediastinal widening, haemoptysis, first rib or clavicular fractures. An urgent thoracic surgical opinion should be sought, as surgical repair is usually required.

Haemothorax
This requires early drainage. Once clot becomes well established it becomes difficult to drain and thoracotomy may be required later. Drainage > 600 ml/h needs urgent surgical referral. (See Practical procedures: Chest drainage, p. 353.) Ensure good venous access, as decompression of a vascular tear can sometimes occur, resulting in massive haemorrhage. Use a large drain size, 32 Fr. Apply low-pressure suction.

Rib fractures
These are significant because of the potential for injury to the underlying viscera. Elderly patients with brittle ribs may have impressive rib fractures with little underlying injury. Conversely, younger patients with more flexible ribs may have severe visceral injury without obvious fractures.

- Apical rib fractures are associated with injury to great vessels.
- Mid-zone rib fractures are associated with pulmonary contusions.

- Basal rib fractures are associated with abdominal visceral injury (liver, spleen, kidneys).

Simple rib fractures without major visceral injury can often be managed conservatively. Adequate analgesia (thoracic epidural or patient-controlled analgesia ± NSAIDs), supplemental oxygen, CPAP and physiotherapy are useful. In the presence of a significant flail segment and underlying pulmonary contusions, IPPV is generally required and should be instituted early before exhaustion and significant hypoxia develop. Typically ventilation will be required for 7–10 days in such cases. Severe life-threatening ARDS may also develop.

There is little place for surgical fixation of the rib cage. Assisted ventilation (IPPV and PEEP) will usually restore reasonable alignment of a distorted rib cage over a few days. (See ARDS, p. 128.)

Mediastinal injury

Rapid deceleration injuries can result in injury to the mediastinal contents; in particular, traumatic transection of the aorta or other great vessels. Many patients with such injuries will die before reaching hospital but some develop a contained rupture which is at risk of massive rebleeding at any time hours or even days ahead. The typical finding is that of a widened mediastinum on CXR. Typical features are shown in Figure 12.1.

Investigations include aortic angiography and spiral CT scan. Transoesophageal echocardiography may have a role but does not provide all the information required for surgery. Some cases of bleeding into the mediastinum will be venous, which does not require surgery, rather than arterial. Immediate management includes controlled hypotension (e.g. GTN or esmolol infusion). Refer the patient to cardiothoracic/vascular surgeons.

Cardiac contusions

Blunt trauma to the anterior chest wall can result in injuries to the myocardium, coronary arteries, valves and other related structures. The presence of a fractured sternum should raise suspicion. Typically myocardial contusions may result in dysrhythmias and ischaemic injury patterns on ECG. These are often transient and not significant but dysrhythmias may require appropriate intervention. Rarely, injury to the anterior descending coronary artery may lead to myocardial infarction. Perform serial 12-lead ECGs and send blood for cardiac enzymes and troponin. Echocardiography will indicate the presence of

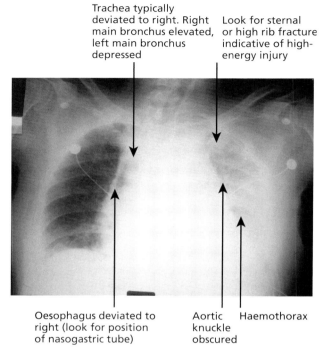

Trachea typically deviated to right. Right main bronchus elevated, left main bronchus depressed

Look for sternal or high rib fracture indicative of high-energy injury

Oesophagus deviated to right (look for position of nasogastric tube)

Aortic knuckle obscured

Haemothorax

Fig. 12.1 Chest X-ray appearances of possible mediastinal haematoma ('widened mediastinum').

myocardial contusions, myocardial dysfunction and pericardial effusions. Seek specialist advice.

Ruptured diaphragm

Blunt trauma to the abdomen may cause the diaphragm to rupture. This usually occurs on the left, due to the protection afforded by the liver on the right. The diagnosis is suggested by abdominal visceral gas shadows in the chest. Check the position of the NG tube. Surgical repair is indicated via the chest or abdomen. Occasional patients have a missed ruptured diaphragm and present later with strangulation of hernia contents. Rupture of the diaphragm may also occasionally be a long-standing, incidental finding. In this situation do not confuse X-ray appearances with pleural fluid/gas collections needing a chest drain!

ABDOMINAL INJURIES

Any intra-abdominal structure can be damaged. Major visceral injury is usually obvious, but more minor injuries such as mesenteric tears are easily missed. Pain, guarding, distension, and presence or absence of bowel sounds cannot be reliably elicited in the unconscious, sedated and ventilated patient. If previously unrecognized injury or continued intra-abdominal bleeding is suspected, seek immediate surgical opinion. Diagnostic peritoneal lavage, plain abdominal films, ultrasound and CT scan may be helpful. If doubt remains, laparotomy should be considered.

Ruptured spleen

Following splenectomy there is greatly increased risk of life-threatening infection (particularly pneumococcal). Patients require long-term prophylaxis with penicillin (2 years minimum) and immunization against *Pneumococcus, Meningococcus*, and *Haemophilus influenzae* in the convalescent phase. (See BNF and local guidelines.)

Ruptured liver

If it is impossible to suture tears adequately, surgeons may pack the liver bed and close the abdomen, with the aim of returning to theatre after 48 hours. If haemodynamically stable, patients with liver rupture should be transferred to a specialist unit.

Abdominal compartment syndrome

If intra-abdominal pressure rises above venous pressure (e.g. as a result of intra-abdominal haemorrhage) then perfusion to the abdominal organs is impaired. The first indication may be a falling urine output in the presence of an increasingly tense and quiet abdomen. Intra-abdominal pressure can be measured by connecting the urinary catheter to a pressure transducer. The management is surgical exploration. Patients may bleed torrentially when the abdomen is opened and become haemodynamically unstable following visceral reperfusion. In some cases it may be necessary to leave the abdomen 'open' after decompression. Closure may be achieved either after a few days, when the cause of the abdominal distension has subsided, or much later after the primary defect has closed by granulation. Abdominal distension can impede diaphragmatic function and make weaning from ventilation difficult (see p. 111).

SKELETAL INJURIES

Pelvic injuries

Pelvic injuries can result in major blood loss. Unstable pelvic injuries are managed by early external fixation, which is typically performed in A&E. This helps to reduce bleeding and ultimately allows for earlier mobilization.

Urethral injury should be considered in all cases of pelvic injury. Suspect if there is bleeding from the urethral meatus or an abnormal rectal examination. Do not attempt urethral catheterization. Seek help from urologists. Diagnosis is by urethrogram, which can be performed in A&E. Management is by suprapubic catheter, with definitive repair at a later date.

Long bone injuries

Look for obvious limb deformity and check for neurovascular integrity. Early reduction of deformity and splinting reduces bleeding and pain. (See also Fat embolism, Compartment syndrome and Rhabdomyolysis below.)

Spinal injuries

(See Spinal cord injury, p. 251.)

FAT EMBOLISM

Fat embolism classically presents with dyspnoea, hypoxaemia, petechial rash and acute confusional state following long bone fracture or orthopaedic instrumentation. The signs are non-specific and can be caused by pneumonia, sepsis and other complications of trauma and surgery.

The mechanisms by which fat embolism occurs are not clear. The simplest explanation is embolization of fat from long bone marrow into the circulation, and then to the lungs and other organs. This does not explain how fat droplets cross the lungs into the systemic circulation to produce CNS effects, or why most patients do not develop the condition despite the common presence of fat droplets in the circulation after long bone injury. Although operative intervention may precipitate fat embolism, trauma studies suggest that early orthopaedic fixation of fractures reduces the overall incidence of clinically significant fat embolism.

Investigations

The diagnosis is often one of exclusion. Fat droplets may be seen in retinal vessels, sputum or urine: none of these findings is specific for the condition. CT scan of the brain is usually normal or shows mild diffuse cerebral oedema; MRI scans show areas of microinfarction in severe cases.

Treatment

Management is essentially supportive. Respiratory insufficiency may progress to severe ARDS. The CNS signs usually settle over time but occasional patients develop severe brain injury, with long-term damage or even death.

LIMB COMPARTMENT SYNDROME

After initial resuscitation, injured areas often become swollen. Swelling of soft tissues in the calf or forearm, where muscle groups are restricted by fascial layers, may result in increased pressure inside the compartments. This restricts blood flow to and from the muscles, which become ischaemic. If left untreated, necrosis, rhabdomyolysis and ischaemic contractures may develop.

Compartment syndrome may be caused by any process that leads to soft-tissue swelling, including infection, haemorrhage or ischaemia. Typical causes are shown in Table 12.2.

Look for swollen, tense and painful muscles (particularly on extension) in the calf and forearm. Remember pain may be masked by epidural/regional anaesthetic blocks. Pulses may be absent but are not invariably so. Compartmental pressure is measured by inserting a 21-gauge (green) needle connected to a flush device and pressure transducer (as for any intravascular monitoring). Pressures greater than 40 mmHg are an indication for fasciotomy and debridement of dead muscle. This can be performed in the ICU. Wounds are left open, and closed subsequently when swelling subsides.

TABLE 12.2 Typical causes of limb compartment syndrome

Forearm fracture
Lower limb fracture
Vascular injury (including surgery)
Pressure from any cause (including crush injury/coma)
Local infection
Local haemorrhage

RHABDOMYOLYSIS

This classically occurs after lower limb crush injury but can occur following injuries to any muscle group or even from necrotic muscle in surgical wounds. It may follow a missed compartment syndrome. It also occurs with prolonged immobility, e.g. following drug overdosage, epilepsy or head injury. Muscle breakdown (rhabdomyolysis) releases toxic products into the circulation. These produce a systemic inflammatory response syndrome, which may progress to multiple organ failure. In addition, myoglobin specifically precipitates in renal tubules and causes ARF.

Management

The management involves prevention, recognition of the problem and supportive care. Measure creatinine kinase (CK), which is usually greater than 5000 units, and urinary myoglobin (rapidly disappears after a few hours). Exclude and treat compartment syndromes and excise dead muscle (amputation may be required).

Myoglobinuria

Fluid loading and diuretics help maintain urine output. An alkaline diuresis may prevent myoglobin precipitation in the renal tubules. Replace the hourly urine output + 50 ml with alternating hours of 1.4% bicarbonate solution and 5% dextrose. In addition give 0.5 g/kg mannitol. Measure serial urine pH and aim to keep in alkaline range. Continue this regimen until resolution of myoglobinuria. (See Forced alkaline diuresis, p. 192.)

Should renal failure occur, supportive treatment is required. Once renal failure is established, the course typically follows that of ATN, with gradual complete recovery of renal function. (See Indications for renal replacement therapy, p. 158.)

BURNS

Patients with extensive burn injuries (> 20% body surface area) are usually managed in regional burns centres. You may, however, be called to help in the initial resuscitation of a burns victim or may be required to manage the patient in the general ICU because of other coexisting problems. A typical chart for the assessment of burn area is shown in Figure 12.2.

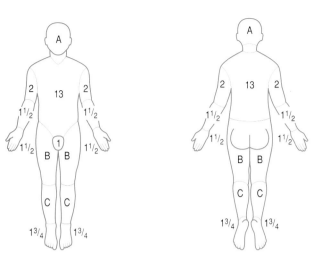

Relative percentage of body surface area affected by growth

Area	Age 0	1	5	10	15	Adult
A=$^1/_2$ of head	$9^1/_2$	$8^1/_2$	$6^1/_2$	$5^1/_2$	$4^1/_2$	$3^1/_2$
B=$^1/_2$ of one thigh	$2^3/_4$	$3^1/_4$	4	$4^1/_2$	$4^1/_2$	$4^3/_4$
C=$^1/_2$ of one leg	$2^1/_2$	$2^1/_2$	$2^3/_4$	3	$3^1/_4$	$3^1/_2$

Fig. 12.2 Assessment of burns. Lund and Browder charts.

Resuscitation

The basic principles of resuscitation of the burn victim are the same as for any other patient. The main problems relate to the potential for thermal injuries to the airway, large fluid losses and potential for infection.

- Give humidified oxygen by face mask. If there are extensive facial burns, or any evidence of thermal injury to the airway, the airway should be secured by endotracheal intubation. This should be performed electively before oedema and swelling make intubation impossible.

TABLE 12.3 Examples of fluid regimens for the resuscitation of burns victims

Mount Vernon formula	Parkland formula
4.5% Albumin	Ringer lactate
Volume (ml) = 0.5 × weight (kg) × % burn	Volume (ml) = 4 × weight (kg) × % burns
Given over six consecutive periods of 4, 4, 4, 6, 6 and 12 hours each	Given over 24 hours

- Establish i.v. access. Where possible, avoid siting cannulae through burned skin, to reduce the risk of infection. (Use ultrasound to guide central venous cannulation if burns are extensive.)
- Give i.v. analgesia and commence fluid resuscitation.

The fluid requirements depend on the size of the burn. This is estimated from the rule of nines or from burns charts. A number of regimens are described for fluid replacement based on either crystalloid or colloid infusion. Examples are shown in Table 12.3.

You should follow local protocols. It is important to realize that such formulae are a guide only and frequently underestimate fluid requirements, particularly if there are other injuries present. The aim of fluid resuscitation is to restore plasma and extracellular volumes and thus adequate tissue and organ perfusion. Urine output and core–peripheral temperature gradient provide a guide. Many burns units avoid central cannulation because of the risk of infection. However, CVP monitoring and pulmonary artery catheterization may be required. If there is a clear clinical indication, these are justifiable.

- Monitor electrolytes and haemoglobin/haematocrit.
- Blood may be required to maintain an Hb > 10 g/dl.
- Circumferential burns may require emergency incision (escharotomy).
- Burns should be covered in sterile drapes or plastic film to reduce infection and fluid loss.
- Major burns may cause SIRS (see p. 277).

Smoke inhalation

Smoke inhalation is common in fires occurring in an enclosed environment, such as house fires. Patients may or may not have accompanying burns. Significant smoke inhalation frequently leads to acute lung injury (see p. 128).

Carbon monoxide and cyanide poisoning

Smoke inhalation may be accompanied by the effects of carbon monoxide and cyanide poisoning (see p. 197).

ELECTROCUTION

Electrocution may occur from the domestic mains supply, from high-tension power supplies or occasionally from a lightning strike. Effects depend upon current strength and duration. These include:

- tachyarrhythmias, particularly ventricular tachycardia, ventricular fibrillation
- asystole
- respiratory arrest secondary to prolonged contraction of the diaphragm
- external burns and internal tissue destruction
- other trauma, e.g. from being thrown clear.

Management is largely supportive:

- Ensure adequate airway and ventilation.
- Appropriate fluid resuscitation for burns and other injuries.
- Manage dysrhythmias appropriately. Check ECG, cardiac enzymes and troponin.
- Early surgical debridement of burns and fasciotomy for compartment syndrome. (See Limb compartment syndrome, p. 267.)
- Management of other injuries as appropriate

NEAR DROWNING

There is no real distinction to be made between the effects of fresh water and salt water drowning. The problems associated are similar in each case. These include:

- hypothermia
- dysrhythmia
- aspiration/acute lung injury
- trauma
- hypoxic brain injury.

The degree of hypoxic brain injury is the main factor in quality of outcome following near drowning. Severe hypothermia can, however,

provide significant brain protection, particularly in children, and
therefore it can be difficult to predict outcomes. Good outcomes can
occasionally be achieved despite prolonged periods of immersion and
prolonged cardiac arrest.

Management
- Ensure adequate airway and ventilation.
- Establish invasive cardiovascular monitoring (arterial line and
  CVP) and support circulation as necessary.
- Treat any dysrhythmias. Actively rewarm and correct electrolyte
  disturbances.
- If evidence of aspiration on CXR, consider broad-spectrum
  antibiotics (seek microbiological advice). Otherwise await cultures.
- Manage acute lung injury as appropriate.
- Look for and manage other injuries as appropriate.

(See also Hypothermia, p. 188.)

OUTCOME AFTER TRAUMA

The outcome following major trauma is critically dependent on the
site of trauma. Significant brain or spinal cord injury greatly increases
the risk of disability and death. There is clear relationship between
increasing number and severity of injuries and death. Age is an
important independent variable. Mortality increases with age and the
very elderly often die after apparently minor chest or long bone injury.
A number of scoring systems have been described in trauma.

Injury Severity Score (ISS)
An anatomical scoring system based on six body areas. For each area
of the body (head and neck; face; chest; abdomen; extremity; skin) an
abbreviated injury score (AIS) from 1 to 6 is assigned (1 = minor
injury; 5 = severe injury; 6 = unsurvivable injury). The abbreviated
injury scores for the three worst affected body areas are squared and
added together to give the ISS. (Any injury which is deemed
unsurvivable (AIS of 6) is assigned an ISS of 75.) The ISS scores
range from 0 to 75 and correlate linearly with outcome.

Revised Trauma Score (RTS)
A physiological scoring system based on the Glasgow Coma Scale,
systolic blood pressure and respiratory rate. Scored from the first set
of observations recorded from the patient. Values range from 0 to
7.8408 (0 = low probability of survival; 7.8408 = high probability of
survival). RTS correlates well with outcome.

Trauma Score – Injury Severity Score (TRISS)

TRISS combines the ISS (anatomical scoring system), RTS (physiological scoring system) together with the patient's age, to predict the probability of surviving either blunt or penetrating trauma. (See also Prediction of outcome, p. 7, and APACHE score, p. 7.)

CHAPTER 13

INFECTION, INFLAMMATION AND MULTIORGAN DYSFUNCTION SYNDROME

INFECTION

Infection is common in the ICU and may be the primary cause of a patient's admission or may occur as a secondary phenomenon in patients who are already critically ill and whose normal barriers to infection are impaired. Factors which predispose to infection in critically ill patients are shown in Table 13.1. (See also Infection control, p. 17, and Stress ulcer prophylaxis, p. 53.)

TABLE 13.1 Factors predisposing to infection in critical illness

Chronic disease states
Effects of acute illness
Effects of sedative and analgesic agents (suppressed cough reflex, GI stasis, etc.)
Endotracheal tube
Vascular catheters, urinary catheters and drains
Increased gastric pH
Poor nutrition and impaired tissue healing
Immune suppressive effects of drugs
Increased risk of cross-infection

INFECTION VERSUS INFLAMMATION

It has been claimed that infection is responsible for up to a quarter of all deaths in intensive care. Early identification of developing infection, drainage/removal of septic foci and the instigation of appropriate antibiotic therapy are therefore vital. Typical signs of infection in critically ill patients include pyrexia, tachycardia, hyperventilation (failure to wean), non-specific deterioration in overall condition and a rise in white cell count. These changes are not specific, however, and similar changes may be produced by any inflammatory process, such as those produced by endotoxaemia, ischaemia reperfusion syndromes, liver failure and pancreatitis.

It is now recognized that many processes (including infection) may trigger activation of endothelial cells, white cells, platelets and other cells, leading to the release of proinflammatory mediators, including platelet-activating factor (PAF), tumour necrosis factor (TNFα), interleukins and other inflammatory cytokines. These have effects such as increased vascular permeability (capillary leak), vasodilatation, and sequestration of neutrophils, platelet adhesion and activation of complement systems. Simultaneous activation of the coagulation and fibrinolytic pathways may lead to disseminated intravascular coagulation (DIC) and failure of the microcirculation.

The inflammatory response produced may range from relatively mild, with minimal sequelae, to severe with resultant multiple organ dysfunction syndrome, multiple organ failure and death. Useful definitions are given below.

SEPSIS, SIRS AND MODS

Systemic inflammatory response syndrome (SIRS)

The systemic inflammatory response syndrome can be said to exist when two of the criteria listed in Table 13.2 are present in the absence of a documented infection.

TABLE 13.2 Definition of SIRS

Requires the presence of two or more of the following features:

Temperature >38°C *or* <36°C
Heart rate >90 beats/min
Respiratory rate >20 breaths/min *or* $PaCO_2$ <4.3 kPa
White blood count >12 000 cells/mm^3 *or* <4000 cells/mm^3 *or* presence of greater than 10% immature neutrophils

---

Sepsis

Features of SIRS together with a documented infection. The infection may be bacterial, viral, fungal, parasitic or other organism. Difficulty may sometimes arise in patients with positive cultures in distinguishing between insignificant colonization and true infection (see below).

Both SIRS and sepsis may vary in severity from mild to severe and both may progress to multiorgan dysfunction. Parallel definitions may be used, as shown in Figure 13.1.

Multiorgan dysfunction syndrome (MODS)

MODS is described as abnormal function of more than one organ such that normal homeostasis cannot be maintained without intervention. In this context 'organ' can be taken to include the respiratory or cardiovascular system, gastrointestinal tract, kidneys, liver, brain (altered conscious level), bone marrow and immune system. MODS may respond to general supportive measures and resolution of the underlying condition or may progress to established multiple organ failure.

SEPTIC SHOCK

The clinical features are those of SIRS, with significant hypotension and end-organ dysfunction (see above). Initially patients may be

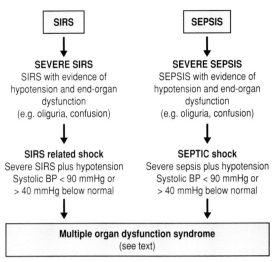

Fig. 13.1 SIRS and sepsis of increasing severity.

hyperdynamic with an elevated CO and reduced systemic vascular resistance, so-called 'warm septic shock'. At this stage patients exhibit warm peripheries, flushing and visible cardiac pulsation. This may rapidly progress, however, to 'cold septic shock' with reduced CO and cold, poorly perfused peripheries. This is frequently accompanied by marked metabolic acidosis.

The first imperatives are resuscitation and stabilization. This is followed by investigation of the underlying source of sepsis. The third stage involves management of specific underlying problems and complications.

Resuscitation
- Give high flow oxygen.
- Consider the need for intubation and ventilation.
- Secure venous access.
- Take blood for culture and give i.v. antibiotics as appropriate.
- Give i.v. fluid challenge.

If end-organ failure is compromising respiration (respiratory failure, severe confusion, etc.), early consideration should be given to securing the airway and instituting artificial ventilation. There is a risk, however, that the drugs used to facilitate intubation may cause circulatory collapse. (See Intubation, p. 337.) Therefore, where ventilation is not required immediately it is often wiser to institute fluid resuscitation and the placement of an arterial line, prior to attempting intubation. Peripheral arterial cannulation is not always feasible and in any case may give a poor guide to central arterial pressures. Consider femoral or brachial cannulation.

Small incremental bolus doses of a catecholamine may be necessary to maintain haemodynamic stability. The drug and dose used will depend on individual circumstances. Consider:

- Adrenaline (epinephrine) 1:10 000. Give 0.5 ml (50 µg) increments.
- Phenylephrine 0.01 mg/ml. Give 0.5 ml (5 µg) increments.

Ongoing management

The principles of managing septic shock are similar to other forms of shock. (See Optimization of the haemodynamic system, p. 61.)

Patients with sepsis and septic shock are often grossly hypovolaemic because of vasodilatation and capillary permeability changes leading to third-space fluid loss. This situation may well be exacerbated by pyrexia and fluid loss related to any underlying pathology. Vigorous fluid resuscitation may, therefore, be required. There is controversy over whether colloid or crystalloid solutions are most appropriate. You should follow local guidelines.

- Give 2–3 litres fluid as initial resuscitation volume (0.9% saline or colloid).
- Establish invasive monitoring, arterial line and CVP. Consider pulmonary artery catheter or alternative (see p. 327).
- Optimize volume loading. Initially aim for a CVP or PAOP of 10–15 mmHg depending on patient's condition and response. Above this level it is unlikely that further fluid loading will produce a further elevation in left ventricular stroke volume index (see p. 66).
- Maintain adequate cardiac output (CI 4–4.5 $1/min/m^2$). Consider addition of an inotrope to increase cardiac output. (See Cardiovascular system, p. 66.)
- Maintain adequate tissue perfusion pressure (MAP ≥ 70 mmHg). If MAP remains low despite adequate volume loading and cardiac output, add a vasoconstrictor, e.g. noradrenaline (norepinephrine).
- Vasopressin levels become rapidly depleted in septic shock. Consider vasopressin infusion at physiological replacement doses (see p. 68).
- If significant metabolic acidosis, pH < 7.1, consider bicarbonate.

- If serum ionized calcium < 0.8 mmol/l, consider calcium supplement.
- If hypotension persists despite resuscitation, consider functional adrenal insufficiency.

Therapeutic end points involve adequate clinical organ and tissue perfusion, e.g. warm pink peripheries, adequate urine output, mentally alert (if not sedated). Ensure all relevant microbiological investigations have been sent and appropriate antibiotics started.

Role of haemofiltration in sepsis

There is anecdotal evidence that the clinical condition of some patients with septic shock may improve significantly when haemofiltration is commenced. This effect is independent of improvements in acid–base status and is possibly due to the removal of proinflammatory mediators. Further studies are awaited. Seek local advice.

Role of anti-inflammatory agents

There has been a great deal of research over recent years on the use of agents to block or modulate the effects of proinflammatory mediators in the inflammatory cascade, in the hope of reducing the inflammatory response to sepsis and improving outcome. Clinical trials of antiendotoxin antibodies, anti-TNFα antibodies and anti-PAF receptor antibodies have failed to show any benefit.

Activated protein C

More recently a worldwide trial of recombinant human activated protein C (PROWESS Trial) has reported an overall 6% reduction in mortality in patients with severe sepsis. While encouraging, further studies are required. Activated protein C is now licensed and available for use in the UK, although its use remains controversial. Follow local protocols and seek senior advice.

Complications

The specific complications and pattern of organ dysfunction will vary from patient to patient. Many patients will require renal support, some may develop prolonged GI tract failure, and a large proportion will develop ARDS or coagulopathy. Some patients will develop multiple organ dysfunction and multiple organ failure. Specific supportive measures for each system are required. (See relevant sections.)

Prognosis

Overall, the mortality from severe sepsis with shock remains high, ranging from 30 to 70% in various studies. Best results are likely to be obtained by early recognition, aggressive resuscitation and attention to detail.

INVESTIGATION OF UNEXPLAINED 'SEPSIS'

Markers of infection

In view of the similarities in the clinical picture produced by SIRS and sepsis, the problem may arise as to how strongly to suspect infection. C-reactive protein (CRP) is a commonly used marker of infection but is not specific. Procalcitonin is an alternative marker that is thought to be more specific for infection.

Investigations

Any patient in the ICU with unexplained 'sepsis' or rising markers of infection should have a thorough examination to identify possible sources. Appropriate microbiological samples should be obtained prior to the institution of antibiotic therapy. These should ideally include 'clean stab' blood cultures from a peripheral vein (in addition to cultures from any existing cannulae), sputum or BAL for microscopy and culture. Urine and any drain fluids should also be cultured. Critically ill patients who develop new episodes of sepsis may have catheter-related infections. Consider changing existing arterial and venous lines and send the tips for culture. (See catheter-related sepsis below.)

Additional investigations will be guided by the clinical picture and may include those listed in Table 13.3.

Intra-abdominal sepsis

Intra-abdominal causes of sepsis account for a significant number of cases of unexplained sepsis. Abdominal ultrasound and CT scan are likely to be the most valuable investigation. If pus or abscesses are confirmed, these should be drained and cultured. In the absence of an identifiable cause of sepsis, and in the face of a deteriorating clinical picture, laparotomy may be warranted. Seek senior advice and a surgical opinion. (See Acalculous cholecystitis, p. 140, and Pancreatitis, p. 149.)

Pyrexia of unknown origin

If the cause of sepsis is not apparent, consider investigation for other causes of pyrexia. Pyrexia of unknown origin may be associated with myocardial infarction, autoimmune inflammatory processes (autoantibodies and vasculitic screen), malignancy, drugs and rare infectious diseases. Seek advice.

TABLE 13.3 Investigation of unexplained sepsis	
Apparent source	*Investigation*
Catheter-related	Blood cultures form catheters/peripheral stab
	Request differential cultures
	Change indwelling vascular catheters and culture tips
Embolic	Serial blood cultures
	Precordial or transoesophageal echocardiography
Chest	CXR
	Tracheal aspirates culture
	Bronchoscopy + BAL
	Tap and culture pleural fluid
	CT scan
Abdomen and pelvis	Amylase
	Culture drain fluids (fresh samples)
	Tap and culture ascites
	Plain abdominal X-ray
	Abdominal and pelvic ultrasound/CT scan
	Laparotomy
Urinary tract	Urine microscopy and culture
	Plain abdominal film/ultrasound/CT renal tract
Wounds/soft tissues	Pus/tissue/swabs for culture
	Re-exploration
CNS	CT scan/MRI scan for spine and soft tissues
	Lumbar puncture
Joints	X-ray/ultrasound/CT scan
	Needle aspiration
Sinuses	X-ray/ultrasound/CT scan

EMPIRICAL ANTIBIOTIC THERAPY

In general, unless patients are at high risk (e.g. immunocompromised), antibiotic therapy is best withheld until a positive microbiological diagnosis is made. In up to 50% of cases of severe sepsis and septic shock, however, no positive microbiological sample is ever obtained and antibiotics may have to be started on an empirical basis. Table 13.4 is a guide only. You should follow your hospital antibiotic policy or ask advice from your hospital microbiologist.

TABLE 13.4 Empirical first-line antibiotic therapy in sepsis

Source	Common pathogens	Suggested antibiotic
Community-acquired pneumonia	*Strep. pneumoniae* *H. influenzae*	Cefuroxime
Including possible atypical pneumonia	*Legionella* *Mycoplasma* *Chlamydia* *Coxiella*	Cefuroxime and clarithromycin
	If *Staph. aureus**	Add flucloxacillin
Nosocomial pneumonia	*Strep. pneumoniae* *H. influenzae*	Cefuroxime (If previously treated ciprofloxacin or ceftazidime)
	Enterobacteria	
Intra-abdominal sepsis	Staphylococci Enterobacteria Anaerobes	Cefuroxime and metronidazole
Pelvic infection	Anaerobes Enterobacteria	Cefuroxime and metronidazole or carbapenem
Urinary tract	*Escherichia coli* Proteus species Klebsiella species	Cefuroxime or gentamicin
Wound infection	*Staph. aureus** Streptococci Enterobacteria	Amoxicillin, flucloxacillin (add metronidazole for traumatic wounds)
Necrotizing fascititis	Mixed synergistic flora	Benzylpenicillin, gentamicin and metronidazole
	If group A strep.	Benzylpenicillin + clindamycin
i.v. line sepsis (remove line)	*Staph. aureus** Coag. neg. staph.* Streptococci Enterococci Gram-neg. species	Flucloxacillin and ceftazidime
Meningitis	*Neisseria meningitidis* *Strep. pneumoniae* *H. influenzae*	Cefotaxime

*If MRSA or Coag. neg. staph. possible, consider vancomycin (see below).

PROBLEM ORGANISMS

> Always seek advice from microbiologists and hospital
> infection control teams who will be aware of local resistance
> patterns and advise on infection control procedures.

GRAM-POSITIVE ORGANISMS

Methicillin-resistant *Staphylococcus aureus* (MRSA)

Colonization of skin and wounds with MRSA is increasingly
common. Patients are usually isolated in side rooms and barrier
nursed to prevent cross-infection. Eradication can be difficult and
antibiotic treatment is often pointless. The patient's flora will
generally change over time as the condition improves.

If treatment is required, vancomycin or teicoplanin are usually the
antibiotics of choice. Alternatively, combinations of synergistic agents
can be used.

Coagulase-negative staphylococci

Coagulase-negative staphylococci (e.g. *Staph. epidermidis*) are part of
the normal skin flora. They adhere to plastic devices and commonly
colonize indwelling central venous lines. They may cause systemic
infection and are often multiply resistant to antibiotics. If suspected,
remove or change indwelling lines and discuss with a microbiologist.
Community-acquired strains may be sensitive to flucloxacillin but
vancomycin or teicoplanin are often required.

Enterococci and vancomycin-resistant enterococci (VRE)

Enterococci are part of the normal flora of the GI tract and female
genital tract, but in ICU patients they may be responsible for
bacteraemia, endocarditis, urinary tract and wound infections. They
are usually sensitive to ampicillin or a combination of ampicillin and
aminoglycoside but there is increasing incidence of antibiotic
resistance. Vancomycin-resistant enterococci are an increasing
concern.

Clostridium difficile

Anaerobic Gram-positive bacillus. Main cause of antibiotic-associated
'pseudomembranous colitis', following broad-spectrum antibiotics.
Presents with profuse diarrhoea (may be blood-stained). *Clostridium
difficile* toxin can be identified in stools. Treatment is with oral (or
i.v.) metronidazole or vancomycin.

GRAM-NEGATIVE ORGANISMS

Escherichia coli, Klebsiella and coliforms

These Gram-negative bacteria are normal commensals in the gastrointestinal tract but are a significant cause of infection on the ICU. They typically infect the respiratory tract, urinary tract and wounds, and may lead to bacteraemia, septicaemia and septic shock. Cephalosporins can be used as first-line treatment, but again there is increasing antibiotic resistance. Seek advice.

Pseudomonas species

The overall incidence of *Pseudomonas* infection in ICUs seems to be declining; however, it remains a serious problem, particularly affecting the respiratory tract. Antibiotic resistance is widespread, but aminoglycosides, ceftazidime, imipenem and ciprofloxacin are useful agents.

Acinetobacter species

Widespread in the environment. They are increasingly recognized as an important pathogen in ICU patients, particularly causing respiratory tract and wound infection and occasionally bacteraemia. They are often multiply resistant to antibiotics.

FUNGAL INFECTIONS

Fungal infection on the ICU is increasingly recognized, particularly among patients who are immune compromised and who have received multiple courses of broad-spectrum antibiotics. *Candida albicans* is the most common species. Diagnosis is difficult, but the presence of topical *Candida* infection at more than one site (e.g. oral, genital, wounds) should raise suspicion of systemic candidiasis. Fungi grow poorly in conventional blood culture bottles, and serological markers (e.g. *Candida, Aspergillus* antigen and antibody tests) may be helpful, although this may not distinguish colonization from infection. Empirical treatment with antifungals may be appropriate.

CATHETER-RELATED SEPSIS

Catheter-related sepsis is a common problem on the ICU and should be considered in all patients with suspected sepsis in whom vascular catheters have been in place for more than 48 hours.

Following catheter insertion, thrombus forms around the puncture site of the vessel and may propagate along the length of the catheter.

This provides an excellent culture medium for bacteria, which may rapidly colonize all catheters either via the puncture site in the skin or following bacteraemia. In addition, catheters may be colonized by bacteria introduced via the access ports when the catheter is used, for example to administer drugs.

Colonization is common and does not necessarily warrant removal of the catheter or treatment. Infection is difficult to diagnose. Cultures taken through the catheter do not distinguish between colonization, infection and unrelated bacteraemia. Brush specimens taken from the lumen of the line are semiquantitive and can suggest infection. Alternatively, paired cultures can be taken from the suspect catheter and from a peripheral vein (clean stab), and the shorter time taken for development of positive cultures from the catheter used to suggest the presence of catheter-related infection.

If there is a strong suspicion of catheter-related sepsis the catheter should be removed and the tip cut off (sterile scissors) and sent for culture. In most cases the diagnosis is made retrospectively after removal of the suspect catheter, positive tip culture and resolution of the clinical condition.

- Ideally catheters should be replaced at a new clean puncture site.
- Ideally there should be a 'line-free' interval between removing and replacing catheters but this is often impractical.
- If necessary, provided the entry site is not obviously infected, catheters can be changed over a guide wire at the same site. This should only be considered when a clean puncture site is not available or is high risk.
- There is no evidence that changing catheters on a regular basis (e.g. 7 days) is of any benefit.

NECROTIZING FASCIITIS

This is a rapidly spreading soft-tissue infection, which often follows relatively minor trauma. It may be caused by a synergistic infection with a mixture of Gram-negative and anaerobic organisms (e.g. *Bacteroides* species, *Clostridium* species and anaerobic streptococci) or by infection with group A streptococcus alone. Infection spreads along fascial planes causing necrosis of skin and subcutaneous tissues. Muscle layers are usually spared. The infection may spread rapidly and can be fatal within a few hours. Treatment is by urgent surgical excision of necrotic and infected tissue together with appropriate antibiotics. Seek microbiological advice. (See also Empirical antibiotic therapy, p. 282.)

MENINGOCOCCAL SEPSIS

Neisseria meningitidis is a Gram-negative diplococcus, which approximately 10% of the population carry as a nasal commensal. It causes a spectrum of illness from meningitis (without systemic sepsis) to a severe septicaemia illness with multiple organ failure and death.

Although meningococcal sepsis is more common in paediatric intensive care, occasional cases occur in young adults. It can be a devastating illness resulting in death within a few hours. You should always seek senior help.

Diagnosis

Early symptoms of systemic infection include fever (often > 40°C), arthralgia, myalgia, headache and vomiting. The diagnosis of meningococcal sepsis is made on the basis of the typical non-blanching purpuric rash together with evidence of hypotension, tachycardia and poor perfusion.

> ⚠ **The diagnosis of meningococcal sepsis is based initially on clinical signs. Life-saving antibiotic treatment (cefotaxime or benzylpenicillin) and resuscitation should be commenced immediately. This must not be delayed by investigations.**

Management

- Antibiotics should be given as soon as the diagnosis is suspected.
- Give high-flow oxygen by face mask. May require intubation and ventilation. Beware of cardiovascular collapse!
- Establish i.v. access. Give fluids, crystalloid/colloid, to support the circulation. Large volumes are usually required to maintain blood pressure and improve peripheral circulation.
- Establish invasive arterial blood pressure monitoring, CVP/pulmonary artery catheter or alternative.
- Commence inotropes as required. Typically adrenaline (epinephrine) is first-line.
- Peripheral and digital ischaemia. If blood pressure is adequate consider epoprostenol (prostacyclin) infusion 5–10 ng/kg/min. This improves microvascular perfusion and may reduce risks of digital ischaemia.
- Coagulopathy and DIC are common. Send coagulation screen. Avoid giving FFP, platelets and cryoprecipitate unless there is active bleeding as these may increase the tendency to microvascular thrombosis and worsen digital ischaemia.

- Hypocalcaemia is common. Consider calcium bolus and possible calcium infusion.
- Metabolic acidosis is normal. This will improve as the patient's condition improves. Do not give bicarbonate unless extreme (pH < 7.1) or inotropes ineffective.
- There is no evidence for the routine use of steroids in meningococcal shock but if adrenal insufficiency is suspected then replacement steroid therapy is appropriate. (This is in contrast to meningococcal meningitis in which recent evidence suggests that steroids are of benefit. See Meningitis, p. 244.) Waterhouse–Friderichsen syndrome (adrenal haemorrhage/infarction) is rare and is usually a postmortem finding.
- Activated protein C may have a specific beneficial role in meningococcal sepsis in reducing the microvascular thrombosis and tissue ischaemia. As yet this is unproven, trials are currently ongoing. (See Activated protein C, p. 280.)

There is increasing use of haemofiltration and plasma exchange in meningococcal sepsis to remove endotoxin, cytokines and other factors, in an attempt to improve overall survival and also to reduce the incidence of sequelae such as digital ischaemia. The benefits of these treatments are as yet not proven. You should seek senior advice.

Microbiological diagnosis
Although treatment is based on clinical suspicion, it is helpful to attempt to establish a microbiological diagnosis. Blood should be sent for culture and polymerase chain reaction (PCR). Skin lesions should be scraped onto a glass slide for microscopy and sent for culture. Seek microbiological advice.

Antibiotics
Meningococcus is usually sensitive to benzylpenicillin in the UK; however, other severe infections, most notably pneumococcal sepsis, may occasionally produce a similar clinical picture and purpuric rash, so high-dose cefotaxime is the first-line agent of choice. When meningococcal disease is confirmed later and the sensitivities are known, benzylpenicillin may be substituted. Neither of these antibiotics eradicates nasal carriage of meningococcus and the patient should receive rifampicin or ciprofloxacin for this purpose during the recovery phase. (See Prophylaxis below.)

Prophylaxis
Most cases of meningococcal disease are sporadic and 'outbreaks' of infection are rare. However, the index patient, direct family contacts

and other close contacts require prophylactic treatment with rifampicin (or ciprofloxacin) to abolish nasal carriage of meningococcus. This is organized by the public health department and the case should be reported to them as soon as possible. (See Notifiable infectious diseases below.)

It is generally considered that there is no need for medical or nursing staff involved in the care of these patients to receive prophylaxis unless direct contamination has occurred.

NOTIFIABLE INFECTIOUS DISEASES

In the UK there is a statutory duty to report a number of infectious diseases to the public health services. This is either to enable disease surveillance or because of the broad risk posed to contacts or the public generally. Notifiable infectious diseases are shown in Table 13.5.

TABLE 13.5 Notifiable infectious diseases

Relatively common in UK	Uncommon in UK
Acute encephalitis	Acute poliomyelitis
Food poisoning	Anthrax
Leptospirosis	Cholera
Measles	Diphtheria
Meningitis	Dysentery
Meningococcal septicaemia	Malaria
Mumps	Paratyphoid fever
Ophthalmia neonatorum	Plague
Rubella	Rabies
Scarlet fever	Relapsing fever
Tetanus	Smallpox
Tuberculosis	Severe acute respiratory syndrome (SARS)
Viral hepatitis	Yellow fever
Whooping cough	Typhoid fever
	Typhus fever
	Viral haemorrhagic fever

POSTOPERATIVE AND OBSTETRIC PATIENTS

THE POSTOPERATIVE PERIOD

Patients are frequently admitted to ICU following prolonged or complex surgery for a period of monitoring, ventilation, cardiovascular support and stabilization, prior to discharge to a high-dependency area or ward. Admission to the ICU may be planned, due to pre-existing disease and/or the nature of the surgery, or may be unplanned as a result of unexpected difficulties in the perioperative period or the emergency nature of the surgery.

Problems in the postoperative period may include the effects of prolonged surgery, massive fluid/blood loss, delayed recovery from anaesthesia and the effects of the stress response to surgery and trauma.

Perioperative optimization

There is ongoing interest in so-called 'perioperative optimization' of cardiovascular variables in order to minimize the physiological disturbances and stress responses caused by surgery. In some centres patients may be admitted to ICU or HDU preoperatively, invasive haemodynamic monitoring instituted and fluids and inotropes used judiciously to optimize the cardiovascular system. The process is similar to that described previously in Chapter 4. (See Optimization of cardiovascular system, p. 61) There is some evidence that perioperative optimization reduces perioperative complications and reduces the need for unplanned ICU admission (or length of ICU stay) after major surgery.

COMMON POSTOPERATIVE PROBLEMS

Effects of prolonged surgery

Anaesthesia and surgery may be prolonged because of the extensive nature of the procedure or because of technical complexity. Problems may include hypothermia, atelectasis, dehydration and fluid loss, anaesthetic drug accumulation, and the effects of pressure, including the development of compartment syndromes. (See Hypothermia, p. 185, and Compartment syndrome, p. 267.)

Delayed recovery of consciousness

The causes of delayed recovery of consciousness following anaesthesia are often multifactorial. It may be impossible initially to determine which is the predominant problem. Typical causes are shown in Table 14.1.

Most patients with delayed recovery of consciousness will require a period of supportive care on ICU. CT scan of the brain and EEG

TABLE 14.1 Causes of delayed recovery from anaesthesia

Residual effects of anaesthetic drugs
Hypoxia
Hypercarbia
Hypotension
Hypoglycaemia
Metabolic encephalopathy
Hypothermia
TIA/CVA

may be helpful to identify pathological causes. In most cases the problem will resolve gradually over hours or days.

Prolonged neuromuscular block

Muscle relaxants are used extensively in anaesthesia to facilitate tracheal intubation, provide relaxation for surgical procedures, and allow lighter planes of general anaesthesia. In the ICU, patients are usually left to clear muscle relaxants without use of reversal agents. Following anaesthesia, the recovery of neuromuscular function is often hastened by the use of anticholinesterase drugs (e.g. neostigmine). These increase the concentration of acetylcholine at the neuromuscular junction and reverse the effects of non-depolarizing neuromuscular blocking drugs (competitive antagonists at the acetylcholine receptor). They are used in combination with glycopyrrolate, which reduces the undesirable (muscarinic) effects of acetylcholine. Typical doses are:

● neostigmine 2.5 mg + glycopyrrolate 0.5 mg.

Problems relating to residual neuromuscular blockade have become less common since the introduction of newer shorter-acting drugs like atracurium. Occasionally, however, there may be delayed recovery of neuromuscular function. Factors which may contribute to this are shown in Table 14.2.

TABLE 14.2 Factors contributing to delayed recovery neuromuscular blockade

Elderly, frail, medically unfit patients
Relative overdose
Renal or liver dysfunction
Underlying neuromuscular disease
Effects of ether drugs (e.g. aminoglycosides)
Electrolyte abnormalities
Hypothermia

Patients exhibit jerky movements, make poor respiratory effort and have marked fade on train of four. (See Muscle relaxants, p. 37.)

- Give oxygen. Support ventilation if necessary.
- If the patient has some neuromuscular function it may be appropriate to administer a second dose of reversal agent and reassess the situation.
- If this fails to improve the situation or if there is minimal neuromuscular function, the patient should be resedated, intubated and ventilated until return of neuromuscular function. Remember to explain to the patient what is happening. He or she may be paralysed but aware of the surroundings.

Hereditary cholinesterase deficiency (1:3000 population) is a specific cause of delayed recovery of neuromuscular function resulting from the delayed metabolism of suxamethonium (and mivacurium). Muscle function usually returns in 2–6 hours. FFP repletes cholinesterase and speeds return of motor power, but is not usually necessary. Send blood to regional centre for identification of particular pattern of cholinesterase deficiency. (See Suxamethonium, p. 37.)

Airway obstruction

Common in the immediate postoperative period while patients are still in the recovery room and the effects of anaesthetic drugs wear off. Usually transient and not severe and can be managed by support of the chin, jaw thrust or the use of an artificial airway (e.g. oral Guedel airway or nasal airway). More severe or prolonged cases or those with associated respiratory depression may require intubation and ventilation.

Following surgical procedures in the neck (e.g. thyroidectomy), postoperative bleeding into the tissues of the neck may occasionally produce airway obstruction by direct compression. In an emergency, you should open the surgical wound and decompress the bleeding to relieve pressure on the airway. The wound can then be formally explored by a surgeon in order to achieve haemostasis. If this fails to relieve the problem the patient will require intubation.

Patients with fractured mandibles frequently have their jaws wired together to ensure correct dental occlusion while the fracture heals. These patients should only be extubated once full consciousness and respiratory effort has returned. They are often admitted to intensive care in the immediate postoperative period for observation and monitoring. If airway obstruction occurs (e.g. due to vomiting), you should cut the wires to gain access to the airway and manage the situation as appropriate. (See Airway obstruction, p. 113.)

Respiratory insufficiency

Postoperative respiratory insufficiency may be predictable in patients with pre-existing respiratory disease and this may be an indication for elective postoperative ventilation. In other patients respiratory insufficiency may arise for a number of reasons and the problem is often multifactorial. Typical causes are shown in Table 14.3.

Many of these problems are resolved by a short period of ventilation in the ICU combined with simple measures. (See also Respiratory failure, p. 96.)

TABLE 14.3 Causes of postoperative respiratory insufficiency

Residual effects of anaesthetic drugs
Residual effects of neuromuscular blockade
Airway obstruction
Bronchospasm
Pre-existing respiratory disease
Pulmonary collapse/consolidation/ARDS
Pneumothorax
Pulmonary oedema
Cardiovascular instability
Sepsis
Hypothermia

Cardiovascular instability

Cardiovascular instability may arise due to pre-existing cardiovascular disease, from the predictable effects of the surgery, particularly when large fluid losses are expected, or as a result of untoward cardiovascular events. Typical causes are shown in Table 14.4.

Many of these problems are solved by simple attention to details of fluid balance as the patient warms up after surgery. More difficult cases may require full invasive monitoring and cardiovascular support. (See Optimizing haemodynamic status, p. 61.)

TABLE 14.4 Causes of postoperative CVS instability

Pre-existing CVS disease
Myocardial ischaemia/infarction
Myocardial depression (effects of drugs/sepsis, etc.)
Fluid losses and bleeding
Fluid overload
Effects of drugs
Effects of epidural/spinal anaesthesia
Sepsis
Hypothermia

Oliguria

Oliguria in the postoperative patient is often multifactorial, with cardiovascular instability, hypovolaemia and the stress response to surgery all contributing. This often improves with fluid loading as the patient rewarms and haemodynamic stability improves. (See Oliguria p. 155, and Stress response to surgery and critical illness, p. 298.)

ICU MANAGEMENT OF THE POSTOPERATIVE PATIENT

The postoperative admission of patients to intensive care allows for:

- controlled recovery from the effects of anaesthesia and surgery
- a period of rewarming
- optimization of respiratory function and controlled weaning from ventilation
- optimization of cardiovascular function
- monitoring of other organ function, e.g. renal output
- adequate analgesia.

When an elective postoperative patient is admitted to the ICU you should be sure that the management plan is agreed with the referring anaesthetist and surgeon. A typical approach is given below:

- Continue ventilation.
- Maintain sedation and analgesia by infusion using short-acting drugs such as propofol and alfentanil. Muscle relaxants are generally discontinued unless there is an indication to continue them.
- Assess the patient fully and decide on priorities for management. Send blood for FBC, clotting screen, U&Es and arterial blood gases. Correct abnormalities as necessary.
- Rewarm patient using warm-air blanket if necessary. As temperature increases, the peripheral circulation will open up (reduction in core–peripheral temperature gradient). Give fluid (colloid or blood) as necessary to maintain adequate circulating volume.
- Metabolic acidosis usually improves as the patient rewarms and circulation improves. Persistent metabolic acidosis usually indicates either inadequate fluid resuscitation or ongoing tissue ischaemia (e.g. gut) requiring further investigation.
- Any inotropes/vasopressors can be gradually reduced as the patient's condition improves.

The aim is to achieve a warm, cardiovascular stable patient, requiring minimal inotropic support, with minimal fluid/blood requirements, adequate urine output and satisfactory arterial blood gases. Depending on the premorbid condition of the patient and the nature of the surgery, this can often be achieved over 6–24 hours. Sedation can then be reduced and the patient woken up and extubated as appropriate.

Aortic aneurysm repair

Following elective aortic aneurysm repair, patients can generally be allowed to warm up and extubate after a few hours as described above. Emergency aneurysm repairs may be more unstable and the management will depend upon individual circumstances. Control of blood pressure is important. This should be maintained at a level which is normal for the patient to ensure adequate perfusion of vital organs, in particular the kidneys. At the same time significant hypertension should be controlled to prevent undue strain on both the myocardium and the vascular anastomosis. This may require use of nifedipine or GTN infusion, especially during the phase of emergence from sedation. Renal dysfunction is common, particularly after suprarenal cross-clamping of the aorta. Spinal cord ischaemia and lower limb paralysis may also occur.

Persistent ischaemia of the lower limbs despite optimization of haemodynamic status may require embolectomy or exploration of the graft. Persistent or worsening metabolic acidosis may indicate gut ischaemia. Seek surgical opinion. (See Hypertension, p. 72.)

Free tissue transfer (free flap)

The management of patients following free tissue transfer is similar to that described above. In addition, however, the adequate perfusion and survival of the graft is paramount.

The normal mechanisms controlling blood flow in the grafted tissue are inactive. The circulation to the graft is essentially passive and depends predominately on the flow through the feeding vessels. Therefore, colloid should be used to maintain the patient's circulation as full as possible. This should be balanced, however, against the deleterious effects of increased oedema in the graft, caused by increased endothelial permeability resulting from reperfusion injury and the absence of lymphatic drainage. Fluid management should therefore be guided by CVP, urine output and core–peripheral temperature gradient. The usual response to any deterioration in these parameters should be to give further fluid.

At the same time the denervated vessels of the graft are highly sensitive to circulating catecholamines (endogenous or exogenous). Adequate analgesia is, therefore, essential. The patient should be kept as warm as possible and inotropes/vasopressor agents should be avoided except in extremis. Inodilators such as dopexamine may be of value in improving graft blood flow and survival. Seek advice.

If despite these measures graft perfusion appears impaired (dusky/congested/swollen), call the surgical team immediately. The vascular pedicles and anastomosis may need surgical exploration.

Transplants

Transplants are a special form of free tissue transfer. The principles are similar to those described above, with particular management issues depending on the particular organ involved. These procedures are only carried out in specialist centres and you should seek senior advice.

STRESS RESPONSE TO SURGERY AND CRITICAL ILLNESS

The local and systemic inflammatory responses to tissue injury and illness vary between patients and may vary from mild pyrexia to systemic inflammatory response syndrome (SIRS), multiple organ failure and death. The clinical magnitude of this response depends in part on the extent of the injury, although other factors including infection, immune status, genetic predisposition and physiological reserve are also important. In addition to these inflammatory responses mediated by cytokines, there are a number of physiological hormonal and metabolic responses to injury and critical illness, which are collectively known as the stress response. (See SIRS and MODS, p. 277.)

Hormonal responses

The secretion of the pituitary hormones antidiuretic hormone (ADH), adrenocorticotrophin (ACTH) and growth hormone (GH) is increased. ADH causes salt and water retention and also has vasopressor activity. ACTH leads to increased secretion of adrenal corticosteroids, cortisol and aldosterone, which further lead to salt and water retention. Growth hormone has a hyperglycaemic effect but this effect is variable.

There is a generalized increase in sympathetic activity and the adrenal secretion of catecholamines adrenaline (epinephrine) and noradrenaline (norepinephrine) is increased. These have predictable cardiovascular effects. Adrenaline also has metabolic effects, most notably hyperglycaemia. Increased production of renin from the kidney leads to activation of the renin–angiotensin–aldosterone pathway. Angiotensin II is a potent vasoconstrictor which increases blood pressure, while aldosterone increases renal salt and water retention.

Metabolic effects

The primary metabolic effects of the stress response are those of salt and water retention and catabolism. Salt and water retention is multifactorial in origin. The degree of water retention may exceed that of sodium retention, such that hyponatraemia is common.

Catabolic effects of catecholamines, steroids and growth hormone include increased glycogenolysis and gluconeogenesis resulting in hyperglycaemia. Endogenous insulin production is increased in response but an insulin infusion is often required to control the blood sugar. Fat and protein are broken down to provide energy substrates for tissue repair.

Role of the stress response

The stress response has evolved to provide survival advantages following severe injury or during critical illness. There is evidence that those that fail to mount an appropriate physiological response to critical illness have a poor outcome despite maximal support (e.g. elderly patients following trauma, burns or minor head injury). At times, however, the stress responses can be detrimental. For example, exaggerated cardiovascular responses can lead to myocardial ischaemia and impaired tissue perfusion. Increased salt and water retention can lead to oliguria. Extreme catabolic responses can lead to severe wasting. For these reasons there has been a great deal of interest in attempting to reduce the stress response.

The most important factors in reducing the stress response are ensuring good quality anaesthesia, where possible preventing or minimizing tissue injury (e.g. laparoscopic surgery), careful fluid resuscitation, and good postoperative pain relief. (See Postoperative analgesia below.)

POSTOPERATIVE ANALGESIA

Patient-controlled analgesia (PCAS)

These techniques are extensively used to provide analgesia particularly in postoperative patients. Typically the patient will be established on such a device prior to transfer to a general ward. Although not intended for operation by nurses, they have been used safely and conveniently in this way in an ICU setting.

Care should be taken in setting devices up; a dedicated line or non-return valve should be used. There have been a number of

TABLE 14.5 Typical PCAS regimen

50 mg morphine in 50 ml 0.9% saline
1 mg bolus
5-minute lockout time
No background infusion

problems due to excessive background dosing, surges of morphine on unblocking i.v. lines, and siphoning of contents under gravity from syringes. Avoid background infusions if possible. Position syringe drivers below the level of the patient to avoid siphoning and use antireflux valves on giving sets. A typical PCAS regimen is shown in Table 14.5.

Regional blockade

An increasing number of patients undergoing major surgery have analgesia provided by the epidural and spinal route. These techniques may also be used to relieve pain from trauma (e.g. fractured ribs) and ischaemic limbs.

Potential advantages include the avoidance of centrally acting sedative analgesic drugs, resulting in awake, co-operative and pain-free patients, better able to cough and clear airway secretions. In addition, in patients with ischaemic limbs, neuroaxial blockade (which includes sympathetic blockade) may provide both analgesia and improvement in perfusion of the ischaemic limb.

Detailed description of epidural techniques is beyond the scope of this book. When a patient is admitted with an epidural catheter in situ you should make sure that you confirm the analgesic regimen with the responsible anaesthetist. Local anaesthetic and opioid drugs may be used alone or in combination. Typical regimens are:

- bupivacaine 0.01–0.25% by infusion at 5–10 ml/h
- ± fentanyl 4 µg/ml.

If breakthrough pain occurs and the patient is otherwise stable give a 5–8 ml bolus of the epidural solution (or 0.25% plain bupivacaine) and then increase the infusion rate. This is normally effective within 10–15 minutes. Beware of hypotension.

> ⚠️ **Great care must be taken to avoid injection of the wrong drugs or wrong doses into epidural catheters. If you are not familiar with epidural techniques, seek help.**

TABLE 14.6 Complications of epidural blockade

Local anaesthetics	Opioids
Potential local anaesthetic toxicity	Itching
Hypotension (sympathetic blockade)	CNS depression including
Muscle weakness (including respiration)	apnoea
Bradycardia (block >T4 level)	Urinary retention
Urine retention	Nausea and vomiting
Complete or high spinal block (cardiovascular collapse, respiratory paralysis, loss of consciousness)	

Complications of epidural blockade

The complications of epidural blockade are shown in Table 14.6.

- Hypotension usually responds to fluid loading (500 ml colloid) and reducing the rate of epidural infusion. If significant hypotension develops, reduce or stop infusion and consider use of vasopressors.
- Muscle weakness is often unavoidable. If the block is too high (e.g. involving arms), reduce the rate of infusion and/or reduce the concentration of local anaesthetic. If respiratory muscle weakness occurs, ventilation may be necessary until the effects of the local anaesthetic wear off.
- At the doses used, the addition of opioids to epidural infusion may significantly improve analgesia without significant increase in the side effect profile. Nausea and itching may be helped by low-dose naloxone without loss of analgesia. CNS depression may require ventilation.
- Epidural techniques carry a small but serious risk of epidural haematoma or abscess formation, which unrecognized can lead to spinal cord compression and paralysis. In routine practice this risk is very small. In ICU patients, however, the risk may be higher because of the effects of coagulopathy and sepsis. The magnitude of this risk is unquantifiable, although overall it remains very low.

ANAPHYLACTOID REACTIONS

Anaphylactoid is a term which encompasses all life-threatening acute 'allergic' reactions, regardless of their exact pathogenesis. It includes true immune-mediated type 1 or anaphylactic hypersensitivity reactions. These reactions are relatively uncommon and are clearly not confined to the perioperative period. Causes include nut allergy and bee stings. In the hospital setting, however, drugs, contrast media, intravenous colloid solutions and latex are common precipitating agents.

Clinical manifestations

The onset of symptoms may occur within 1–2 minutes of exposure to the precipitating agent or may be delayed up to 1–2 hours and may be modified by the effects of general or regional anaesthesia. The clinical manifestations include:

- cutaneous flushing urticaria, angio-oedema
- abdominal pain, nausea, vomiting and diarrhoea
- laryngeal oedema, bronchospasm, increased airway pressure
- acute pulmonary oedema
- tachycardia, hypotension, cardiac arrest.

Life-saving treatment depends on early recognition and appropriate management. The differential diagnoses are given in Table 14.7.

> ⚠ **A spectrum of reactions exists, from mild hypotension with bronchospasm to profound shock and cardiac arrest. Response must be measured against the condition of the patient.**

Management

- Stop precipitating drugs.
- Give oxygen. If airway compromised by facial oedema, laryngeal oedema or bronchospasm, secure airway by endotracheal intubation as soon as possible. Ventilate and commence external cardiac massage if necessary.
- Establish i.v. access if not already done, and give rapid fluid load, e.g. 2–4 litres crystalloid or colloid (remember that synthetic colloids may be the cause of the reaction!).
- Give adrenaline (epinephrine) titrated against response:
  — 0.5–1.0 mg i.m. or 50–100 µg bolus i.v. for moderate hypotension

---

TABLE 14.7 Differential diagnosis of anaphylactoid reactions

Vasovagal reaction
Dysrhythmia
Myocardial infarction
Effects of drugs (including illicit drugs)
Pulmonary embolism
Bronchospasm
Pulmonary oedema
Aspiration
Hereditary angioneurotic oedema
Idiopathic urticaria
Carcinoid tumours

   — 0.5–1.0 mg bolus i.v. for profound collapse, followed by
     adrenaline infusion.

- Establish central venous, pulmonary artery and arterial catheterization when appropriate. Take blood (EDTA and serum) for later analysis.
- Measure arterial blood gases. If significant acidosis consider 50–100 mmol sodium bicarbonate. (See Metabolic acidosis, p. 176.)
- If persistent bronchospasm consider:
  — nebulized salbutamol 2.5–5 mg
  — aminophylline 5 mg/kg i.v. (loading dose) followed by 0.5 mg/kg/h.
- Glucocorticoids may reduce late sequelae. Consider:
  — hydrocortisone 200 mg followed by 50 mg 6-hourly
  — methylprednisolone 1 mg/kg initially repeated every 6 hours.
- Antihistamines are of no proven benefit.
- Following resuscitation these patients should be managed in the ICU. Late reactions can result in clinical deterioration even some hours after initial stabilization. Cancel surgery/other interventional procedures unless life-saving.

Evaluation of cause of anaphylactoid reactions

Following an anaphylactoid reaction it is important to try and establish the cause so that future reactions may be avoided. Take a detailed history of this and other previous allergic reactions. Blood samples taken as soon after the reaction as possible and at regular intervals thereafter can be analysed for immune markers, including antibodies (IGE), complement and mediator levels. These may help elucidate the nature of the reaction rather than the causative agent. Radioallergosorbent tests (RAST) and interval skin-prick testing may determine the causative agent but this is often inconclusive.

- Seek advice from laboratory services/immunology department.

It is essential that patients and their relatives are made aware of the reaction. In the case of nut allergy or bee sting anaphylaxis, patients are now given prefilled adrenaline (epinephrine) injectors for emergency use.

MALIGNANT HYPERPYREXIA

Malignant hyperpyrexia (MH) is a rare inherited life-threatening condition in which there is an abnormality of ionic calcium transport in muscles. Following exposure to trigger agents (including volatile anaesthetic agents and suxamethonium) susceptible individuals may

---

TABLE 14.8 Clinical Features of MH

Increased muscle tone
Increased metabolic rate
Hyperthermia (typically increase >2°C/h)
Rising ETCO$_2$
Falling SaO$_2$
Mixed respiratory/metabolic acidosis
Hyperkalaemia/hypocalcaemia
Myoglobinuria and renal failure
Cardiac failure/dysrhythmia/cardiac arrest

---

develop increased muscle tone, increased metabolic rate and hyperpyrexia. The clinical features of MH are shown in Table 14.8.

Management

- Discontinue trigger agents. Monitor ECG, SaO$_2$ and core temperature.
- Intubate if not already.
- Ventilate with 100% oxygen.
- Monitor ETCO$_2$. Manage hypercarbia by hyperventilation.
- Paralyse and ensure adequate sedation and analgesia.
- Institute active cooling measures.
- Give dantrolene 1 mg/kg i.v. over 10 minutes; repeat as necessary up to 10 mg/kg.
- Monitor blood gases, potassium and calcium. Treat metabolic acidosis, hyperkalaemia and hypocalcaemia as appropriate.
- Measure urine output and myoglobin. Give fluids and consider dopamine to maintain urine output. Mannitol and sodium bicarbonate increase the clearance of myoglobin. (Note: Dantrolene also contains mannitol to improve clearance of myoglobin).

Following stabilization, these patients must be monitored in the ICU. The half-life of dantrolene is approximately 5 hours. Hyperpyrexia may recur, requiring further doses of dantrolene. Seek advice from national/regional MH centre. (See Hyperthermia, p. 185.)

THE OBSTETRIC PATIENT

All pregnant women over 20 weeks' gestation must be nursed in the lateral position or with lateral tilt to avoid hypotension and uterine hypoperfusion due to compression of the inferior vena cava by the gravid uterus.

Any medical condition can present in pregnancy and a small number of obstetric patients are admitted to the ICU each year. The principles of management are the same as in the non-pregnant female, although the physiological changes associated with pregnancy and the safety of the fetus in utero are important considerations.

> ⚠ **Obstetric patients admitted to the ICU are by definition young and critically ill and the management issues are complex. You should always seek senior advice.**

Obstetricians and neonatologists should be involved in decisions regarding the viability of the unborn child and the appropriateness and timing of early termination of the pregnancy/delivery of the child.

There are some specific conditions associated with late pregnancy that may precipitate admission to ICU. In most cases patients will be admitted post delivery, as the primary management of most specific obstetric problems is urgent delivery of the fetoplacental unit.

PRE-ECLAMPSIA/ECLAMPSIA

Pre-eclampsia is a condition characterized by proteinuria, oedema and hypertension. Eclampsia, which may be preceded by pre-eclampsia or present acutely, is a more severe manifestation of the same disorder in which there are seizures. These conditions usually occur in late pregnancy but may occasionally present immediately post delivery. The exact pathogenesis of the condition is not known but urgent delivery of the fetoplacental unit, usually by caesarean section, initiates resolution. Hypertension and seizures may, however, continue for 48 hours.

● Give oxygen by face mask. Intubate and ventilate if necessary. Beware of rises in blood pressure and intracranial pressure on laryngoscopy/intubation. Bolus alfentanil 10 µg/kg may modify this. Subsequently ensure adequate sedation.
● Control hypertension. Hypertension results from vasoconstriction and is accompanied by reduced plasma volume. Vasodilatation and restoration of plasma volume should proceed synchronously. Use labetalol/nifedipine/hydralazine to control blood pressure. (See Hypertension p. 72.)

- Control seizures. Simple measures include benzodiazepines. Consider prophylactic anticonvulsant therapy with phenytoin or magnesium. Magnesium sulphate 4 g (16 mmol) over 20 minutes followed by infusion of magnesium sulphate 1 g (4 mmol) every hour. Monitor magnesium levels: aim for 2.5–3.5 mmol/l.
- Plasma volume is reduced and oliguria is common. Volume expansion is appropriate but can exacerbate hypertension and lead to pulmonary oedema. Use invasive monitoring to guide fluid challenges (CVP and PA catheter or equivalent).

Complications include DIC, HELLP syndrome, pulmonary oedema, cerebral oedema, cerebral haemorrhage and renal failure. These should be managed as necessary.

PERIPARTUM HAEMORRHAGE

Peripartum haemorrhage remains a significant cause of mortality in the obstetric patient. Control of the bleeding will usually require delivery of the fetoplacental unit and/or surgical repair. Occasionally packs will be placed in the uterus in an attempt to control bleeding in the hope that hysterectomy can be avoided. These patients are usually then admitted to ICU for continued management. Arterial and CVP monitoring is usually required. Large quantities of blood and blood products are often necessary and DIC is common. Seek senior help.

HELLP SYNDROME

HELLP syndrome (haemolysis, elevated liver enzymes, low platelets) is a distinct condition occurring in the peripartum period but frequently accompanies pre-eclampsia/eclampsia. There are abnormalities of the microvascular circulation associated with red cell destruction and increased platelet consumption. The liver is particularly affected, resulting in some cases in hepatic necrosis and rupture. The clinical features are primarily those of abdominal (right upper quadrant) pain and mild jaundice. Thrombocytopenia may result in bleeding. The diagnostic criteria are shown in Table 14.9.

Management is largely supportive. Adequate resuscitation, volume loading and epoprostenol (prostacyclin) infusion may improve microvascular circulation. Platelets are generally unnecessary unless there is active bleeding. Plasma exchange may be of value in severe cases. Seek advice.

TABLE 14.9 Diagnostic criteria HELLP syndrome	
Haemolysis	Abnormal blood film Hyperbilirubinaemia
Elevated liver enzymes	LDH >600 units/l AST >70 units/l
Low platelets	<100 × 10^9/l

PREGNANCY-RELATED HEART FAILURE

Pregnancy and delivery are characterized by increased physiological demands on the heart. In patients with pre-existing heart disease or pregnancy-related cardiomyopathy the heart may be unable to meet these demands and heart failure supervenes. Management is supportive, as for other causes of heart failure. Pregnancy-related cardiomyopathy usually improves after delivery. (See Cardiac failure, p. 87.)

CHAPTER 15

PRACTICAL PROCEDURES

GENERAL INFORMATION

Patients in intensive care often require large numbers of practical procedures. The information in this chapter is intended only as a guide. The advice is generalized; you should always read the instructions provided with the equipment that you use, and follow your local hospital guidelines.

 Always seek senior help if you are not familiar with a procedure.

Consent
Formal consent/assent may be appropriate for some procedures, such as tracheostomy, while consent/assent may be implied for minor or life-saving procedures. In any event, always explain to patients, even if apparently 'unconscious', what you intend to do and keep relatives informed. (See Consent to treatment, p. 25.)

Local anaesthetic
Paralysed and sedated patients in ICU may still feel pain from invasive procedures. Use local anaesthetic for all painful procedures.

Universal infection control precautions
Contamination with blood imposes significant risk to staff from blood-borne infection, particularly hepatitis and HIV infection. Universal precautions should be adopted for all invasive procedures. These are intended to prevent the spread of infection, to protect you, your patients and colleagues. It is not always possible to know who has an infection; universal infection control precautions apply to everybody, all of the time:

- Wash your hands thoroughly.
- Cuts or grazes on the hands or forearms should be covered with a waterproof dressing while at work. Seek medical advice about any septic or weeping areas.
- Single-use gloves should be worn for direct contact with blood or body fluid, broken skin or mucous membranes. Face protection and plastic aprons should be worn if there is a risk of blood or body fluid splashing the face or clothing.
- Place all sharps directly into a sharps bin; do not manually resheath or break needles. Do not overfill sharps bins, and ensure that the bin is securely fastened before disposal.

- If you do accidentally cut, scrape or puncture your skin, follow the 'accidental inoculation procedure', i.e.
  — encourage bleeding, wash with warm soapy water, dry and cover with a waterproof dressing
  — report the incident to the senior person in charge and ensure a report is completed
  — seek advice from the occupational health department or from A&E.
- Clinical waste should be discarded into colour-coded bags for incineration.
- Blood or body fluid spills should be disinfected immediately; follow instructions.

Always follow guidelines and safety information that apply to your department. If you need further information, talk in the first place to a senior member of staff. Where necessary, further advice can be obtained from specialists in microbiology, infection control, occupational health, COSHH (Control of Substances Hazardous to Health), health & safety, etc.

Aseptic technique

ICU patients are generally severely debilitated and at increased risk of infection; therefore, when performing procedures, no matter how minor, good infection control procedures are important. For all invasive procedures strict aseptic technique is required:

- Collect all necessary equipment before starting.
- Ensure assistance is available to open packs, etc.
- Wash hands with disinfectant (generally chlorhexidine or iodine).
- Dry hands on towel provided in gown pack.
- Put on gown.
- Put on gloves using closed technique.
- Prepare the equipment on the trolley.
- Prepare the patient by washing with spirit or iodine.
- Place sterile towels around the proposed site to make a sterile field.
- Remember to keep hands up to avoid contamination.

> ⚠️ **It is the responsibility of the person performing a procedure to dispose of all sharps safely and correctly at the end of the procedure. Remember: never resheath needles. Deposit needles and other sharps directly in the appropriate bins.**

ARTERIAL CANNULATION

Arterial cannulation is one of the most commonly performed
procedures in the ICU. There is, however, an associated risk of
morbidity and the indication for arterial cannulation in the individual
patient should be considered carefully.

Indications

● Haemodynamic monitoring: particularly in situations where non-
  invasive measurements are inadequate, e.g. where changes in
  arterial blood pressure are likely to be sudden or profound, at
  extremes of blood pressure and in the presence of arrhythmias.
● Repeated blood sampling. Especially for repeated arterial blood gas
  sampling. The complications associated with arterial cannulation
  are outweighed by the morbidity and inconvenience of repeated
  arterial puncture.

Contraindications

These are relative. Exercise caution in arteriopaths and do not
recannulate an artery where previous vascular compromise has
occurred. Where possible avoid areas of local sepsis and trauma,
limbs with dialysis fistulae and end arteries such as the brachial artery.

Procedure

Arterial cannulation. You will need:

Universal precautions; sterile gloves
Minor dressing pack
Skin disinfectant
Syringe of local anaesthetic/needle
Syringe of heparinized saline flush
Arterial cannulae (usually 20 gauge or 22 gauge)
Extension line and three-way tap
Suture
Dressing

Decide which artery to cannulate. The radial artery of the non-
dominant hand is usually preferred in the first instance. Alternatives
include the ulnar, dorsalis pedis and posterior tibial arteries. It is
pointless, however, to persist with attempts at peripheral arterial
cannulation in patients who are hypotensive and 'shut down'. The
femoral and brachial arteries are useful during resuscitation of
profoundly shocked patients.

⚠ **Allen's test has been suggested as a way to establish the adequacy of ulnar collateral circulation to the hand before cannulation of the radial artery. The test is of no proven value. If there is any evidence of vascular compromise the arterial line should be removed and surgical exploration of the artery considered where perfusion is not rapidly restored.**

- Arterial cannulation often results in blood spillage. Universal precautions should be used.
- Clean the puncture site and establish a sterile field.
- Gently palpate the artery and inject local anaesthetic to raise a small intradermal bleb at the puncture site 1 cm distal to the proposed cannulation site.
- A Seldinger technique or a direct cannulation technique may be used.

Seldinger technique
- Advance needle through the puncture site towards the artery at a shallow angle. As the vessel is punctured, a flashback of arterial blood is seen in the hub. Pass the guide wire through the needle into the artery. Withdraw the needle and pass the cannula over the guide wire. The guide wire is then discarded.

Direct cannulation
- Either: advance the cannula and needle through the puncture site towards the artery at a shallow angle. As the vessel is punctured a flashback of arterial blood is seen in the hub. Holding the needle still, advance the cannula over the needle into the artery. This should be a single smooth movement without resistance.
- Or: advance the cannula at a steeper angle and, after observing the flashback, continue through the artery to transfix it. Withdraw the needle slightly from the cannula and then pull the cannula back gently until the tip is in the artery and flashback is again observed. Advance the cannula into the artery.

- Attach extension tubing and three-way tap.
- Aspirate blood from the line to confirm placement and to remove any air bubbles, then flush line with heparinized saline.
- Secure in place and cover with occlusive dressing.
  (If using stitches, do not place stitches too deeply. It is possible inadvertently to damage peripheral arteries.)

- Attach the arterial catheter to a pressure transducer and flushing device.

Sampling from arterial lines
- Clean sample port with alcohol swab and attach syringe.
- Aspirate 1–2 ml blood into the syringe and then discard this syringe.
- Aspirate sample into fresh syringe or vacuum container.
- Samples for blood gases should be drawn into preheparinized syringes to prevent damage to the blood gas analyser. Any air in the syringe should be expelled. If not analysed immediately in the ICU, the syringe should be capped and placed on ice.
- Flush the line with heparinized saline and place a clean cap on the sampling port.

Complications
Complications of arterial cannulation are shown in Table 15.1.

Vascular compromise may occur at any stage. Inadvertent injection of drugs into an arterial catheter is an important avoidable cause of morbidity and all cannulae and lines should be clearly labelled. Risk of infection increases with time. Any manifestly infected catheter should be removed. After removal press firmly for at least 5 minutes. Occasionally persistent bleeding may require a suture (5/0 nylon) to close the skin wound and then further pressure.

TABLE 15.1 Complications of arterial cannulation

Immediate	Early	Late
Bleeding	Arterial embolism	Infection
Haematoma	Vasospasm	Ulceration
Arterial damage		Thrombosis
		Arteriovenous fistulae

PRESSURE TRANSDUCERS

A transducer converts one type of energy (e.g. arterial pressure) into another (e.g. electrical impulse). There are a number of different types of transducer available but the principle is similar for all:

- The patient's arterial catheter is connected to the transducer by a continuous column of heparinized saline. A pressurized flushing device maintains a small forward flow (approx. 2–3 ml/h) to keep the cannula patent.
- Pressure changes in the vessel are transmitted via the saline to a diaphragm. As this diaphragm moves in response to the pressure

changes, its electrical conductivity changes. This results in fluctuations in electrical signal from the diaphragm, which is interpreted by a monitor and displayed as an arterial waveform and blood pressure values. Systolic, diastolic and mean pressures are usually displayed.

Using transducers

In order for the arterial waveform and blood pressure recording to be accurate, the transducer must be used appropriately. Therefore:

● There must be no air bubble in the connection tubing or transducer chamber. This will damp the trace and produce lower blood pressure values. Flush well before connecting the transducer to the patient.
● The transducer should be maintained at the level of the left atrium and appropriately zeroed. (If raised above this level the recorded pressure will be too low, and vice versa.)

Zeroing transducers

● To zero a transducer turn the three-way tap so the transducer is open to air and the patient connection is switched off. The transducer is now connected to atmospheric or zero gauge pressure.
● Zero the monitoring system according to the manufacturer's instructions. (There is usually a single button to press.)
● When zeroing is complete, turn the three-way tap back to reconnect the patient to the transducer. Check that the trace and values obtained are as expected.

COMMON PROBLEMS: INVASIVE PRESSURE MONITORING

Invasive and non-invasive pressures disagree

If the blood pressure displayed by the invasive arterial monitoring differs from that obtained by non-invasive methods this is usually the result of either damping or resonance in the invasive monitoring. In most cases the mean arterial pressures are usually in close agreement.

● Check the arterial line is correctly sited and flush the lumen with heparinized saline.
● Check that there are no air bubbles in the connecting tubing or transducer chamber.
● Check zero on invasive monitoring.
● Check that the transducer is at the level of the left atrium.

In some cases, peripheral vasospasm may be a cause of this error. If in doubt, resite the arterial line, or use the non-invasive measurements of blood pressure. In this case, the line can still be retained for arterial blood gas sampling.

CENTRAL VENOUS CANNULATION

> ⚠️ **Do not attempt central venous cannulation without supervision until you have been adequately taught to do so. You must be aware of possible complications and how to manage them.**

Indications
Central venous access is almost universal in intensive care patients. Indications include:

- monitoring of CVP
- drug administration
- total parenteral nutrition
- fluid resuscitation
- insertion of temporary pacing wires
- insertion of pulmonary artery catheters
- dialysis
- lack of peripheral venous access.

Contraindications
These are relative but include inability to identify landmarks, limited sites for access, previous difficulties or complications, severe coagulopathy, thrombocytopenia and local sepsis. In addition, if an awake patient is unable to lie flat, central venous cannulation may be impractical.

Ultrasound guidance for vascular access
It is now increasingly recommended that ultrasound should be used to guide all central venous access. Ultrasound allows:

- direct visualization of the vessels (artery and vein) and their associated structures
- identification of thrombosis, valve or anatomical abnormalities
- identification of best target vessel
- first-pass cannulation in the midline of a vessel directly avoiding other vital structures
- visualization of guide wire and cannulae entering vein
- reduction of puncture-related complications.

Arteries can be distinguished from veins by their round cross-section, non-compressibility and their pulsatility. Veins, by contrast, show respiratory fluctuation and are easily compressible. In order to maintain sterility during vessel puncture the ultrasound probe can be placed in a sterile plastic sheath. (Sterile ultrasound gel is required both inside and outside the sheath.) The use of ultrasound requires practice. You should seek instruction before attempting to use it on a patient. You should also be familiar with the landmark approaches to the central veins described below.

Internal jugular vein

Internal jugular vein cannulation is associated with a lower incidence of complications and higher incidence of correct line placement than other approaches. It is especially appropriate for patients with coagulopathy or those patients with lung disease in whom pneumothorax may be disastrous. It may be best avoided in those patients with carotid artery disease or those with raised intracranial pressure because of the risks of carotid puncture and of impaired cerebral venous drainage. Internal jugular cannulation is associated with a higher incidence of catheter infection than subclavian cannulation but both have a much lower infection rate than the femoral approach.

The internal jugular vein runs from the jugular foramen at the base of the skull (immediately behind the ear) to its termination behind the posterior border of the sternoclavicular joint where it combines with the subclavian vein to become the brachiocephalic vein. Throughout its length it lies lateral, first to the internal and then common carotid arteries, within the carotid sheath, behind the sternomastoid muscle. See Figure 15.1.

Many approaches to the internal jugular vein have been described. Ultrasound will demonstrate the close association of the vein and carotid artery. Choose a site for puncture where the vein does not lie directly over the artery. A typical approach is from the apex of the triangle formed by the two heads of the sternomastoid:

- Slightly extend the neck.
- Turn the head slightly to the opposite side.
- Palpate the carotid artery at the level of the cricoid cartilage.
- Look for the internal jugular vein pulsation. If compressed, the internal jugular can usually be seen to empty and refill.
- To locate the vein, introduce needle from the apex of the triangle at an angle of 30° and aim towards the ipsilateral nipple.
- Often when attempting to puncture the vein it collapses under the pressure of the needle and puncture is not recognized. The vessel

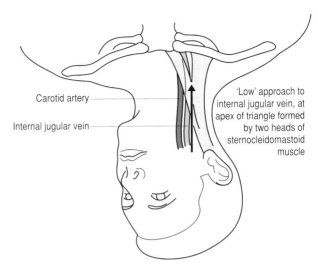

Carotid artery

Internal jugular vein

'Low' approach to internal jugular vein, at apex of triangle formed by two heads of sternocleidomastoid muscle

Fig. 15.1 Approach to the internal jugular vein.

⚠ It is a common mistake to assume the internal jugular vein is deep. Typically it is < 2 cm from the skin and can be easily located with a standard blue 'seeker' needle. Once the vessel has been identified the seeker needle can be left in place as a guide to puncture with the introducer needle.

may then be located by aspirating as the needle is slowly withdrawn. Blood will be aspirated as the needle tip passes back into the vein, which refills once the pressure has been removed.

External jugular vein

The external jugular vein lies superficially in the neck, running down from the region of the angle of the jaw, across the sternomastoid before passing deep to drain into the subclavian vein. It can be used to provide central venous access, particularly in emergency situations when a simple large-bore cannula can be used for the administration of drugs and resuscitation fluids. Longer central venous catheters can be sited via the external jugular but the angle of entry to the

subclavian vein often leads to inability to pass guide wires centrally
and results in a high failure rate.

Subclavian vein

Subclavian vein cannulation is associated with a higher incidence of
complications, particularly pneumothorax, and a higher incidence of
incorrect line placement than internal jugular cannulation. It is,
however, more comfortable for the patient long-term and the site can
more easily be kept clean.

The subclavian vein is a continuation of the axillary vein. It runs
from the apex of the axilla behind the posterior border of the clavicle
and across the first rib to join the internal jugular vein, forming
the brachiocephalic vein behind the sternoclavicular joint. See
Figure 15.2.

- Position the patient supine (some people advocate placing a
  sandbag between the patient's shoulder blades, which allows the
  shoulders to drop back out of the way).
- Identify the junction of medial third and outer two-thirds of the
  clavicle.

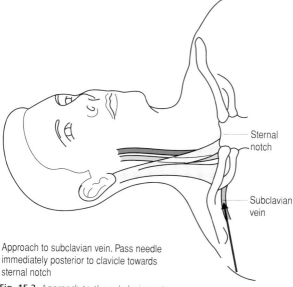

Sternal notch

Subclavian vein

Approach to subclavian vein. Pass needle
immediately posterior to clavicle towards
sternal notch

Fig. 15.2 Approach to the subclavian vein.

- Introduce the needle just beneath the clavicle at this point, and aim towards the clavicle until contact with bone is made.
- To locate the vein, redirect the needle closely behind the clavicle and towards the suprasternal notch.

Ultrasound can be used to guide puncture of the vein using a more lateral approach. The axillary vein can be identified in the apex of the axilla at a depth of 3–4 cm in the average patient. Longer catheters (20 cm left and 25 cm right) are required by this approach.

Femoral vein

The femoral vein lies medial to the femoral artery immediately beneath the inguinal ligament. It is particularly useful for obtaining central access in small children and in patients with severe coagulopathy.

- Palpate the femoral artery.
- To locate the vein, introduce the needle 1 cm medial to the femoral artery close to the inguinal ligament. It is a common mistake to go too low where the superficial femoral artery overlies the vein.
- Ultrasound can be used to identify the vessels and ensure that the vein is punctured near the inguinal ligament where the artery and vein lie side by side.

Procedure

Central venous cannulation. You will need:

Universal precautions; sterile gown and gloves
Skin disinfectant
Sterile towels
5-ml syringe of local anaesthetic
CVP line kit
Three-way taps
Heparinized saline to flush line
Suture
Dressing
ECG monitoring and defibrillator
Ultrasound machine

Central venous catheterization is almost universally achieved using a catheter over a guide wire (Seldinger) technique. This is associated with a lower incidence of incorrect line placement and complications than cannula over needle techniques.

- For internal jugular, external jugular and subclavian veins position the patient supine with 10–20° head down tilt. This distends the vein to aid location and helps prevent air embolism.

- Monitor ECG in case of dysrhythmias (a defibrillator should be immediately available).
- Universal precautions.
- Use aseptic technique, sterile gown and gloves.
- Prepare sterile field.
- Prepare all equipment.
- Check wire passes through the needle freely. Attach three-way taps to all open ports of the cannula. Flush the lumens with heparinized saline.
- Inject local anaesthetic to the entry site. Do not forget to anaesthetize suture sites as well.
- Identify the target vessel by ultrasound and/or landmark technique.
- Using a 10-ml syringe (partially filled with saline) and needle enter the central vein by the chosen approach, maintaining suction on the syringe at all times.

> If you appear to have missed the vein on the first pass, pull back slowly while maintaining suction on the syringe. You often find you have gone through the vein and can find it on withdrawal.

- Pass the Seldinger wire through the needle. This should pass freely and without any force into the vein. Watch for arrhythmias. Never pull the wire back through the needle once it has passed beyond the end of the bevel: it may shear off.
- Use a scalpel blade to make a small nick in the skin. Hold the blade up and cut away from the wire.
- If provided, pass the dilator over the wire into the vein. Then remove it, leaving the wire in situ.
- Pass the cannula over the wire into the vein. Make sure that before you push the cannula forward the wire is visible at the proximal end. Hold on to the wire at all times, to prevent it being lost inside the patient!
- For an average adult patient the central venous cannula does not need to be inserted more than 12–15 cm. Check markings on the cannula. Many are 20 cm long and do not need to be inserted up to the hub.
- Draw back blood, flush all the lumens of the line with heparinized saline and lock off the three-way taps. At this point the patient can be levelled.
- Suture the line into place using the anchorage devices provided and cover with an adhesive sterile dressing.

- Attach a transducer and display the waveform on the monitor.
- Dispose of your sharps and clear away your trolley.
- Obtain CXR to verify position of the line and check for complications, including pneumothorax and haemothorax.
- Document the procedure in the patient's notes.

Position on chest X-ray

The catheter should lie along the long axis of the vessel and the tip should be in the superior vena cava (SVC) or at the junction of the SVC and right atrium but outside the pericardial reflection. The pericardium lies below the carina so ideally catheter tips should be at or above the level of the carina. Catheters below this level may perforate the heart and cause cardiac tamponade. Catheters placed via the left subclavian must not be allowed to lie with the tip abutting the wall of the superior vena cava. This may cause pain, perforation and accelerated thrombus formation. Either advance the catheter to lie in the long axis of the SVC or pull it back to lie in the brachiocephalic vein. See Figure 15.3.

COMMON PROBLEMS: CENTRAL VENOUS ACCESS

Cannot find the vein

Check position (ultrasound and/or landmarks) and try again. If unsuccessful do not persist with repeated passages of the needle in the hope of striking oil! You may have misinterpreted the landmarks or the vein may be absent or occluded (e.g. with thrombus). Seek help.

> ⚠️ **Do not proceed immediately to attempt cannulation on the contralateral side: this increases the risk of complications, such as bilateral pneumothorax!**

Aspirating blood (needle in vein?) but cannot pass wire

Check needle position by drawing back on the syringe; good flow is essential. Adjust the angle of incidence of the needle to the vein to improve flow. Tip the patient further head down to further extend the vein. Try rotating the needle through 180° and draw back again. Remember the wire must pass easily without force. If this doesn't work, repuncture the vein at a slightly different angle.

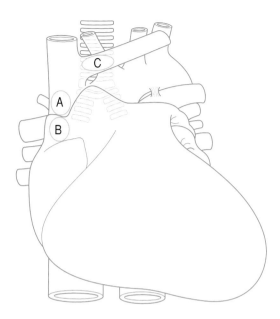

A: Ideal position for tip of all upper body central venous catheters, at or just above the level of carina (outside pericardium)

B: Acceptable position for the tip of right internal jugular catheters (just within pericardial reflection)

C: Acceptable position for tip of left sided central venous catheters that are too short to reach the ideal position A. DO NOT allow the tip of the catheters to abut the wall of the IVC

Fig. 15.3 Acceptable position for tip of central catheters on chest X-ray.

Is it arterial?

Occasionally, particularly if using a technique where the wire passes through the barrel of the syringe, it is difficult to know whether you have hit the artery or the vein. In this case it is important to avoid

passing a large central venous catheter into the vessel until you are
sure. Consider the following:

- Remove the syringe from the needle and observe for pulsatile flow.
- Connect a transducer directly to the needle in the vessel and look at
  the waveform.
- Pass the wire into the vessel and remove the needle. Pass an
  18-gauge i.v. cannula over the wire into the vessel and remove the
  wire. Attach a transducer or manometer set directly to the cannula.
  When venous placement is confirmed, pass the wire back through
  the i.v. cannula and continue as before.

Arterial puncture
- Needle only, then simply remove and press for 10 minutes. (Watch
  clock!)
- If large-bore cannula then action depends on circumstances.
  Usually can remove and press until bleeding stops. If severe
  coagulopathy, leave in situ and give platelets and FFP before
  removing. Seek advice and consider the need for surgical
  exploration and removal under direct vision.

Complications
Complications of central venous cannulation depend in part on the
route used but include those in Table 15.2.

The management of pneumothorax depends upon the size of the
pneumothorax and the patient's condition, particularly whether he or
she is ventilated or not. A small pneumothorax in an unventilated
patient with good gas exchange may be observed, or aspirated using a
small-bore cannula and syringe with three-way tap. Larger
pneumothoraces, those that fail to resolve or those that cause any
impairment of gas exchange and/or haemodynamics require a formal
chest drain. Any significant haemothorax should be formally drained

TABLE 15.2 Complications of central venous cannulation

Early	Late
Arrhythmias	Infection
Vascular injury	Thrombosis
Pneumothorax	Embolization
Haemothorax	Erosion/perforation of vessels
Thoracic duct injury (chylothorax)	Cardiac tamponade
Cardiac tamponade	
Neural injury	
Embolization (including guide wire)	

as soon as possible. Once blood has clotted in the chest, drainage is difficult. (See Chest drainage, p. 353.) Seek cardiothoracic/surgical opinion.

Bleeding around the puncture site can occasionally be a persistent problem. If this does not resolve with pressure, use a suture (5/0 Prolene) to tie a purse string around the puncture site. This usually stops the bleeding.

CHANGING AND REMOVING CENTRAL VENOUS CATHETERS

Line colonization with bacteria and fungi is common and there is no evidence that changing lines on a regular basis (e.g. every 5–7 days) is of benefit. (See Catheter-related sepsis, p. 285.)

Changing catheters over a wire

If new central venous catheters are required these should usually be placed at a clean site. Occasionally it may be necessary to change a catheter over a guide wire using an existing site. The technique is similar to that described above for placing any central venous catheter. The main problem is avoiding contamination of the new catheter.

- Cut sutures on the old line before scrubbing.
- Use universal precautions, aseptic technique, gown and gloves.

> The problem with this technique is keeping the new line sterile. Wear two pairs of gloves and discard the top pair when you have finished with the old line.

- Clean and prep area.
- Pass the wire down the central lumen of the old central venous catheter. (Make sure that the new wire is longer than the old CVP line.)
- Remove the old catheter, leaving the wire in place, and send the tip of the old catheter for culture.
- Clean the puncture site with antiseptic solution.
- Use the wire to site the new line as required.

Removing central venous catheters

Removal of central venous catheters can precipitate air embolism, pneumothorax, haemothorax, embolization of thrombus and bacteraemia/sepsis.

To remove central lines ensure that all drugs and infusions have been stopped or relocated to other lines. Lay the patient down to reduce the risk of air embolism and remove the line smoothly, applying pressure to the puncture site. Sit the patient up. If infection is suspected, send the tip of the line in a dry specimen pot for culture.

LARGE-BORE INTRODUCER SHEATHS/DIALYSIS CATHETERS

Indications
Introducer sheaths are available in a number of sizes for different applications, including insertion of pulmonary artery catheters and temporary pacing wires. In adults 7.5 or 8.5 Fr are generally used. They may be used as large-bore access for volume resuscitation. Smaller sheaths may be used for introducing specialized monitoring such as jugular bulb oximetery.

Large-bore double lumen dialysis catheters are used for haemodialysis, haemofiltration, plasma exchange and rapid transfusion.

Procedure
See Central venous cannulation above.

All these devices are inserted using a Seldinger technique and a large stiff dilator is used to dilate the initial needle track sufficiently to allow the large-bore catheter to be passed easily into the vessel. These dilators do not pass around a tight bend easily and can readily damage or perforate vessels. The left internal jugular vein is best avoided. Introducer sheaths can usually be sited safely at all other sites. Dialysis catheters may be best placed by the right internal jugular or femoral routes (particularly in patients with chronic renal failure, to preserve the venous drainage of the arm for subsequent AV fistulae formation).

- Universal precautions.
- Aseptic technique, sterile gown and gloves.
- Enter vein with needle, as for central venous line, and pass Seldinger wire.
- Make small nick in the skin with a blade.
- Pass the sheath mounted on the introducer/dilator over the wire into the vein. The dilator is generally longer than needed and does not need to be passed right up to the hub. When the dilator has entered the vein, slide the sheath forward without advancing the dilator any further.

> ⚠ The dilators provided are often very stiff and can easily bend guide wires and tear vessels if advanced too far or too aggressively.

- Remove wire and dilator. Draw back and flush with heparinized saline. (For dialysis catheters use heparin 1000 units/ml and flush to the volume of the catheter printed on the hub.)
- When in situ and not in use the sheath port should be occluded with an obturator.
- Get CXR to check position and complications.

PULMONARY ARTERY CATHETERIZATION

The place of pulmonary artery catheters has been questioned recently and their use has diminished. They may be of value, however, in any condition in which haemodynamic instability or shock is unresponsive to fluid and inotrope therapy guided by conventional CVP measurement. Traditional indications and contraindications are shown in Table 15.3. (See Haemodynamic monitoring, p. 61.)

Procedure

> ⚠ Before attempting to insert a PA catheter ECG monitoring must be established and a defibrillator must be immediately available because of the risks of dysrhythmia.

TABLE 15.3 Indications and contraindications for pulmonary artery catheterization

Indications	Relative contraindications
Shock	Severe coagulopathy
Sepsis/SIRS	Unstable ventricular rhythm
ARDS	Heart block
Valvular heart disease*	Temporary transvenous pacemaker (wire dislodgement)
Left ventricular failure	Stenosis tricuspid or pulmonary valve†
Cor pulmonale/pulmonary hypertension	
High-risk surgical patients	

*Relative indication.
†Severe stenosis or mechanical valves absolute contraindication.

PA catheterization. You will need:

Universal precautions; sterile gown and gloves
Sterile towels
Skin cleaning solution
5-ml syringe of local anaesthetic
Introducer sheath (see previous section)
Pulmonary artery catheter
Three-way taps
Heparinized saline to flush line
Transducer and monitor
ECG monitoring and defibrillator

- Use universal precautions.
- Full aseptic technique. Sterile gowns and gloves.
- Insert introducer sheath as above.
- Position the patient flat before inserting the PA catheter. (This reduces the pulmonary artery pressures and reduces the risk of pulmonary artery rupture.)
- Connect 3 three-way taps to the open ports, and flush lumens with heparinized saline.
- Connect 1.5-ml syringe to the balloon port and test the balloon. (Check the size of the balloon before starting.)
- Pass protective sleeve over PA catheter if provided.
- Pass the proximal end of the catheter to an assistant who can connect a pressure transducer to the PA port (yellow) and flush the lumen. Then zero the transducer and check the signal on the monitor. Need to display trace on the monitor (scale 0–75 mmHg) continuously.
- Calibrate fibreoptics if using a fibreoptic PA catheter.
- Insert PA catheter into introducer sheath and pass to 20 cm. Note normal CVP trace.
- Inflate balloon and advance catheter gently to right ventricle at approx. 30–40 cm. Advance further until the pulmonary artery is entered at approx. 40–50 cm.
- Advance the catheter until pulmonary artery occlusion trace or wedge trace is observed, approx. 20 cm from RV (approx. 50–60 cm total). Deflate the balloon and see return of the PA trace (Fig. 15.4).
- Once the PA catheter is in position, perform a CXR
  — check the position of the catheter in the proximal pulmonary artery
  — exclude pneumothorax/haemothorax/knotting of the line.
- While in use ensure that the PA pressure trace is displayed continuously on the bedside monitor so that inadvertent 'wedging'

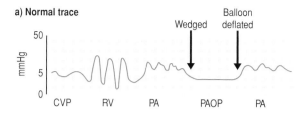

a) Normal trace

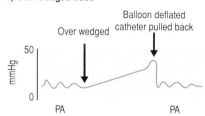

b) Over wedged trace

Fig. 15.4 Waveforms displayed while passing PA catheter. **a** Normal trace;
b over wedged trace.

> ⚠ **Never advance the catheter with the balloon down.**
> **Never force the catheter.**
> **Never pass more than 20 cm of catheter without seeing a change in the trace.**
> **Never overinflate the balloon.**
> **Never pull the catheter back with the balloon up.**

of the catheter can be recognized and the catheter pulled back to prevent pulmonary infarction.

COMMON PROBLEMS: PULMONARY ARTERY CATHETERIZATION

Catheter will not take the correct path
This may be due to a dilated RV or low CO. Do not persist if unsuccessful:

● Remove completely, check direction of curvature of catheter and try again.

- To enter RV place patient head down and left side up.
- To enter PA place patient head up and supine.

Catheter is 'over wedged'

- Always watch the pressure trace when wedging the catheter. If pressure rises then catheter is 'over wedged' (Fig. 15.4.)
- The catheter is too distal within the PA. There is a risk of pulmonary artery rupture. Deflate balloon, pull catheter back and try again.

Catheter will not wedge

- This may be because the catheter is curled up within the PA. Do not pass more than 20 cm without a change in trace. Pull back and try again.
- In the presence of severe mitral regurgitation or pulmonary hypertension it may not be possible to obtain a satisfactory wedge trace and attempts may be associated with increased risk of PA rupture. Accept that the catheter will not wedge and use pulmonary diastolic pressure instead of PA occlusion pressure.
- In low CO states there may be insufficient flow of blood in the pulmonary artery to advance the catheter when the balloon is inflated. Do not persist. Use PA diastolic as above.

Complications

PA catheterization is not without risk and is certainly not a therapeutic manoeuvre in its own right! If patients are to benefit then regular collection and interpretation of haemodynamic and oxygen delivery variables, together with the appropriate therapeutic response, is required.

Potential complications of pulmonary artery catheterization are shown in Table 15.4.

MEASURING PAOP

Most monitoring systems have a specific function key for use when measuring PAOP. These generally display the pulmonary artery pressure trace on a larger scale, allowing changes in the trace to be more easily observed and provide a cursor, which can be positioned to indicate the PAOP:

- Enter PAOP function on the monitor.
- Inflate the balloon and observe the wedge trace.
- Position cursor over the 'wedge trace' at the point corresponding to end expiration (Fig. 15.5).

TABLE 15.4 Complications of pulmonary artery catheterization

Complication	Comment
Central venous puncture	Any complications of central venous cannulation
Dysrhythmia	Usually on passage through tricuspid valve and RV Especially if hypoxia, acidosis, hypokalaemia: withdraw catheter and reposition Complete heart block may occur
Pulmonary infarction	Check catheter is in proximal PA on chest X-ray Never leave balloon inflated Display PA trace continuously
Pulmonary artery rupture	Pulmonary haemorrhage and blood up the endotracheal tube Avoid overinflation of balloon, watch trace and never inflate against resistance, pull back first
Infection	Risk includes endocardial damage and endocarditis Careful aseptic technique and catheter care Remove after 72 hours or ASAP
Knotting	Poor insertion technique Do not insert more than 20 cm without a change in trace Do not attempt to pull back. Call for help

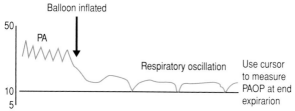

Fig. 15.5 Measuring PAOP.

THERMODILUTION MEASUREMENT OF CARDIAC OUTPUT

Pulmonary artery catheters incorporate a thermistor near the tip to allow thermodilution measurement of cardiac output. A volume of cold 5% dextrose solution (usually 10 ml) is injected through the central venous port of the PA catheter (in SVC or RA) and the temperature change in the PA is detected by the thermistor. The degree and the rate of temperature change is used to calculate cardiac output. (Some catheters incorporate a heated coil and fast reacting thermistor to allow continuous cardiac output measurement.)

- Ensure that the correct cables are connected between the monitor and the PA catheter (one to the distal thermistor and one to measure the temperature of the injectate).
- Enter cardiac output function on monitor.
- Check that the correct computation constant is entered into the monitor. This depends upon the volume and temperature of the injectate and also the type of catheter used. The correct computation constant is found on the packaging information of the PA catheter.

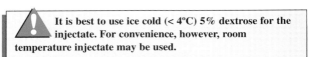

It is best to use ice cold (< 4°C) 5% dextrose for the injectate. For convenience, however, room temperature injectate may be used.

- Enter the patient's height and weight for calculation of body surface area (BSA).
- Set the computer to measure cardiac output, and when prompted inject 10 ml of 5% dextrose into the right atrial (CVP) lumen of the PA catheter. Time the injection at the end of inspiration and inject as rapidly as possible.
- Repeat the measurement. The individual cardiac output values obtained should not vary more than 5% from each other. Discard any inconsistent value and take the average reading for cardiac output.

Having measured the cardiac output and PA occlusion pressure a range of haemodynamic variables can be calculated. This is generally performed by the monitoring system. Normal values for these variables are shown in Table 15.5.

In addition by measuring blood gases on blood drawn simultaneously from the pulmonary artery catheter (mixed venous) and an arterial line, oxygen delivery and consumption variables may be calculated.

TABLE 15.5 Normal values for haemodynamic variables

Central venous pressure (CVP)	4–10 mmHg
Pulmonary artery pressure (PAP) Systolic/diastolic (mean)	15–25 mmHg/5–10 mmHg (10–20 mmHg)
Pulmonary artery occlusion pressure (PAOP)	5–15 mmHg
Cardiac output (CO)	4–6 l/min
Cardiac index (CI)	2.5–3.5 l/min/m^2
Stroke volume (SV)	60–90 ml/beat
Stroke volume index (SVI)	33–47 ml/beat/m^2
Systemic vascular resistance (SVR)	900–1200 dyne.s/cm^5
Systemic vascular resistance index (SVRI)	1700–2400 dyne.s/cm^5/m^2
Pulmonary vascular resistance (PVR)	100–200 dyne.s/cm^5
Pulmonary vascular resistance index (PVRI)	210–360 dyne.s/cm^5/m^2

> ⚠ **Therapy is directed by the results of haemodynamic and oxygen delivery variables. It is important, however, to treat the patient and not commence therapy on the basis of a single abnormal variable in a patient who is otherwise stable and maintaining adequate tissue and organ perfusion.**

(See Optimizing haemodynamic status, p. 61, and Oxygen delivery and consumption, p. 61.)

PERICARDIAL ASPIRATION

Indications
- Cardiac tamponade.
- Large pericardial effusions.
- To obtain diagnostic pericardial fluid.

Small loculated effusions, not causing haemodynamic compromise and without diastolic collapse on echocardiogram, do not require pericardiocentesis. (See Pericardial effusion and cardiac tamponade, p. 90.)

Procedure

Pericardial aspiration. You will need:

Universal precautions; sterile gown and gloves
Skin cleaning solutions
Sterile towels
10-ml syringe of local anaesthetic and needle
Pigtail catheter or 14-gauge single lumen central venous catheter
(including syringe, needle and guide wire)
Three-way tap
50-ml syringe or vacuum drainage bottle
Suture
ECG monitoring, defibrillator and resuscitation equipment

- Place patient supine with 20° of head-up tilt.
- Establish i.v. access if not already present and monitor ECG.
- Provide adequate sedation if necessary.
- Full aseptic technique. Sterile gowns and gloves.
- The point of needle insertion is immediately below and to the left of the xiphisternum, between the xiphisternum and the left costal margin. Infiltrate the skin and subcutaneous tissue with local anaesthetic.
- Using a 10-ml syringe, advance the needle at 35° to the patient, beneath the costal margin and towards the left shoulder, aspirating continuously and observing the ECG (Fig. 15.6).
- Fluid (straw-coloured effusion or blood) is generally aspirated at a depth of 6–8 cm. Hold the needle stationary and pass the guide wire through the needle into the pericardial space.
- Remove the needle, leaving the guide wire in situ and then pass the catheter over the wire into the pericardial space. Attach a three-way tap.
- Use a 50-ml syringe to aspirate pericardial effusion or attach to a closed drainage system such as a vacuum bottle. Aspiration should produce immediate haemodynamic improvement.
- Suture the drain in place.

⚠ In an emergency situation when aspirating presumed cardiac tamponade it is difficult to know whether blood aspirated is from the pericardial space or whether the ventricle has been punctured. Observe the ECG throughout. If the needle touches the ventricle an injury pattern or arrhythmia should be observed.

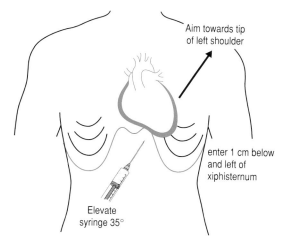

Aim towards tip
of left shoulder

enter 1 cm below
and left of
xiphisternum

Elevate
syringe 35°

Fig. 15.6 Pericardial aspiration.

Complications

Performed carefully, complications are few. They include
pneumothorax, ventricular tachycardia, myocardial puncture and
damage to the coronary arteries. A repeat CXR and echocardiogram
should be performed after the procedure to confirm adequate
placement and drainage and to identify any problems.

Insertion of a pericardial drain should only be considered a
temporary measure. Seek general surgical or cardiothoracic surgical
advice regarding repair of the underlying problem and/or creation of a
pericardial window.

DEFIBRILLATION AND DC CARDIOVERSION

> ⚠ **Defibrillators are potentially dangerous pieces of
> equipment. Make sure you know how to use
> defibrillator equipment safely. It is your responsibility to
> ensure the safety of everyone in the proximity, including
> yourself. Paddles should be either in the safe position or in
> contact with the patient. Do not charge except when ready to
> deliver a shock.**

Indications

Treatment of any life-threatening 'shockable rhythm' according to advanced life support protocols. (See Cardiac arrest, p. 90, and Dysrhythmias, p. 73.)

Procedure

- Prior to 'elective' DC cardioversion, consider the need for anticoagulation (usually unnecessary except in chronic dysrhythmias).
- Check the patient is adequately sedated/anaesthetized. This may require supplementation of sedation and analgesia in a ventilated patient with a small bolus dose of midazolam, opioid or other similar agent. Conscious patients will require anaesthesia, usually with a cardiostable drug such as etomidate.
- Place conducting gel pads over the patient's apex and sternum.
- Select the appropriate mode (asynchronous or synchronous) and select required energy levels (see relevant algorithms) before removing the paddles from the defibrillator.
- Take paddles from the defibrillator and place immediately on to gel pads on the patient. Only charge the paddles once they are in contact with the patient.
- Before charging paddles give an 'all clear' warning to ensure that no-one is touching the patient and check that everyone is clear.
- Before delivering the shock, give a second all clear warning; check that everyone is clear and that any oxygen source is temporarily removed from the patient. Ensure that you yourself are not inadvertently in contact with the patient.
- Deliver shock.
- After delivery of the shock, several seconds may pass before monitors yield an ECG trace. Keep paddles in contact with the patient if you may wish to deliver a further shock, or return them to the safe position on the defibrillator.

If normal rhythm is not restored seek expert help. Consider:

- Higher energy shock.
- Alternative paddle position (e.g. cardiac long axis, anteroposterior).
- Use of antidysrhythmic drug before repeat attempts.
- Many patients on ICU develop atrial fibrillation that does not return to sinus rhythm for more than a very short period after DC cardioversion, until their underlying condition has improved.

INTUBATION OF THE TRACHEA

This is covered at greater length in standard anaesthesia texts; however, there are some aspects of tracheal intubation of particular relevance to patients in intensive care.

> ⚠ **Do not attempt tracheal intubation without senior help if you are not experienced in the technique. In an emergency, ventilate the patient with a bag and mask or via a laryngeal mask and await reinforcements!**

Indications

These fall broadly into three groups: relieving airway obstruction, protection of the airway from aspiration and facilitation of artificial ventilation of the lungs. Typical indications are given in Table 15.6.

Patients requiring intubation in ICU frequently have limited physiological reserve and are liable to haemodynamic collapse. Drugs used to facilitate intubation must therefore be used judiciously. In some cases patients may already have a markedly obtunded conscious level and small doses of benzodiazepines (e.g. diazepam 5–10 mg) may be all that is required. In other patients low doses of i.v. anaesthetic agents may be appropriate (e.g. propofol 1–2 mg/kg or etomidate 0.1–0.2 mg/kg); however, these may be associated with cardiovascular collapse.

Muscle relaxants will usually be required to facilitate intubation. Suxamethonium (1–2 mg/kg) is rapid in onset and relatively short-acting in most patients. It is the drug of choice for rapid sequence

TABLE 15.6 Indications for tracheal intubation

Airway obstruction	Risks of aspiration	Facilitation of IPPV
Tumours	Obtunded conscious level	Anaesthesia and surgery
Head and neck trauma	Bulbar palsy	Cardiopulmonary resuscitation
Epiglottis	Impaired cough reflexes	Respiratory failure
Surgery		Cardiac failure
Airway oedema		Multisystem organ failure
		Major trauma including chest injury
		Brain injury

> ⚠ **Do not use i.v. anaesthetic agents or muscle relaxants unless you are familiar with them. (See Sedation and analgesia, p. 30, and Muscle relaxants, p. 37. For Contraindications to suxamethonium, see p. 38.)**

induction. It has a number of side effects, however, which limit its use. Atracurium (0.5 mg/kg) is an alternative but is slower in onset and has a longer duration of action.

Procedure

Tracheal intubation. You will need:

Skilled assistant
Self-inflating bag (Ambu or similar) and oxygen supply
Face mask
Oral/nasal airways
Suction and suction catheters
2 laryngoscopes (check bulbs)
Selection of endotracheal tubes
Sterile lubricant
Syringe for cuff inflation and tape to tie tube
Gum-elastic bougie, airway exchange catheter or rigid stilette
Laryngeal mask (for use in failed intubation)
Anaesthetic drugs and muscle relaxant
Resuscitation drugs – atropine, adrenaline (epinephrine)

- Preoxygenate the patient. Administer 100% oxygen using a tight-fitting face mask for a period of 3–4 minutes prior to administering any drugs or attempting intubation, if possible. This will wash out nitrogen and fill the functional residual capacity with oxygen, thereby providing an oxygen reservoir and increasing the safety margin in the event of difficulties.
- Check the head is in the 'sniffing the morning air' position (neck flexed, atlantoaxial joint extended, one firm pillow).
- If the patient might have a full stomach, ask your assistant to apply cricoid pressure; if the neck is supported from behind and the cricoid firmly gripped, downward pressure prevents any passive regurgitation. If possible, avoid inflating the lungs with the face mask and self-inflating bag until the tube is in place, as blowing air into the stomach may increase the risks of regurgitation.
- Give sedative anaesthetic and muscle relaxant as appropriate.
- Hold the laryngoscope in the left hand (size 3 or 4 Macintosh scopes are most commonly used). Slide the scope into the right of

the mouth, sweeping the tongue into the groove in the blade, under it and to the left. As you advance the laryngoscope blade over the base of the tongue, the epiglottis pops into sight. With the blade between the epiglottis and the base of the tongue (vallecula), apply traction in the line of the laryngoscope handle, gently drawing the epiglottis forward and exposing the V-shaped glottis behind (Fig. 15.7A, B).

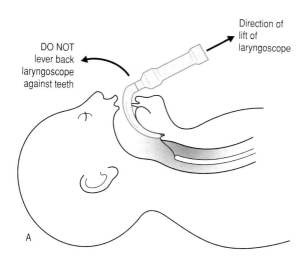

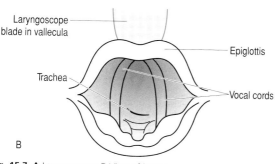

Fig. 15.7 A Laryngoscopy. **B** View of larynx.

- Pass the endotracheal tube between the vocal cords so that the cuff is just distal to them. There is usually a mark on the endotracheal tube above the cuff, which when placed at the level of the cords indicates the correct position of the tube.
- If you can visualize the vocal cords but are having difficulty passing the endotracheal tube into the larynx, pass a gum elastic bougie or airway exchange catheter into the larynx and then try passing a lubricated endotracheal tube over this.
- Inflate the cuff while ventilating through the endotracheal tube with the self-inflating bag until any gas leak just disappears.

> ⚠ If immediate intubation proves to be difficult or impracticable, do not persist with fruitless attempts. Ventilate the patient with 100% oxygen using bag and mask or laryngeal mask and call for help.

- Verify correct positioning of the tube by observation of chest movement, auscultation and if possible by capnography. Secure it, and attach to the ventilator via a suitable catheter mount. Recheck the tube position and chest movement.
- Check the cuff pressure with a standard pressure gauge to reduce the risks of laryngeal mucosal injury.
- Pass a nasogastric tube if this is not already in situ (see p. 357).
- Obtain a CXR to confirm tube position. Check if the tube is too short, too long (endobronchial?). Check for lobar collapse, pneumothorax, etc.

Complications

Potential complications of endotracheal intubation are shown in Table 15.7.

TABLE 15.7 Complications of endotracheal intubation

Immediate	Late
Trauma to teeth	Accidental extubation or obstruction of
Trauma to airway/larynx/	airway
trachea	Complications associated with mechanical
Obstruction of airway	ventilation
Aspiration	Nosocomial pneumonia
Misplacement of tube	Sinusitis
Hypoxia (prolonged	Injury to vocal cords
attempts)	Tracheal stenosis

The commonest and most immediately life-threatening complication is oesophageal intubation. If in doubt, remove the tube, ventilate by face mask, and start again. Nasal intubation may provoke epistaxis or predispose to mucosal injury (e.g. submucosal positioning of the tube). In the longer term, nasal intubation may occlude the maxillary antrum and give rise to sinusitis. It is nevertheless better tolerated than oral intubation, particularly during weaning from ventilation. Long-term complications include erosion and stenosis of local tissues, particularly of the larynx and trachea. This may present as airway obstruction and stridor after extubation. (See Miscellaneous problems: Airway obstruction, p. 113.)

EXTUBATION OF THE TRACHEA

Before you consider extubation, the patient should be breathing spontaneously with a satisfactory respiratory pattern and acceptable blood gases. The patient should have an appropriate conscious level and airway reflexes and not be requiring repeated airway suctioning. (See Weaning from artificial ventilation, p. 111.)

- Check a suitable system for providing humidified oxygen by face mask is available, and you have everything necessary for reintubation.
- Explain to the patient what you are going to do, then aspirate any secretions from the posterior pharynx.
- Insert a wide-bore suction catheter through the endotracheal tube. Deflate the cuff, and simultaneously aspirate through the suction catheter as you withdraw the endotracheal tube. This ensures that any secretions that have collected above the cuff are removed.
- Finally, fit a face mask and encourage the patient to cough out any further secretions.
- Observe the patient closely for signs of respiratory inadequacy or distress developing over the next few hours. Consider the early use of CPAP/BIPAP.

INSERTION OF LARYNGEAL MASK

In the event of being unable to intubate a patient it is vital that oxygenation is maintained. Laryngeal masks are relatively simple to use, provide a clear airway and effectively free the operator's hands. Laryngeal masks come in a range of sizes for all ages. Size 3 is suitable for average adult females and size 4 for average adult males.

- Maintain oxygenation by bag and mask.
- Deflate the cuff of the laryngeal mask.

- Lubricate with aqueous gel.
- Pass into the mouth and push back over the tongue into the oropharynx until the laryngeal mask fits naturally in the posterior pharynx.
- Inflate the cuff with 20–30 ml of air.
- Attach breathing circuit.
- Gently ventilate the patient with 100% oxygen and check for chest movement and end-tidal CO_2.
- Seek senior help to secure airway by endotracheal intubation.

PERCUTANEOUS TRACHEOSTOMY

In recent years tracheostomy has become a common procedure on the ICU. Traditionally, tracheostomy was only performed after patients had been intubated for about 10–14 days because of fear of laryngeal and subglottic injury resulting from continued intubation. The advent of percutaneous techniques has allowed tracheostomy to be performed safely and easily at the bedside without the use of specialized surgical instruments, lighting or diathermy. As a result, many units now perform tracheostomy earlier.

Advantages of tracheostomy
These include:

- More comfortable than naso-/orotracheal tubes, which allows significant reductions in muscle relaxants, sedative and analgesic drugs. This promotes return of GI tract function.
- Patients easily switched from IPPV/assist modes/CPAP/T-piece without the need for extubation and reintubation.
- Easier clearance of tracheal secretions by suction.
- Speech is possible with cuff deflation or speaking tube.
- There may be a lower risk of airway problems after prolonged tracheostomy than after prolonged translaryngeal intubation. Narrowing and scarring of the major airways is a potential risk in both situations.

Indications
- Actual or impending airway obstruction. Tracheostomy should be considered early, before progressive swelling makes reintubation in the event of tube blockage or dislodgement potentially impossible.
- Known difficult intubation.
- The need for prolonged IPPV (see below).
- Aid to weaning (see below).
- Inability of patients to protect or maintain their own airway in the longer term, e.g. severe brain injury, bulbar palsy.

Procedure

> ⚠️ **This procedure requires a separate anaesthetist to manage the patient and airway and an operator to perform the tracheostomy. On no account should percutaneous tracheostomy be attempted by a single operator.**

Percutaneous tracheostomy. You will need:

Anaesthetic assistance ± anaesthetic machine
Nurse to help (not scrubbed)
Universal precautions; sterile gown and gloves
Skin disinfectant
Local anaesthetic (1% lidocaine (lignocaine) + adrenaline (epinephrine), syringe and needle
10 ml normal saline and syringe
Basic surgical instruments (e.g. venous cutdown set)
Percutaneous tracheostomy kit
Appropriate size cuffed tracheostomy tubes (1 size smaller and larger than planned)
Suture and securing tapes
Drugs and equipment for emergency reintubation
Bronchoscope (camera/monitor) and light source

Explain to the patient (and relatives) what you are going to do. Get written or verbal consent. Check the patient's coagulation status. Position the patient flat with the head and neck extended over a pillow. The majority of patients are already intubated and ventilated and are given either an intravenous or volatile anaesthetic. This is supplemented by infiltration of the surgical area with 10 ml of local anaesthetic plus adrenaline (epinephrine), which helps reduces skin edge bleeding.

A bronchoscope can be passed into the larynx during the procedure (through the endotracheal tube or laryngeal mask). This allows the operator to visualize the needle puncture of the trachea and the correct placement of guide wire, dilator and tracheostomy tube. A camera system and monitor make this much easier.

Anaesthetist

● Ensure appropriate monitoring and anaesthetize patient with inhalational or intravenous technique as appropriate. Beware of relying solely on intermittent bolus of propofol, as there is a risk of 'awareness'. A muscle relaxant is usually required.

- Suction trachea and oropharynx.
- Ventilate with 100% oxygen throughout the procedure.
- When the operator is ready, withdraw the endotracheal tube under direct vision using a laryngoscope, until the cuff is visible at the laryngeal inlet. This prevents the endotracheal tube being transfixed by the operator's needle when the trachea is punctured.
- Care must be taken not to lose the airway when the tube is withdrawn. Consider passing a gum elastic bougie or airway exchange catheter down the tube prior to withdrawal to ensure the tube can be replaced if it is pulled back too far. (Equipment must be available to reintubate the patient in case of difficulty.)
- An alternative approach is to remove the endotracheal tube altogether and to use a laryngeal mask to maintain ventilation and oxygenation.
- If a bronchoscope is to be used, pass this down the endotracheal tube or laryngeal mask and into the larynx so that the operator has a view of the trachea at the level at which needle puncture will occur.
- Maintain ventilation until the procedure is complete and then pass the catheter mount to the operator to attach to the tracheostomy tube.

Operator

Tracheostomy may be safely performed through the cricothyroid membrane or in the subcricoid region. In the UK it is recommended that the tracheostomy stoma should be between the 2nd and 4th tracheal rings. At higher levels there may be an increased risk of laryngeal/tracheal stenosis, which may ultimately necessitate tracheal resection. At lower levels there is an increased risk of haemorrhage from major vessels in the thoracic inlet.

There are a number of different percutaneous tracheostomy kits available. Most require that the trachea is punctured by a needle and a guide wire passed through the needle into the lumen of the trachea. This is then used to guide a tracheal dilator, which creates the tracheostomy, allowing the insertion of a tracheostomy tube. The following notes are a guide only, the exact details of the method of insertion will depend upon the system used.

- Check that all necessary equipment is available and prepared.
- Position patient flat with the neck extended over a pillow.
- Examine the neck and ascertain the position of the trachea. Look for anatomical abnormalities, large veins or palpable arterial pulsation. (Ultrasound gives good images of deeper vessels that may be at risk during the procedure.)

- Clean the skin.
- Palpate the cricothyroid membrane and sternal notch. Infiltrate the skin with 1% lidocaine (lignocaine) and adrenaline (epinephrine), midway between the two.
- Make a 2-cm superficial incision horizontally across the midline.
- Use blunt forceps and a finger to dissect the pretracheal tissue until you can feel the tracheal rings and identify the level. If necessary, tie off the anterior jugular veins, which occasionally bleed.
- Ask the anaesthetist to withdraw the endotracheal tube until the tip is just within the larynx.
- Puncture the trachea with the introducer needle below the level of the first tracheal ring and in the midline. Using a saline-filled syringe, confirm the position of the needle by aspiration of air/mucus from the trachea. A bronchoscope passed through the endotracheal tube can also be used to confirm the correct position of the needle tip within the tracheal lumen.
- Pass the guide wire through the needle into the trachea and remove the needle.
- Dilate the trachea according to the manufacturer's instructions supplied with the tracheostomy kit used and insert the tracheostomy tube, again according to instructions.
- Remove the introducer and guide wire.
- Suck out any blood from the trachea. Blood clot in the airway may produce total airway obstruction or act as a ball valve, allowing gas in but not out.
- Inflate the cuff and ventilate the patient through the tracheostomy.
- Correct placement of the tube may be confirmed by bronchoscopy or capnography. Check that chest expansion is symmetrical and that there are bilateral breath sounds, and that oxygen saturations are maintained.
- Tie the tracheostomy tube in place using tracheostomy tapes. In addition, it is advisable to place two stay sutures through the wings of the tracheostomy tube to prevent early accidental decannulation.
- Obtain a chest X-ray to confirm position and exclude any complications.

COMMON PROBLEMS DURING PERCUTANEOUS TRACHEOSTOMY

Bleeding

Heavy bleeding from the wound may sometimes occur, particularly if an anterior jugular vein is damaged. If possible place a clip on the bleeding vessel and tie off. Otherwise pack the wound with gauze, apply pressure and wait. If you are near the end of the procedure insert the tracheostomy tube, as this will often tamponade the bleeding. If bleeding does not stop, consider removing the tracheostomy tube (reintubate the patient via the oral route and pass the endotracheal tube beyond the stoma), pack the wound and seek surgical assistance.

Difficulty ventilating the patient

This usually means that the tracheostomy tube has been misplaced. Do not persist as this may produce a tension pneumothorax! Remove the tracheostomy tube and reintubate the patient by the oral (nasal) route.

Complications

The potential complications of percutaneous tracheostomy are shown in Table 15.8.

Air emphysema is common but, unless accompanied by a pneumothorax, is usually unimportant and will resolve over time. Pneumothorax is generally the result of attempting to ventilate the patient through a misplaced tube, resulting in air tracking down into the mediastinum and pleural cavities.

Care of the patient with a tracheostomy

Patients with tracheostomy tubes should receive adequate humidification of inspired gases to prevent drying, and regular suction to remove secretions. Spare tracheostomy tubes of the same size and one size smaller should be kept at the bedside, together with a pair of tracheal dilators.

Choice of tracheostomy tubes

A wide range of tracheostomy tubes in different lengths and sizes is available. Tubes with adjustable flanges are available to cater for

TABLE 15.8 Complications of tracheostomy	
Early	*Late*
Bleeding (may lead to total airway obstruction)	Tracheal stenosis
Pneumothorax	Tracheo-oesophageal fistula
Tube misplacement or dislodgement	Skin tethering/scarring
Air emphysema	Late haemorrhage from innominate vessels
Mucus plugging/obstruction	
Stomal infection	

patients in whom standard tubes are not suitable (e.g. those with very fat necks, goitres, etc.). Tubes with removable inner sleeves are useful for preventing build-up of secretions on the inner surface of the tube. In long-term patients, fenestrated or valved tubes, which allow speaking, may be useful.

Changing tracheostomy tubes

Tracheostomy tubes can be changed at any time if necessary, but it is more difficult if the tract is not well established. Give the patient 100% oxygen and position as for performing a tracheostomy. Pass a large-bore suction catheter (with the end cut off) or gum elastic bougie through the old tracheostomy tube before removing it and use this as a guide to insert the new tube. Facilities for ventilating the patient with a bag and mask and for reintubation should be available in case of difficulty.

Decannulation

When the patient's condition has improved, the question of when to remove the tracheostomy tube inevitably arises. Consideration should be given to the following:

- respiratory effort
- volume of tracheal secretions and ability to cough
- laryngeal competence and ability to swallow pharyngeal secretions
- general condition and strength
- conscious level.

There is no difficulty in a trial of decannulation, providing the tract is well formed (5–7 days after insertion). It is not routine practice to stitch up stomas: they are usually left to granulate on their own. A simple occlusive dressing should be applied over the stoma. Ideally, patients should be seen in an ICU follow-up clinic. If tracheal stenosis or other problems develop, appropriate referral can be made.

CRICOTHYROIDOTOMY/MINITRACHEOSTOMY

Cricothyroidotomy is a life-saving procedure used to provide emergency access to the airway (e.g. following obstruction of the upper airway) when measures such as bag and mask ventilation and tracheal intubation have failed. It involves the insertion of a small tube through the cricothyroid membrane, through which oxygen/ventilation can be provided until a definitive airway is obtained.

Minitracheostomy is a term used to describe the insertion of a similar small-bore non-cuffed tube through the cricothyroid membrane (4 mm internal diameter), principally to aid the clearance of secretions. The passage of suction catheters stimulates coughing and allows secretions to be aspirated. As a short-term measure these devices may help to prevent the need for naso-/orotracheal intubation and assisted ventilation. The small size of the tube limits its value and the use of minitracheostomy has declined in recent years.

Both cricothyroidotomy and minitracheostomy kits are commercially available. The technique for the insertion of each is essentially the same.

Procedure

Cricothyroidotomy/minitracheostomy. You will need:

Universal precautions; sterile gown and gloves
Skin disinfectant
Sterile drape
Syringe of local anaesthetic/needle/(10 ml of 2% lidocaine (lignocaine) and adrenaline (epinephrine)
Cricothyroidotomy/minitracheostomy kit (containing needle, guide wire, dilator tube and tape)
Suture
Dressing

Explain to the patient what you are going to do. Get written or verbal consent if appropriate. Check the patient's coagulation status. Position the patient comfortably with the head and neck extended over a pillow. Then:

- Palpate anatomy to identify the cricothyroid membrane.
- Clean the neck with antiseptic solution.
- Infiltrate over the cricothyroid membrane with 2–3 ml of local anaesthetic.
- Warn the patient that you are going to make him or her cough and perform cricothyroid puncture with a green 21-gauge needle. Aspirate air to confirm the tracheal position of the needle and rapidly inject 2 ml of lidocaine (lignocaine). Wait for coughing to subside.
- Perform a superficial skin incision.
- Pass the introducing needle into the trachea and aspirate air.
- Pass the guide wire through the needle and then remove the needle.
- Pass the introducer over the guide wire and then slide the cricothyroidotomy/minitracheostomy tube off the introducer. Remove the introducer and guide wire together, leaving the cricothyroidotomy/minitracheostomy in place. Suction to remove any blood.
- Obtain CXR to verify the position.

Complications

The complications of minitracheostomy are the same as for formal tracheostomy. Misplacement and bleeding are particular problems.

BRONCHOSCOPY

Flexible fibreoptic bronchoscopy is a useful diagnostic and therapeutic tool in the ICU. In this situation it is usually performed on patients who have access to their airway via an endotracheal tube or tracheostomy.

Indications

- Fibreoptic intubation.
- Removal of secretions (associated with areas of collapse on CXR).
- Retrieval of sputum samples for microbiology.
- Bronchoalveolar lavage (see below).
- Assessment of airway injury and burns.
- Biopsy of tumours and lung tissue.
- Assessment of endotracheal tube position.
- To guide operator during tracheostomy (see above).

Contraindications

These are relative. Patients with high airway pressures, critical oxygenation, cardiovascular instability or raised intracranial pressure may not tolerate bronchoscopy.

Preparation

The bronchoscope should be leak-tested and sterilized before use. This generally takes about 20 minutes. Most hospitals will have automatic washers for this.

> ⚠️ **Use of the bronchoscope clearly requires knowledge of the endoscopic anatomy of the bronchial tree. If you do not know this you should not be performing a bronchoscopy.**

Procedure

Before commencing the procedure, check that the size of the patient's endotracheal tube is adequate to allow bronchoscopy. Tubes smaller than 8 mm internal diameter may be significantly occluded by the bronchoscope, making ventilation and oxygenation of the patient difficult.

Bronchoscopy. You will need:

Bronchoscope
Light source/battery pack
Bowl of sterile water
Suction
Sputum traps
Sterile saline
Swivel connector with bronchoscopy port
Gown gloves and goggles

- Attach the swivel connector to the patient's endotracheal or tracheostomy tube.
- Ventilate the patient on 100% oxygen prior to and during the bronchoscopy.
- Adequately sedate the patient and then give a small dose of muscle relaxant (such as atracurium) to prevent the patient biting or coughing on the bronchoscope. Instil 3–5 ml of local anaesthetic (e.g. 1% lidocaine (lignocaine)) down the trachea. It is sensible to have an assistant to look after patient sedation and ventilation while you perform the bronchoscopy.
- Bronchoscopy should be a clean procedure to avoid contaminating the patient's airway.
- Lubricate the scope with a small amount of lubricant jelly. Avoid getting it over the lens.

> ⚠ **When handling the scope never allow it to bend or fold at an acute angle, as this will break the fibreoptic components.**

- Pass the bronchoscope through the bung on the swivel connector and into the endotracheal or tracheostomy tube. Continue forward under direct vision.
- Pass the scope forward to the carina. Then explore each side of the bronchial tree in turn. Identify and enter each lobar and segmental bronchus (Fig. 15.8). Take note of any abnormal anatomy and remove any secretions.
- If there are thick secretions that cannot be sucked up the scope, try instilling 10–20 ml of sterile saline down the suction port of the bronchoscope. This may help to loosen them. Large plugs and blood clots may be dragged out on the end of the scope.
- To obtain microbiology specimens place a sputum trap in between the bronchoscope and the wall suction. Use a separate trap for each

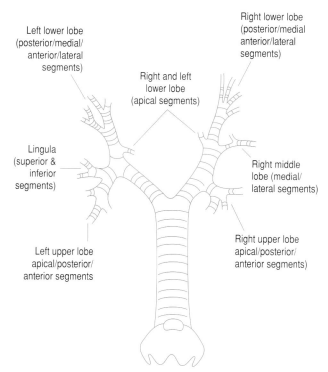

Fig. 15.8 Anatomy of the bronchial tree.

side. Be careful to keep the sputum trap upright to prevent the
secretions disappearing down the suction tubing. Also remove
sputum traps before removing the scope from the patient to prevent
specimens being contaminated with upper airway flora.
- Bronchial biopsy should not be performed by trainees in intensive
  care. Seek help.
- Following bronchoscopy, perform a CXR to exclude pneumothorax
  and look for improvement in lung expansion where large sputum
  plugs have been removed.
- Ensure the scope is washed and sterilized according to your
  hospital policy.

BRONCHOALVEOLAR LAVAGE

Bronchoalveolar lavage (BAL) is a technique for obtaining microbiology specimens from low in the respiratory tree, avoiding contamination of samples with upper respiratory tract flora. It may be performed during bronchoscopy or using specially designed BAL catheters.

Indications

BAL may be used to obtain specimens in any patient with pneumonia. It is of particular value in investigating pneumonia in the immunocompromised patient. In addition to conventional pathogens such as *Streptococcus pneumoniae* and *Haemophilus influenzae*, other likely pathogens in these patients are *Pneumocystis carinii*, either alone or with a copathogen, *Mycobacterium* species including tuberculosis, cytomegalovirus and fungi.

Discuss the clinical situation with a microbiologist before performing the BAL. He or she will advise on appropriate specimens and tests (see below).

BAL during bronchoscopy

This has the advantage that the operator can be highly selective in the area for lavage in the case of localized disease. It is, however, more invasive and operator-dependent.

- During bronchoscopy (see above) the bronchoscope is passed into a subsegmental bronchus until it wedges.
- Up to 100 ml of saline is instilled down the suction channel.
- This is then aspirated and collected into a series of sputum traps.

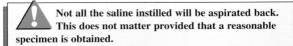

Not all the saline instilled will be aspirated back. This does not matter provided that a reasonable specimen is obtained.

BAL using catheter

BAL catheters consist of a protective outer sleeve and an inner suction catheter. The suction catheter can be connected via a three-way tap to suction and a syringe for instilling saline. This should be a clean procedure and you should wear apron, gloves and goggles.

- Preoxygenate the patient with 100% oxygen.
- Pass the catheter, with inner tube protected, into the airway, beyond the endotracheal tube.

TABLE 15.9 Investigation following BAL

Urgent Gram and Ziehl–Neelsen stain
Microscopy, culture and sensitivity including TB (AAFB)
Differential cell count
Fungi
Viruses
Legionella immune fluorescent antibody test
Pneumocystis carinii

- Advance the inner protected suction catheter forwards until it meets resistance. Do not use undue force.
- Perform BAL according to local protocol. Generally 80–100 ml of saline are instilled down the suction catheter, and then aspirated into 2 or 3 sputum traps. Not all the saline may be aspirated. This does not matter.
- Withdraw the inner suction catheter into the protective sleeve before removing from the patient.

Having performed a BAL, telephone the laboratory and then send samples immediately with full diagnostic information and appropriate requests (Table 15.9).

CHEST DRAINAGE

⚠️ **The emergency treatment of life-threatening tension pneumothorax is large-bore needle decompression. The diagnosis is made on clinical grounds without chest X-ray. A 14-gauge cannula is inserted into the pleural cavity immediately above the second rib in the midclavicular line. This should be followed by placement of a formal chest drain.**

Indications

Chest drains are indicated for the drainage of air (pneumothorax), blood (haemothorax), fluid (pleural effusion), pus (empyema) and lymph (chylothorax) from the pleural cavity. In critically ill patients pleural fluid is a common finding on chest X-rays, CT scan and ultrasound. In most cases unless the effusion is large or ventilation is clearly compromised there is no need to drain this fluid. It will resolve as the patient's condition improves. Blood in the pleural cavity should be drained as soon as possible. Once it becomes clotted it will not drain readily and thoracotomy may be required to remove the clot and allow the lung to re-expand.

Type of drain

Chest drains are of two types. Traditionally large-bore tubes, particularly suitable for draining blood or pus, have been placed manually through an incision made in the chest wall directly into the pleural cavity. More recently, Seldinger versions have become available. Seldinger drains should only be used blindly to drain obvious large collections because of the risk that the introducer needle may damage the lung. For smaller collections, Seldinger drains should be placed under ultrasound guidance to reduce the risks of needle damage.

Site of drain

This is partly dictated by the position of the collection clinically and radiographically. In the case of long-standing collections, which may be loculated, ultrasound guidance may be helpful. In all other cases the drain should be sited in the 5th intercostal space, just anterior to the midaxillary line, and can be directed cephalad for air and caudally for fluid or blood. All drains should be placed immediately above the rib to avoid damage to the neurovascular bundle, which lies underneath.

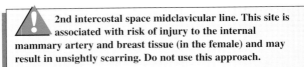

> ⚠️ **2nd intercostal space midclavicular line. This site is associated with risk of injury to the internal mammary artery and breast tissue (in the female) and may result in unsightly scarring. Do not use this approach.**

Procedure

Chest drainage. You will need:

Universal precautions; sterile gown and gloves
Skin disinfectant
Sterile drape
10-ml syringe, local anaesthetic and needles (lidocaine (lignocaine) 1–2%)
Basic instruments: scalpel, blade, large arterial clamps
Chest drain
Strong silk sutures, adhesive strapping and dressings
Underwater seal, low-pressure vacuum (wall vacuum or pump)

Insertion of drain through thoracostomy

- Explain procedure to the patient.
- Position the patient (supine with arm lifted, a pillow behind back).

- Prepare a sterile field.
- Infiltrate superficial structures down to rib with local anaesthetic.
- Make a 2–4 cm incision.
- Palpate through skin incision and perform blunt dissection down to rib and through pleura.
- Push finger into pleural cavity and sweep around to ensure no viscera are adjacent.
- Insert drain and direct into appropriate position.

 Trocars should not be used to insert drains. They are sharp and may cause injury to underlying viscera.

- Connect to underwater drain and confirm position by drainage of collection and respiratory swing.
- Secure drain in position with suture. Purse-string sutures result in very unsightly scarring when chest drains are removed and are best avoided. Use mattress sutures to close the skin edges and a simple tie to hold in the drain.
- Order a chest X-ray.

Insertion of Seldinger drains and pigtail catheters
- Explain procedure to the patient and position as before.
- Ideally determine and mark the optimal position for drain site using ultrasound.
- Prepare a sterile field.
- Infiltrate superficial structures down to rib with local anaesthetic.
- Advance needle through chest until blood/fluid/air aspirated.
- Feed guide wire into pleural space.
- Pass chest drain/pigtail catheter over guide wire.
- For large drains attach underwater seal as above, for pigtail catheters aspirate and/or attach drainage bag.
- Order a CXR.

DO NOT CLAMP CHEST DRAINS. If moving a patient, simply keep the underwater drain bottle below the level of the chest. Clamping drains may produce a tension pneumothorax.

COMMON PROBLEMS DURING INSERTION OF CHEST DRAINS

Lung will not expand
- Reassess diagnosis and position of tube.
- Is tube 'swinging' or is it blocked/kinked? Is the effusion loculated?
- Consider low-pressure suction (wall suction or pump 10–20 mmHg).
- Increase tidal volume or add 10 cm of PEEP.
- Consider need for surgical referral (see below).

Persistent air leak
- Check the drain and reposition if necessary (it may have come out of the chest and be entraining room air). If air leak persists, attempt to minimize airway pressures.
- In trauma patients, consider bronchoscopy to exclude airway rupture.
- Wean patient onto spontaneous breathing modes.
- If ventilated, ensure adequate sedation, analgesia and muscle relaxation.
- Use pressure-controlled ventilation and reduce PEEP.
- Accept a degree of hypercapnia, e.g. $PaCO_2$ 8 kPa.
- Consider high frequency jet ventilation.
- Consider thoracic surgical opinion (see below).

Indications for urgent thoracic surgical opinion
The combination of persistent air leak and non-compliant lungs (e.g. ARDS) may make adequate ventilation and gas exchange impossible. Urgent thoracic surgical opinion may be required (Table 15.10).

Removing chest drains
- Chest drains can be removed when they are no longer needed. In practice, this means that if the clinical and CXR findings that required a chest drain have resolved, and the drain is no longer bubbling or draining fluid, it can be removed.
- There is no need to clamp drains before removal.

TABLE 15.10 Indications for surgical opinion/thoracotomy

Collection not fully drained or lung not fully re-expanded
Massive air leak (bronchopleural fistula/ruptured bronchus)
Continued bleeding
Presence/suspected presence of other intrathoracic injuries

- Clean the site with antiseptic solution. Cut the retaining suture, remove the drain and occlude by pressing.
- Close the wound with a suture. If this is already in situ it can be tied as the drain is removed to reduce any air entrainment. (Avoid purse strings, as above.)
- Obtain a CXR.

PASSING A NASOGASTRIC TUBE

All patients in the ICU who require ventilation require a nasogastric tube, initially at least, to ensure gastric drainage and early enteral feeding (Table 15.11).

Procedure

Passing a nasogastric tube. You will need:
Gloves and mask
NG tube
Lubricating jelly
Laryngoscope
Magill forceps

- Explain to the patient what you are going to do, even if he or she is apparently unconscious. Position the patient supine with head neutral.
- Lubricate the NG tube and, keeping alignment with the long axis of the patient, introduce through the nose. Do not force. If resistance is met, try the other side.
- If the patient is co-operative ask the patient to swallow the tip of the tube when he or she feels it in the back of the throat. In

TABLE 15.11 Indications and contraindications for nasogastric tube

Indications	Contraindications
To deflate the stomach after ventilation with a bag and mask	Base of skull fracture (use orogastric tube)
To aspirate gastric contents which might otherwise reflux and soil the airway	Recent gastric or oesophageal surgery (discuss with surgeon)
To provide a route for enteral feeding and drugs	Oesophageal varices (relative contraindication)
	Severe coagulopathy (consider oral route to avoid nose bleed)

unconscious patients the tube may pass directly into the
oesophagus but often coils up in the mouth.

- In this case, use a laryngoscope to examine the pharynx and pass the
  tube manually into the oesophagus using a pair of Magill forceps.
  (Be careful not to traumatize the uvula and pharyngeal mucosa.)
- Confirm the position of the NG tube in the stomach by aspiration
  of gastric contents (turns litmus paper red), auscultation (gurgling
  when air blown into tube) or by CXR. The presence of a cuffed
  endotracheal or tracheostomy tube does not prevent feeding tubes
  entering the lung.
- Secure the NG tube in position with adhesive tape.

Nasojejunal feeding tubes

Nasojejunal feeding tubes are fine-bore soft tubes designed for long-term
use. They are usually provided with the feeding tube mounted on a wire
insert, which stiffens the tube during placement and allows X-ray
determination of position. This is removed once the tube is in place.

The main difficulty in passing nasojejunal feeding tubes is getting
them to pass through the pylorus. The simplest approach is to pass a
reasonable length of tube into the stomach (as for NG tube above) and
leave for a few hours before getting an abdominal X-ray. Some tubes
will simply migrate into the duodenum/jejunum. Alternatively, jejunal
tubes can be placed using X-ray screening, ultrasound or endoscopic
guidance. Seek advice.

PASSING A SENGSTAKEN–BLAKEMORE TUBE

A number of tubes have been designed to apply pressure to
oesophageal varices in order to compress the vessels and reduce
bleeding while the patient is resuscitated and definitive treatment
carried out. The Sengstaken–Blakemore tube has three lumens. Two
are used to inflate balloons, one in the stomach and the other in the
oesophagus, while the third is used to aspirate gastric contents.

Procedure

Passing a Sengstaken–Blakemore tube. You will need:

Universal precautions
Suction apparatus
Sengstaken–Blakemore tube (usually kept in a fridge)
500 ml saline
50-ml syringe
Traction (string and 500-ml bag of fluid)

- Read instructions for the specific device you are using.
- Explain to the patient what you are going to do.
- Position the patient comfortably. Left lateral is best if the patient is vomiting.
- Check the patency of the tube lumens and integrity of the balloons.
- Pass the tube orally into the oesophagus and down into the stomach. (Local anaesthetic spray to the pharynx may make this more tolerable in the awake patient.) Insert the tube to at least 30 cm.
- Inflate the gastric balloon with 250 ml of saline. You should not feel any resistance.
- Pull the tube backwards gently until resistance is felt as the gastric balloon meets the gastro-oesophageal junction.
- Inflate the oesophageal balloon with air or saline (approximately 100 ml). The pressure in the oesophageal balloon can be measured using a sphygmomanometer and should be 25–35 mmHg. Chest pain, respiratory difficulty and cardiac arrhythmias may occur during inflation of the balloon.
- Apply traction to the tube by tying a piece of string to the end and suspending a 500-ml bag of fluid over a fulcrum. Traction should be released at regular intervals to prevent pressure necrosis of the gastro-oesophageal junction.
- The position of the tube should be checked by CXR. The point where the tube exits the mouth should be marked in order to detect subsequent migration. Check the pressure in the oesophageal balloon regularly.

Removing the tube

After 24 hours the traction should be removed and the oesophageal balloon deflated to assess for bleeding. If bleeding recurs, the balloon can be reinflated for a further period of 24 hours; however, the need for surgery becomes increasingly likely. If there is no bleeding the tube is generally left in situ deflated for 24 hours in case bleeding recurs. After this time the tube can be removed.

TURNING A PATIENT PRONE

Patients may be turned prone when oxygenation is critical despite ventilation and high inspired oxygen concentrations. (See ARDS, p. 128.) Turning large adult patients prone can be hazardous both for the staff and the patient. Where possible, hoists or other aids to handling patients should be used. The nursing staff will advise on the best approach. In general terms, whatever approach to physically turning the patient is adopted, there must be adequate numbers of staff available to ensure patient safety, and security of airway, vascular cannulae and drains, etc.

- Temporarily discontinue all non-essential drug and fluid infusions.
- Ensure that all lines and monitoring cables are positioned such that they will not be trapped under the patient when he or she is turned.
- Remove ECG electrodes from the patient's front and replace on the back.
- Designate specific individuals to be responsible for maintaining the security of the endotracheal tube, vascular access and lines. Designate other individuals to turn the patient.
- Position pillows so that they will be under the patient's chest and pelvis when the patient is prone. Alternatively, position them afterwards. They are to ensure that the abdomen is not compressed, which can impair venous return and CO.
- When everyone is ready, use the commands 'ready, steady, move'. Turn the patient on 'move'.
- Ensure the patient is comfortably positioned and that there is no pressure on the tip of the nose, eyes or any peripheral nerves. The arms should be positioned towards the patient's head (not unduly extended) to ensure there is no tension on the brachial plexus.
- Re-establish any monitoring or drugs and fluid infusions that were previously discontinued.

TRANSPORTING CRITICALLY ILL PATIENTS

Critically ill patients in intensive care often require transport either within the hospital (for example for investigations or surgery), or between hospitals (for example for specialist care). You are therefore likely to be involved in transporting a patient at some stage, even if only within your own hospital.

The standards of care during transport, whether intrahospital or interhospital, should be the same as that provided within the ICU. Before moving the patient, it is important that the patient is fully resuscitated and stable. If there is any doubt regarding the adequacy of resuscitation, this should be addressed before transfer. The general principles are as follows:

- Full monitoring should be continued. This should include blood pressure monitoring (preferably invasive), ECG, oxygen saturation, and end-tidal CO_2 for intubated/ventilated patients. If a PA catheter is in situ the pressure trace must be displayed, or the catheter should be pulled back into the SVC to prevent inadvertent pulmonary artery occlusion.

- Ensure that the airway is secure; this usually means endotracheal intubation.
- Ensure adequate supplies of oxygen to complete the transfer. In case the supply fails, an alternative means of ventilating the patient should be available. This should be a self-inflating bag, rather than an anaesthetic breathing circuit.
- Ensure that a portable suction unit is available.
- Ensure adequate intravenous access, usually at least two secure intravenous cannulae.
- Discontinue non-essential drug infusions. Ensure that essential infusions are delivered using syringe pumps with fully charged batteries.
- Ensure any drugs or resuscitation equipment that you are likely to need during the transfer are available.

During the transfer you should be accompanied by an intensive care nurse or an operating department assistant. The transfer should be fully documented, including a record of pulse, blood pressure, ventilation and other vital signs. Departure and arrival times should be notified to the receiving hospital sufficiently in advance to enable suitable preparation to be made.

END OF LIFE ISSUES

INTRODUCTION

Mortality rates on ICUs range from 15 to 35%, depending on case mix, and are typically about 20%. In addition, significant numbers of patients will die soon after leaving the ICU. The ability to deal with death and the issues surrounding it is therefore an important part of work on an ICU. The dying patient must be afforded respect and allowed to die with dignity, while relatives must also be treated sympathetically. If handled appropriately, relatives will often gain great comfort from the peaceful passing of a loved one and be grateful for all that has been done.

It is particularly important to be honest and to recognize when patients are deteriorating such that death is inevitable. Once recognized, the family can be warned and relatives from further afield given the opportunity to travel to the hospital. Decision regarding the continuation or withdrawal of treatment can be made in a timely unhurried manner, avoiding the need for frantic telephone calls in the middle of the night when the patient arrests.

Do not resuscitate (DNR) orders

Patients on the ICU may die unexpectedly (e.g. from sudden cardiac arrest) but, more commonly, death is anticipated and often occurs as result of a decision that active treatment should be limited or withdrawn. Such decisions are much more common than standard 'do not resuscitate' (DNR) orders as practised on general wards. If a DNR order is considered appropriate, this should wherever possible be discussed with the patient and/or the relatives. The DNR order and the reasons for it should be clearly documented in the notes. DNR orders should be reviewed regularly and revoked if the situation or condition leading to them changes.

WITHDRAWAL OF TREATMENT

Patients are often admitted to the ICU for a period of stabilization and assessment. Over time, however, it may become clear that the patient has no prospect of meaningful recovery. Under these circumstances a decision may be made to withdraw treatment or limit further escalation of treatment. In this setting it is important to understand that there is no medicolegal obligation to continue treatment that is futile and, indeed, to do so could be considered as assault on the patient.

In general:

- There should usually be a consensus from all clinicians and nursing staff involved with care of the patient that continuation of life-sustaining treatment is inappropriate. If there is any doubt, it is better to continue treatment until consensus is reached.
- The final decision to withdraw treatment should be made by the consultant intensivist and the referring consultant.

Intensive care patients will frequently be unconscious or sedated and are rarely therefore competent to be involved in decisions regarding withdrawal of care. Where appropriate, however, the decision to withdraw treatment should be discussed with the patient. Where this is not possible, there is no legal requirement in the UK to obtain consent from family members or relatives regarding withdrawal of treatment. Nevertheless, it is fundamental to good clinical practice to involve the family as far as possible and to be open and honest. Most relatives appreciate time spent in explanation and will accept the concept of withdrawal of treatment. Discussion with relatives should be led by an appropriate consultant, either from the referring team or from the ICU.

The best approach to the actual process of withdrawal of treatment will vary from case to case. From a legal point of view there is no distinction drawn between, for example, the withdrawal of vasoactive drugs and assisted ventilation. Commonly:

- Inotropes and vasopressor agents may be discontinued.
- Artificial ventilation may be withdrawn.
- Endotracheal tubes may be removed.
- The inspired oxygen concentration may be reduced.
- The patient should be kept comfortable throughout the process. (See Euthanasia below.)
- Fluids and nutrition are usually continued, as hydration is considered an important aspect of patient comfort.

Euthanasia

UK law does not allow the practice of euthanasia. Patients who are dying should not, however, be allowed to suffer needlessly. It is

> ⚠ **The withdrawal of life-sustaining therapy such as nasogastric feeding from patients in persistent vegetative state (PVS), who do not otherwise require any form of organ support, is a complex legal issue. This would normally take place outside the ICU and is beyond the scope of this book.**

permissible to administer sedative or analgesic drugs to relieve patient distress, accepting that in some cases the administration of these drugs will speed up the process of death. This is known as the principle of double effect. Most units would prescribe benzodiazepines or opioids for this purpose and many relatives gain comfort from the fact that the dying patient is not allowed to suffer unnecessarily.

Other aspects of managing death

Consideration should be given as to when and where is the best place for a patient to die.

The process is often best managed in intensive care, where staff can support the patient and relatives. Some units have developed so-called 'tender loving care' rooms specifically designed for this purpose. If the patient's bed is likely to be required in the near future it may be more appropriate to transfer the patient to a general ward. Occasionally, particularly when patients are aware of their surroundings and what is happening, it may be appropriate to transfer the patient somewhere else, such as a hospice, or even home, in order that he or she may die in peaceful surroundings.

Consideration should also be given to the timing of withdrawal of therapy in order that relatives visiting from afar may be present. Relatives will also often ask how long death will take. This can be very difficult to predict. Some patients may survive a few minutes, others a few hours. Occasionally a patient may even apparently improve temporarily following withdrawal of inotropes. Therefore, be honest and say that you do not know, but will be in a better position to judge once life-sustaining therapy has been withdrawn.

CONFIRMING DEATH

When a patient dies, death must be confirmed by a doctor. Interestingly there is no legally agreed definition of death in the UK (other than brainstem death); however, it is generally taken to include cessation of breathing and the absence of a heartbeat. Note the following and record findings in the medical records along with the date and time of death:

- Absence of palpable pulse. Absence of heart sounds.
- Absence of respiratory effort (disconnect ventilator). Absence of breath sounds.
- Pupils are fixed and dilated.

> ⚠ **Confirming death in severely hypothermic patients is very difficult.** In general, patients should not be declared dead until they are warm and dead. This may require heroic attempts at resuscitation and rewarming, for example in victims of cold water immersion. If in doubt, seek help. (See Hypothermia, p. 185.)

Who to inform

Once death is confirmed you must make sure that the relatives have been informed (see below). You should also inform the people listed below, although this can often wait until the next morning if the patient has died out of hours; actions will depend upon the circumstances and, in particular, whether or not the death was expected:

- Referring clinician(s).
- Consultant in charge of intensive care.
- The patient's general practitioner. (This is especially important. It fosters good relations between the hospital and the community and allows the GP an opportunity to offer counselling and support to the relatives.)
- Coroner's officer, if appropriate (see below).

BREAKING BAD NEWS

This is never an easy task, particularly if the death has occurred unexpectedly or if the patient was very young. If the relatives are not present at the time of the death they will generally be called by a senior nurse and asked to come into the hospital. Try to avoid talking on the telephone if at all possible. When they are present or when they arrive you should speak to them in a quiet side room. It is worth checking that all relevant members of the family are present, as different branches of families may not communicate.

- Follow the basic guidelines on talking to relatives (see Chapter 2, p. 24).
- Be honest but not brutal! Avoid euphemisms such as 'he slipped away' as these may not be interpreted in the way you expect. Clearly say that the patient has died.
- Relatives often find it helpful to know that their loved one was not in any pain or distress, if this is true.

The stages of bereavement include denial, anger and gradual acceptance. Any of these emotions may be expressed. It is not uncommon for the initial response to take the form of anger if they believe that things have gone badly for their relative. Such anger will often subside over time as the realities of the situation become apparent. Sympathetic handling, honesty and compassion with relatives will avoid many later complaints.

Many units now offer relatives the chance to return at a later date to revisit the sequence of events surrounding a patient's death and to ask any questions they may have. This is a valuable part of the grieving process for relatives. Formal grief counselling may benefit some relatives.

ISSUING A DEATH CERTIFICATE

In the UK the whole area of death certification, including the role of the coroner, is currently under review. The following notes reflect the death certification process at the time of writing. The death certificate asks you to give information about the cause of death. You can issue a death certificate if:

- You have attended to the patient during the last illness, and you have seen the patient alive within 14 days of the death (28 days in Scotland and Northern Ireland).
- You are satisfied that the death was due to natural causes (see below).
- You are reasonably sure of the cause of death.
- There is no specific requirement to inform the coroner.

If you can issue a death certificate, then complete the relevant sections. The death certificate is then given to the patient's family so that they can register the death. In many hospitals a bereavement liaison officer will handle these matters. Ensure that you fill in the form accurately, as it is very distressing for relatives if the certificate is rejected by the registrar:

- Write legibly. If your writing is difficult to read, it is best to print the details.
- Do not use terms such as heart failure as a sole cause of death. (Strictly this is a mode of death rather than a cause.) If used, these terms must be backed up by an underlying diagnosis, e.g. ischaemic heart disease.
- Avoid using terms such as alcohol, drugs or HIV where these are not strictly necessary, as this can be upsetting for relatives. (Additional information can be provided to the registrar at a later date where necessary.) Seek senior advice if unsure.

- Print your name next to your signature so that you can be easily identified in case of difficulty.

POSTMORTEM EXAMINATIONS

Where the cause of death is known but information from a postmortem examination would be of interest, you may ask the family for permission to perform a hospital postmortem. Where a death occurs after major surgery, most surgeons will require a postmortem. This may help clarify the events leading up to the death. There is space on the death certificate to record that more information may subsequently be available from a postmortem. In this case the registrar's office will write to you once the result of the postmortem is available.

> ⚠ **If you do not know the cause of death then you cannot ask for a hospital postmortem. In this instance the death must be reported to the coroner.**

Consent to postmortem examination

Following a number of high profile legal cases relating to retention of organs and tissues during postmortem examinations, new guidelines have been issued relating to consent for postmortem examinations. Fully informed consent should be obtained from relatives for both the examination and for the retention of any samples. You must therefore be aware of what the postmortem examination will entail and what samples may be retained. This may require you to discuss the details of the postmortem with the pathologist. Follow your hospital guidelines and ask if in doubt.

REPORTING DEATHS TO THE CORONER

If you are unable to issue a death certificate you must report the death to the coroner (procurator fiscal in Scotland). The commoner indications for reporting a death to the coroner are given in Table 16.1. If in doubt, ask.

   If in any doubt you should discuss the death with the coroner. You will generally deal with the coroner's officer. These are usually specially trained policemen with variable degrees of medical knowledge, but are nevertheless a useful source of advice. When speaking to the coroner's officer you will need the following information:

TABLE 16.1 Indications for reporting death to the coroner

Death cannot be certified as due to natural causes
Deceased not seen by a doctor within the last 14 days
Death occurred within 24 hours of hospital admission
Death occurred in suspicious circumstances or following an accident or violence
Death occurred during or shortly after imprisonment or while in police custody
Death occurred while deceased was detained under Mental Health Act
Death may have been contributed to by actions of deceased, including self-injury or drug abuse
Death associated with neglect, including self-neglect
Deceased was receiving any form of war pension or industrial disability pension
Death could be in any way related to the deceased's employment
Death associated with abortion, spontaneous or induced
Death occurring during an operation or before full recovery from the effects of an anaesthetic or in any way related to an anaesthetic*
Death was related to a medical procedure or treatment*
Death may be due to lack of medical care*

*It is advisable to discuss any death following surgery or other procedure with the coroner. There is no formal time limit laid down for this.

- deceased patient's name, date of birth, address
- address and telephone number of next of kin and GP
- brief summary of the patient's last illness, including date of admission, diagnosis, operations, complications, and date and time of death
- reason for reporting death
- suggested cause of death if prepared to offer a death certificate.

If the cause of death is not suspicious, or unnatural, the coroner may give permission for you to issue a death certificate (initial box 'A' on the reverse of the death certificate). In this case the cause of death cited on the form is agreed with the coroner's officer, who then issues a covering slip to the registrar's office.

If the cause of death is unknown, or is suspicious or unnatural, then the coroner's officer will take over. Generally a coroner's postmortem will be performed, and if necessary an inquest convened.

Situation in Scotland

In Scotland the situation is slightly different. The procurator fiscal investigates deaths reported to him or her. The main concern is to establish evidence of negligence or criminality rather than the cause of death. If satisfied that the death is natural, the procurator fiscal may instruct a doctor to examine the body and issue a death certificate. If the cause of death is suspicious, an application must be made to the sheriff for a postmortem examination. The cause of death is then certified by the pathologist. If there is evidence of negligence or criminality, then the lord advocate may order that a fatal accident enquiry be held.

BRAINSTEM DEATH AND ORGAN DONATION

The brainstem is responsible for the maintenance of life-sustaining functions within the body, in particular the maintenance and adequacy of respiration. With the advent of modern intensive care it is possible for patients in whom brainstem death has occurred to be on a ventilator and still have a heart beat and pulse. These patients are not capable of sustaining life on their own. Therefore brainstem death is now a legally accepted definition of death, the diagnosis of which is governed by strict guidelines and protocols. (See Brainstem death, p. 246.)

Patients who are brainstem dead and on a ventilator may be suitable for organ donation. Although organ donor cards may be considered an advanced directive, it is good practice to discuss the issue of organ donation with the relatives and ask them for permission to remove organs from their relative. You may also need to ask permission of the coroner if the case would normally have been reported to the coroner (see above).

Not all relatives will give consent to organ donation, some religious groups in particular find it difficult. You must accept their wishes, no matter what your own views. (See Organ donation, p. 250.)

NON-HEART BEATING ORGAN DONATION

The shortage of donor organs from cadaveric, heart beating (brainstem dead) donors has led to renewed interest in the use of non-heart beating (asystolic) donors. A number of UK centres are now developing asystolic donor programmes. There are, however, still a number of medicolegal and ethical issues that require clarification, including issues of consent, timing and definition of death, and the time elapsed between death and organ procurement.

In general, organs may be suitable for organ donation after asystole, if the time interval between death and retrieval is short, so that irretrievable damage to the organs does not occur. Four categories of patients who might be suitable have been described. These are shown in Table 16.2.

TABLE 16.2 Maastricht categories for non-heart beating donors

Category 1: Dead on arrival at hospital	Death needs to have been witnessed and the time documented Adequate 'resuscitation' between asystole and admission
Category 2: Unsuccessful resuscitation	Patients who suffer a witnessed cardiac arrest (usually in A&E Dept) in which the interval of resuscitation and the efficiency of resuscitation has been well documented
Category 3: Awaiting cardiac arrest	Patients, typically on ICU, for whom death is inevitable but who do not fulfil criteria for brainstem death
Category 4: Cardiac arrest following confirmed brainstem death	Patients already on ICU declared brainstem dead. May be awaiting arrival of retrieval team

Typically patients on ICU are in category 3. The patient does not fulfil criteria for brainstem death, but death is inevitable, withdrawal of treatment is planned and the family wish their relative to become an organ donor. Following discussion and consent from relatives, there may be a planned withdrawal of supportive treatment. Following asystole, there is a 'stand off' period during which relatives may 'say goodbye' to their loved one, after which the organs are cold perfused in situ by cannulation of the femoral artery and vein before being removed for transplant.

DEATH AND DIFFERENT CULTURAL VIEWS

Different religious groups have different ways of dealing with death. This may clash with your own religious or cultural beliefs. Some groups may have large extended families and publicly display their grief. A number of religious groups are unhappy about postmortem examinations and some prefer to remove the body from the hospital as soon as possible after death. This can sometimes be arranged. You should respect the views of others.

Table 16.3 gives a brief guide to the beliefs and practices of the more common religious groups. The information has been compiled from a number of sources and every effort has been made to ensure that it accurately reflects religious and cultural beliefs. Any errors or admissions are unintentional and no offence is intended.

- Routine care of the dying and last offices are appropriate unless otherwise stated.
- No religious objection to postmortem examination or organ donation unless otherwise stated.

TABLE 16.3 Beliefs and practices of common religious groups

Anglicans	May request Baptism, Eucharist, or Anointing
Roman Catholics	May request Baptism, Holy Communion and Sacrament of the Dying
Members of Christian Free Church	Christians who do not conform to the Anglican or Catholic tradition Generally less emphasis on the sacraments May request a minister for informal prayers
Jehovah's Witnesses	Unrestricted access family and friends and church elders (There are no formal ministers, all Jehovah's Witnesses are ministers) There are no ceremonial rites at death
Christian Scientists	Believe in the power of God's healing and avoid conventional medicine May accept conventional medicine due to family or legal pressure without loss of faith and allow medical care of children No specific ceremonial rites at death Would not wish to consent to postmortem or organ donation
Afro-Caribbean Community	Extended family and church visits More emphasis on prayer than sacraments May prefer body to be handled by staff of same cultural background Older members of the community may believe in the sanctity of the body and not wish to consent to postmortem or organ donation
Rastafarian	May prefer alternative therapy to conventional medicine Distinctive hairstyle, may not want hair cut Second-hand clothes are taboo, may be reluctant to wear hospital gowns No specific ceremonial rites at death Unlikely to consent to postmortem or organ donation
Buddhists	State of mind is important Require peace and quiet for meditation and chanting May request counselling from local Buddhists No specific ceremonial rites at death A Buddhist monk should be informed of the death

Cont'd

TABLE 16.3 Cont'd

Jews	Orthodox Jews will wish to maintain customs of dress, diet, prayer and observe the Sabbath while in hospital
	May object to any intervention which may hasten death (e.g. withdrawal of treatment)
	Relatives may wish to consult a rabbi
	No specific ceremonial rites at death but may recite special prayers
	There is a wish that dying Jews should not be left alone
	Ritual laying out of the body by Jewish burial society with burial arranged ideally within 24 hours. Postmortem not permitted except where law requires it. Unlikely to consent to organ donation
Muslims	Muslim women will not want to be seen by male doctors
	Prayers ritual may be continued
	Cleanliness important and running water required for washing
	Friends and family may recite prayer, dying patient may wish to be turned towards Mecca (south-east)
	Body should not be touched by non-Muslims (if necessary wear gloves) and should be prepared according to the wishes of the family or priest
	Funerals should take place within 24 hours where possible
	Believe in the sanctity of the body
	Unlikely to consent to postmortem or organ donation
Hindus	Hindu women will prefer female doctors
	Prayer ritual may be continued
	Dying patients may wish to lie on the floor to be close to 'Earth'
	Rites including tying of a holy thread and sprinkling with water from the River Ganges
	Religious tokens should not be removed
	Body should not be touched by non-Hindus (if necessary wear gloves) and should be prepared according to the wishes of the family or priest
	Ideally cremation should be arranged within 24 hours, often not practicable
	No specific religious objection to postmortem or organ donation, although these are not liked

Cont'd

TABLE 16.3 Cont'd	
Sikhs	Sikh women will prefer female doctors
	Sikh men will wish to keep their hair covered at all times
	The five symbols of faith should not be disturbed in life or death
	Running water preferred for washing
	No specific ceremonial rites at death
	Traditionally Sikh families will lay out the body but no specific objection to others touching the body

DEALING WITH DEATH AT A PERSONAL LEVEL

Working on an ICU can be both very satisfying and very demanding. Doctors and other health care professionals working on the ICU, who frequently deal with dying patients and bereaved relatives, often develop robust coping mechanisms to help them deal with death on a day-to-day basis. There are times, however, when even the most seasoned professional will find it hard to deal with a particular patient's death or a particular set of circumstances. The effects may even be felt some considerable time after the event and staff may even feel guilty about their feelings. It is important at these times to seek support.

If you find yourself affected by anything you come across on intensive care, do not keep it to yourself. Discuss it with friends, colleagues or senior medical or nursing staff, or make use of the support groups and counselling services that are available.

DRUG
INFORMATION

The following drug/prescribing information is for guidance only. Doses are based on an average 70-kg adult. Requirements will vary according to patient age, weight and condition. It is the responsibility of the prescriber to ensure that drugs are prescribed and used appropriately. For further information refer to the ward pharmacist or consult the *British National Formulary (BNF)*.

Drug	Method of administration	Notes
N-Acetylcysteine	Continuous infusion 100 mg/kg in 250–1000 ml 5% dextrose over 16 h	
Adrenaline (epinephrine)	5 mg in 50 ml 5% dextrose 0.1–1 µg/kg/min	Increase concentration and dose according to response
Aminophylline	Loading dose 5 mg/kg over 20 min Maintenance 0.5–0.8 mg/kg/h	Omit loading if already receiving theophyllines Increase dose in smokers Reduce dose if receiving concurrent erythromycin or cimetidine Check levels
Amiodarone	300 mg in 250 ml dextrose over 1 h followed by 900 mg in 500 ml over 24 h then 1200 mg in 500 ml over 24 h	Half dose after 48 h
Calcium gluconate	10 ml 10% calcium gluconate slow i.v. bolus, or infusion in 5% dextrose	Precipitates with sulphates, bicarbonates and phosphates
Digoxin	Loading dose 0.5–1 mg in 50 ml 5% dextrose over 30 min Maintenance 62.5–250 µg over 30 min daily	Check levels
Dobutamine	250 mg/50 ml 5% dextrose 0–20 µg/kg/min	Increase concentration and dose according to response

Drug	Method of administration	Notes
Dopamine	200 mg/50 ml 5% dextrose 2.5–5 µg/kg/min renal dose	
Dopexamine	50 mg/50 ml 5% dextrose 0–5 µg/kg/min	
Enoximone	100 mg/40 ml 0.9% saline loading up to 90 µg/kg/min maintenance 5–20 µg/kg/min	Beware hypotension Loading dose often avoided. Max. 24 h 24 mg//kg
Epoprostenol (prostacyclin)	250 µg in 50 ml 0.9% saline 5–10 ng/kg/min	
GTN	50 mg/50 ml (neat) 0–0.5 µg/kg/min	
Heparin	5000 units i.v. loading dose 500–2000 units/hour i.v. according to indication	Monitor APTT
Hydralazine	5–10 mg i.v. bolus repeated as necessary. If required continuous infusion 50 mg/500 ml 0.9% saline 0.05–0.3 mg/min	
Insulin	50 units in 50 ml 0.9% saline continuous infusion as required	Monitor blood sugar
Isoprenaline	10 mg/100 ml 5% dextrose 0–0.5 µg/kg/min	
Labetalol	100 mg/20 ml (neat) i.v. bolus 5–20 mg Infusions start at 15 mg/h Double every 30 min to maximum of 160 mg/h according to response	
Lidocaine (lignocaine)	i.v. bolus 1 mg/kg (100 mg) infusion 1 g/500 ml 5% dextrose at 2–4 mg/min	
Noradrenaline (norepinephrine)	4 mg/50 ml 5% dextrose 0.1–0.5 µg/kg/min	Increase concentration and dose according to response
Phenylephrine	100 mg in 100 ml 5% dextrose 0–10 µg/kg/min	

Drug	Method of administration	Notes
Potassium chloride	10–20 mmol/20–50 ml 0.9% saline over 30 min	Give via central line Monitor ECG
Phenytoin	15 mg/kg loading slow i.v. injection Maintenance 3–5 mg/kg daily	Do not exceed 50 mg/min
Salbutamol	200–300 µg i.v. bolus repeated if necessary, infusion 5 mg/500 ml 5% dextrose 5–20 µg/min	
Streptokinase	1.5 mega units in 0.9% saline over 60 min	

DRUG LEVELS

Drug	When to take sample	Desired levels
Cyclosporin	Predose	100–250 ng/ml
Digoxin	>6 h postdose	1–2.6 nmol/l
Gentamicin	Predose 1 h postdose	<2 mg/l 5–10 mg/l
Phenytoin	>4 h postdose	10–20 mg/l
Tacrolimus	Predose	5–20 ng/ml
Teicoplanin	Predose 1 h postdose	10–15 mg/l up to 40 mg/l
Theophylline	2 h postdose (unless on continuous infusion)	10–20 mg/l
Tobramycin	Predose 1 h postdose	<2 mg/l 5–10 mg/l
Vancomycin	Predose 2 h postdose	5–10 mg/l 18–26 mg/l

In general:

- If the trough level is too high, omit until a random level is within the desired range. Give further doses at increased intervals.
- If peak level is too high, reduce the dose given.

USEFUL LINKS

British Association of Critical Care Nurses	www.baccn.org.uk
British Blood Transfusion Society	www.bbts.org.uk
British National Formulary (BNF)	www.bnf.org.uk
European Resuscitation Council	www.erc.edu
European Society of Intensive Care Medicine	www.escism.org
ICNARC (Intensive Care National Audit and Research Centre)	www.icnarc.org.uk
Intensive Care Society	www.ics.ac.uk
Intensive Care Society of Ireland	www.icmed.com
Resuscitation Council UK	www.resus.org.uk
Scottish Intensive Care Society	www.scottishintensivecare.org.uk
Society of Critical Care Medicine	www.sccm.org
UK Department of Health	www.doh.gov.uk

These web sites contain useful information and many have downloadable guidelines. Most also contain links to related areas of interest.

INDEX